Praise for A

"*Abundantly Well* is literally the most honest guide for healing I've ever seen. Susun invites you on a journey through disease, healing, and wellness with simple profound truths at every turn that are at once powerfully accessible and revealing of the inner healer within all of us."
Dr. Christopher Hobbs, PhD, LAc.

"Susun S. Weed is a true original. She has never wavered from her natural approach to medicine and healing. I have learned a great deal from her deep wisdom. This new book is a real treasure of healing medicine."
Christiane Northrup, MD, New York Times best-selling author of "Goddesses Never Age," "The Wisdom of Menopause," and "Women's Bodies, Women's Wisdom"

"*Abundantly Well* is an amazingly thoughtful and unique resource. One of the best of the 'coyote teachers,' Susun instructs us to think for ourselves, make our own decisions, and empowers people to make their own choices about health and healing."
Rosemary Gladstar, founder of United Plant Savers, director of Sage Mountain, herbalist, best-selling author

"I always appreciate Susun's ability to make people squirm, living on that edge of uncomfortable, questioning our agreed upon belief systems, this is where change happens. *Abundantly Well* challenges us to think critically on how to assess and guide people along the good medicine road. Her Seven Medicines is the most inspiring perspective on therapeutic, regenerative herbalism that I have encountered yet, a truly integrated approach to the complex human-earth-evolutionary-technology dynamic. This book above all the rest, is her legacy."
Sarah Wu, clinical herbalist, permaculture design consultant

"It is almost unbelievable that Susun has fit so much information, knowledge, experience, and wisdom into just over 300 pages. An essential handbook for care of the bodymind."
Charlene Spretnak, author "Relational Reality"

Abundantly Well

"Susun inspires me to ever greater health and vitality! Even after 30 years, I'm still awed. A must-have for every kitchen table."
Ann Drucker, herbalist

"Filled with compassionate counsel, illuminating stories of healing, and step by step guidance through the daunting maze of the modern medical system."
Robin Rose Bennett, "The Gift of Healing Herbs"

"A truly remarkable and comprehensive resource, amazingly complete, well researched and clear. A super valuable guide."
Betzy Bancroft, core faculty Vermont Center for Integrative Herbalism

"Instructive, inspiring, filled with insight and love. Medical doctors: This book offers a profound vision of what your practice could become. Should be on the shelf of anyone healing themselves or others."
Sharol Tilgner, ND

"A unique and comprehensive guide brilliantly formatted in an unusually friendly way to galvanize you to take your health into your own loving hands."
Vajra Ma, GreatGoddess.org

"Beautifully written and a pleasure to read, *Abundantly Well* is now my first 'go to' reference. I simply cannot say enough about it. Buy two copies and give one to a friend. This book will change the way that you consider your health and well being and the way that you approach your health care options."
Barbara WhiteHorse Volk, woman living with the earth

"Being unwell is frightening and lonely. Throughout your journey into wellness, allow Susun, through this book, to be your knowledgeable and compassionate guide."
Heather Níc an Fhleisdeir, clinical herbalist, apothecary

"Susun Weed has gifted us with an impressive, extensive, intensive compendium of information and inspiration for living a happy, healthy life based on her fifty years of experience and knowledge. She is an herbalist and healer supreme."
Mama Donna Henes, urban shaman, "Bless This House"

Abundantly Well

"Wisdom, love, clarity and compassion shine through *Abundantly Well.* Wellness is a revolution. Let Susun be your guide."
Astrid Grove, founder: Mountain West Women's Herbal Gathering

"Part reference book, part spiritual guide, and brimming with down-to-earth, practical wisdom, *Abundantly Well* gives us a well-researched road map for navigating health in these complex times. There is no one I trust more than Susun to help me understand how to take responsibility for my own wholeness. As a woman and mother, I came across *Herbal for the Childbearing Year* 30 years ago. In the intervening years, I've counted on her research, knowledge, and wisdom to help guide me through health challenges, large and small. As a researcher and educational psychologist, I am constantly amazed by the breadth and depth of the resources Susun curates for us and the effective way she integrates insights from myriad times and places with her own extensive, home-spun experience. *Abundantly Well* creates an effective new paradigm for understanding and making use of the often confusing choices we face as we strive to optimize wholeness and maintain health. Make room for *Abundantly Well* on your nightstand – you'll want to turn to it often – for reassurance, facts, inspiration, encouragement, and ideas."
Cheryl MoonEagle Arndt, PhD

"A book for those who want health and are willing to say 'No' to what they don't want. Brilliant."
Larch Hanson, the seaweed man

"Here is a beautifully wise book that takes us to the deepest core levels of healing that brings about true transformation."
Brigitte Mars, herbalist, author, "Natural First Aid"

"Susun is a visionary in health. There is really only one medicine, whether it be natural, alternative, or standard. Either it works or it does not. Either it has some degree of risk, or it does not. It has credibility from studies or a long tradition of effectiveness and safety, or it does not. This is what Susun gives you."
Wayne Dillard, DO, formerly of Tufts School of Medicine

"A delight. Every page is filled with so much information, makes you want to engage in your own health that much more."
Feather Jones, herbalist, creator of Sedona Teas

Abundantly Well

"You will want this in your library for generations to come. Susun's unique approach saved my life. I am forever grateful and you will be too."
Linda Conroy, founder: Midwest Women's Herbal Conference

"A heart-felt, information-packed resource guide for navigating your unique path to greater health. If you only read one book this year, let it be this one. For everybody interested in the deep medicine of life."
EagleSong Evans Gardener, herbalist, earth keeper

"An insightful guide to authentic, powerful health care. Susun's clear thinking, deep wisdom, and joyful voice shine through."
Lisa Natoli, shamanic herbal apprentice

"This book bursts with *joie de vivre*, fascinating information, thought-provoking ideas, and – in an age where the word is so often diminished – a truly empowering spirit."
Molly Hall, honey bee

"Susun Weed offers yet again a book jam-packed with concise, practical, ageless wisdom and a plethora of viewpoints. Certain to expand your perspective on wellness."
Suzy Meszoly, homeopath

"Susun's work remains for me a powerful stable reference point in areas of health that are often full of confusion, fear, and incomplete information."
Sasha Daucus, retired midwife, Golden Light Center

"An amazing book, so knowledgeable and very interesting."
MaDonna Maree Adams, retro shop owner

"Susun's books speak from the heart, awaken the wise woman in all of us, yet contain conventional medicine for when we need that too. This book empowers me to take control of my health and well-being, and reminds me I am perfect as I am."
Sam Lacey, holistic therapist, trainer, hedgerow herbalist

"An exceptional book. A wealth of information for your health. Highly recommended."
Alicia McCord Charmbury, mother

Abundantly Well

"Finally a road map to navigating medical issues and feeling empowered throughout the process. *Abundantly Well* is accessible and useful to everyone. It includes physical, mental, and spiritual health, the invisible as well as the visible. Buy two copies: one for yourself and one for a loved one. This *is* a book you need on your shelf."
Tonya Lemos, Blazing Star Herbal School

"It's never too late to return to the earth for the healing you need. Let her call you home from the pages of this book."
Raewyn McColley, community herbalist

"This book is amazing! It is incredibly accessible to all levels of knowledge. I read it to my youngest son as he falls asleep at night and he stays tuned in, even at 3½."
Ashley Marie Manix, office manager, Heart of Wellness

"Loving this book. Lots of needed info."
Susan Lynn Bozarth-Staff, mother, herbalist, empath

"I feel like I've been waiting my whole life for this book!! Thank you Susun, for putting all the puzzle pieces together and making them so easily referenced!! I can hardly wait to add this gem to my table. This book should be in every household."
Ursula Krieger, green thumb, grandmother

"The knowledge in this book allows me to go out into the world with the confidence that I am the most knowledgeable expert when it comes to facilitating wellness in myself and my family. My daily health choices matter; and I make those choices mindfully. The sort of caring-confidence I exude is truly contagious."
Mary Jo Greenwood, CSW

"This book reminds me that what is healthy/healing for me is also healthy/healing for the world around me. Inspiring."
Holly Hughes, E.ART.H, environmental artist

"A beautifully written manual which gently guides the reader through the Seven Medicines. Each page oozes wisdom. Sentences flow like syrup and make reading a joy. Highly recommended, if you want control of your health and well-being."
Tracy Miller, grandmother, medical herbalist in training

Abundantly Well

"Susun Weed's newest book, *Abundantly Well,* is a truly remarkable guidebook chock full of magical, potent wisdom. A tapestry of facts and folklore, science and stories, wise counsel and vivid color. Empowering medicine for body, mind, spirit, soul, and roots. No better moment exists than right now to deepen our connection with our wholeness. Highest recommendation."
Rosemary Clare Woodward, herbalist, culinary artist

"As someone who struggles with retaining new information, I was pleasently surprised with how quickly I was able to pick this up. Very easy to read. Susun has a beautiful way with words."
Sarah G, student

"*Abundantly Well* is a wealth of information. An absolute must-have book for anyone who wants to make informed decisions about their health, healthcare, and well-being. I feel so fortunate to be a part of this empowering, integrated medicine revolution."
Vickie Quillian Schulz, nemophilist

"*Abundantly Well* is a great read for anyone looking to deepen their understanding on how to approach health. Deep wisdom to keep at your fingertips. Every home needs a copy."
S. Marie Carlson, publisher: "Home Herbalist Magazine"

"What an amazing book! Such wisdom and knowledge. Practical, useful information for any stage of illness and wellness. There is something in here for everyone."
Leela Ehrhart, therapist

"Timely, wise, and useful from cover to cover."
Lori Jarema, mother, wildlife conservationist, herbalist

"It is no surprise that Susun Weed has done it again: another comprehensive, easy to read, and richly illustrated book on health and wellness to help us navigate the complicated, confusing, and sometimes scary medicine choices at our avail. Susun gently and expertly takes our hand and guides us to optimal health. Truly a book we need on our shelf, on our coffee table, and in our hands. Brava!"
Justine Smythe, graphic artist, chef, mother, videographer

Abundantly Well

"The genius that is Susun Weed shines through. A wealth of information not found anywhere else. I can't wait to hold it in my hands and have it nearby. Susun has changed the way we view healthcare. I feel abundantly blessed!"
Bettie McLawhorn Thomas, MA, CCC-SLP, herbalist, grandmother

"As soon as I began to read this book, I felt a peacefulness come over me. The style is so different from other books on mind, body, and spirit wellness. Step by step, Susun brilliantly leads us away from guilt and body shaming, to intuitive self-care and self-love. She shows us how to enjoy increased pleasure, sensual self-indulgence, and ambient living. As with all of her books, she delivers a broad scope of scientific wisdom and practical resources."
Donna Virgilio, fitness specialist BS, Goddess Spirituality Tours

"I have been traveling the Wise Woman medicine path for the past few years and resonate deeply with the offerings + wisdom in *Abundantly Well.*"
Ashley Dohe, earth whisperer

"Had this book been available to me when I was 22, or even 42, instead of 82, I would have lived a much healthier life, and not endured so much deep medicine on the advice of my doctors."
Gretchen Gould, herbalist, author, composer

"Susun weaves a path forward for any woman looking to maintain or restore her health."
Bevin Clare, professor: Maryland University of Integrative Health, herbalist, nutritionist, president: American Herbalists Guild

"A beautifully written book, thought provoking and well planned. It made me feel good to see how she thinks about food and encourages me to stay on my path. I cherish her words."
Diane Cornwell, author, herbalist

"This loving, sage, and powerful book is so all-encompassing, it may well be the only book anyone, of any gender, needs."
Cassendre Xavier, founder: Philadephia's Annual Black Women's Arts Festival

Abundantly Well

"I'll be referring back to *Abundantly Well* time and time again! Susun Weed has created a map that integrates her Wise Woman knowledge all in one place. The book also includes valuable pages of references and studies providing evidence-based support. Thank you for getting this book out into the world now! It's a must-own."
Sherry Fuhler Phoenix, gardener, herbalist, nature lover

"Gratitude. We are gifted once again with wisdom gathered from the ancients and decades of interaction with people and plants. In *Abundantly Well*, Susun holds a lantern for our healer within and guides us graciously through the Seven Medicines. Integrated healthcare shines brightly and nurtures deeply. Àse. Blessed be!"
Lucretia Lukaya, wise woman herbalist, artisan, mother

"A fun read."
Linda Gregory, mother of three

"A joy to read. Like a tool box, with the steps to a logical path, and strong supporting research. A reference guide of sequential steps to support body and mind on life's journey. Thank you Susun!"
Chan Siefert, business professional, auntie

"I went to the seventh river when I was a teenager, for breast augmentation. Instead of healing my dysphoria, it gave me Breast Implant Illness. *Abundantly Well* found me ten years later, just as I was considering removing my toxic implants. I couldn't put it down. Susun's wise words are with me and my partner as we interview surgeons, get anxious in waiting rooms, and endure sales pitches to further modify my body. I am going in without fear because I invested a few hours reading this wonderful resource."
Samantha JoAnn Stolle, student

"Indispensable for empowered, pro-active health care."
Vic Hernandez, MD, researcher, activist

"Let Susun take you on a comprehensive journey through the Seven Medicines leading you to be abundantly well."
Dr. JoAnn Quattrone, DDS, herbalist, acupuncturist

"A wise and thoughtful roadmap for the healing journey."
Doug Elliott, herbalist, author, story-teller

"This message came when I needed to hear it."
Mika Holt, herbalist

"A must have for any one feeling at a crossroads with how to handle their own health changes. With *Abundantly Well - Seven Medicines*, I feel confident that I have ways to protect myself even if I need to seek invasive medical help. A well written and easy to understand guide."
Erica Paquette Schveighoffer, herbalist and certified aromatherapist

"Susun weaves a path forward for anyone looking to maintain or restore their health."
Bevin Clare, MS, RH, CNS, clinical herbalist, nutritionist

"A new paradigm in medicine! Absolutely everything you can do, and not do, to be abundantly well. A survival guide and the crowning achievement of one of America's best-kept secrets (not much longer!) – Susun Weed – my hera!"
Sabine Ehrenfeld, Wise Woman teacher, herbalist

"Gorgeously, shamelessly, Susun makes green magic accessible and practical. Not an airy tome but a real guide to dancing with your own abundant health ... on your own time! The amount of information would be staggering – if it wasn't presented in such a digestible format. I will reference this book for the rest of my life!"
Samantha Caplan, former apprentice, farm hand

Abundantly Well

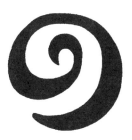

Susun S. Weed

Other Books by Susun S. Weed

Wise Woman Herbal for the Childbearing Year
   English, French, German, Spanish, Dutch, ebook

Healing Wise, the second Wise Woman Herbal
   English, German, Japanese

Breast Cancer? Breast Health! The Wise Woman Way
   English, German, Dutch

New Menopausal Years the Wise Woman Way
   English, Dutch

Down There, Sexual and Reproductive Health the Wise Woman Way
   English

Abundantly Well

The Complementary Integrat~~ive~~ ed
Medicine Revolution

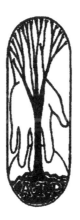

Ash Tree Publishing
PO Box 64
Woodstock NY 12498
AshTreePublishing.com

Abundantly Well

All information in this book is based on the experiences and re-search of the author and other professional healers. This information is shared with the understanding that you accept complete responsibility for your own health and well-being. You have a unique body, and the action of each remedy is unique. Health care is full of variables. The result of any treatment suggested herein cannot always be anticipated and can never be guaranteed. The author and publisher are not responsible for any adverse effects or consequences resulting from the use of any remedies, procedures, or preparations included in this Wise Woman Herbal. Consult your inner guidance, knowledgeable friends, and trained healers in addition to the words written here.

© 2020 by Susun S. Weed
Ash Tree Publishing
PO Box 64, Woodstock, NY, 12498, USA; 845-246-8081
www.ashtreepublishing.com

Illustrations © 2020 by Durga Yael Bernhard, except pages 17, 36, 41, 53, 60, 63, 137, 144
Cover design by Justine Smythe

Publisher's Cataloging-in-Publication Data
provided by Five Rainbows Cataloging Services

Names: Weed, Susun S., author.
Title: Abundantly well : the complementary integrated medical revolution / Susun S. Weed. Description: Woodstock, NY : Ash Tree Publishing, 2019. | Series: Wise woman herbal series. | Includes bibliographical references and index.
Identifiers: LCCN 2018912912 | ISBN 978-1-888123-22-7 (paperback)
Subjects: LCSH: Alternative medicine. | Integrative medicine. | Dietary supplements. | Herbs— Therapeutic use. | Drugs—Effectiveness. | Cancer—Alternative treatment. | BISAC: MEDICAL / Alternative & Complementary Medicine. | BODY, MIND & SPIRIT / Healing / General. Classification: LCC R733 .W434 2019 (print) | DDC 615.5—dc23.

⑥ Table of Contents ⑨

Step 0: Do Nothing   Serenity Medicine   1
Do nothing; benefits; how to; relaxation; to remove trauma; rest cure; safety; sleep; breathing; meditate; be silent; know nothing; release linear time; be alone; fast; references & resources

Step 1: Collect Information   Story Medicine   25
Gather information/access wisdom; benefits; diagnosis as story; access wisdom; non-invasive diagnosis; gather information; kinesiology; iridology; diagnosis by the skin; a second opinion; become your own expert; diagnosis the Wise Woman way; mind-opening diagnosis; tell your story; safety; references & resources

Step 2: Engage the Energy   Mind Medicine   47
Imagine health; benefits; belief/faith; how to pray; embrace your unique life; placebo; homeopathy; Bach flower essences; intention; positive thought; affirmation; visualization; guided meditation; trance; hypnosis; color therapy; art therapy; mandalas; archetypes; energy; vitalism; earth energy; forest bathing; minerals; wisdom of Asia; touch; Alexander technique; aten stunde; biodynamic craniosacral therapy; Feldenkrais; hugs; laying on of hands; mudras; non-dual therapies; Reiki; Rosen method; therapeutic touch; chakras; psychic surgery; vibrational medicine; dowsing, electro-medicine/Rife machines; magnetic therapy; orgonomy; radionics; references & resources

Step 6: Break & Enter   Deep Medicine 223

Benefits; dive into deep medicine; Step 6 as metaphor.

Scientific tradition: screening tests; Step 6 for diagnosis; radiation tests/therapies (x-rays, mammograms, DEXA, CT, PET scans); protect yourself from radiation damage; adaptogens aid radiation therapy; non-radiation tests (sonograms/ultrasound, thermography, MRI, blood tests); surgery; increase your personal health; time for Step 6?; your advocate; choose the best surgeon; choose the best hospital; the consent form; anesthesia; close to surgery allies; right before & during surgery allies; immediately after surgery allies (nausea, pain, stroke, pneumonia); fear as an ally.

Heroic tradition: humoral theory; poking/bloodletting; puking/vomiting; purging/colonics, enemas, implants; body modification.

Wise Woman tradition: change your mind; power plants; psychedelic agent dosage guide; psilocybin; peyote; ergot; ayahuasca,; witch's garden nightshades; tobacco; poppy; mistletoe therapy. References & resources for all three traditions

⑥ Foreword ⑨

The book you are holding has taken me thirty years to write. Twenty years ago, I almost published it. I'm so glad I didn't.

Abundantly Well was originally called *Healing Well*, and was slated for publication right after *Healing Wise* (in the late 1980s). Didn't happen. More than a decade later, after my own menopause and *Menopausal Years the Wise Woman Way*, which did happen, I rewrote *Healing Well*, intending to see it in print by 2001. Didn't happen again. (But *Breast Cancer? Breast Health! the Wise Woman Way* and *Down There the Wise Woman Way* and *NEW Menopausal Years the Wise Woman Way* did.)

Much has happened in the intervening decades, both in my own growth and understanding, and in the broadening of science's horizon. The words I wrote twenty years ago, based on experience, intuition, and understanding are now supported by serious scientific study. The reference and resource sections of this book have more than doubled in size: my old favorites now intermingle with websites and twenty-first-century studies.

During those decades, my desire to restore herbal medicine as people's medicine has succeeded and birthed thousands and thousands of green beings who are teaching and spreading the news: You can be abundantly well with simple, safe, no- or low-cost remedies and the Seven Medicines. You can integrate medicines for optimum health. You can be part of the complementary integrated medicine revolution.

It's a non-violent revolution, and it draws upon the best of all worlds to nourish your unique abundant health.

The most important person in this revolution is you. You are the one who can choose a healthy lifestyle. You are the one who can use simple herbal remedies instead of drugs for everyday health concerns. You are the one who can integrate complementary medicines when undergoing cancer treatment. You are the one who can use and benefit from the Seven Medicines.

The Seven Medicines are the basis of *Abundantly Well,* which brings together my fifty years of experience and expertise in health and healing, science and spirit. It is a guide to integrated medicine. Hands-on examples and easy-to-follow recipes let you take immediate charge of your own health, whether you want to regain or maintain health.

I intend for it to amuse you and horrify you, empower you and make you think. Like all my work, I intend for it to clarify relationships among things and to simplify your decision-making process. Whether you are healthy and want to stay that way, looking for the best way to deal with a new health problem, investigating new views on your old problems, coping with a chronic illness, facing a frightening diagnosis, or healing from an accident – there is something here for you.

I want *Abundantly Well* to be a road map for you when you are faced with health-care choices. I believe *Abundantly Well* will make it easy for you to become your own expert, so you can achieve the health results you want on your best terms. I trust that *Abundantly Well* will help you work well with any medical professional you seek out or encounter when you need or want their expertise.

This book supports a revolution, a patient centered, client empowered, nature loving revolution. Let *Abundantly Well* spark a revolution in your health and your health care. Take the hand of your curiosity and let's explore the Seven Medicines together.

Green blessings
Susun, Laughing Rock Farm, 11 Jan 2019

More on the Seven Medicines:
Seven Medicines video course at wisewomanschool.com
Seven Rivers of Healing also at wisewomanschool.com
Seven Medicines MP3 at wisewomanbookshop.com

And here's Patch Adams MD, in his "professional attire" – big red nose and an underwear hat – to introduce me to you all:

⑥ Introduction ⑨

I turn down so many introductions I feel I have to say why I'm doing this one. Susun has grit! It made sense at the first gathering of herbalists I ever went to, that we would gravitate toward each other. We dress as if we had no idea what others are wearing. I noticed and liked her carriage. In our current society self confidence with compassion sticks out.

Before I heard the term "Wise Woman," I was prejudiced to think that woman already meant wise. So here was a woman calling herself a wise woman in a society that seems to be fully disconnected from the idea of wisdom in any form. I watched her protect wisdom by insisting on engagement if someone asked her a question. I saw her give wisdom as if it were a precious thing, and a fragile thing, needing the protection a mother gives to her children. I went to a long workshop and saw her courage to be controversial and committed to a minority opinion. She seemed to insist that each of us has to digest incoming wisdom through our own filters.

I saw her have tenderness for other opinions, even contradictory ones, from healers she respected. I saw a combination of love, great strength, and sweet softness. I got an invitation to visit her home/school, where she tends goats and students. The students are there for her mentorship of all parts of their lives in becoming a wise woman. I saw the attention she gave both goat and student and I wished nature and humanity were so cared for.

She wasn't just easy, I saw tough love. She seemed so devoted to the task of mentor, to choose wisdom over being liked, a rarity in many compassionate healers.

All this swims in my head while I read her new book, *Abundantly Well*. Whoever you are, you will disagree, even be angry at some of what is said: good experiences when reading about such broad subjects. When I look at the many books in my library on these subjects, I wonder if there is a limit on what can be said – even Hippocrates' material covers them. So why will I add (and be excited to add) Susun's book?

Healing is an art form made up of all of one's input and intentions. No two healers or patients are alike. The healer needs to be surrounded by many points of view (conflicting views) to keep their intelligence humble and open to diversity. In primary care one quickly finds out how little they really cure, how inadequate even the most elaborate and most touted healing techniques are when spread over many patients. We need many voices so that at least one will open the needed doors toward health for the patient.

This is especially true in the modern climate of corporate medicine, where patient and healer have so little time to learn or listen to anything. Economics so influences health-care delivery now that it is a lie to call it a healing interaction even if it works out great. One good outcome of this pernicious direction has been the patient's moving away from a paternalistic mechanistic surrender to the healer, and towards a consideration of self care.

Enter Susun's book: Whichever books you have, this one will add to them. No paternalism here. She leads with the perfect beginning – do nothing, relax. First, be with your great self. Of course, ideally, you would not first read it while sick, rather read it through to take an inventory and to have a sense of direction if you need a healing interaction. As a book worm, I delight at her lush bibliography and quotes for deeper reflection. Like all good books on wellness, it doesn't rest on being fully comprehensive, rather it's a teaser for just how complicated we might be.

An important thing about Susun is that she invites you to a whole-world utopia where your health may be a political act. If we are to find solutions to all the horrors in the world, they (the solutions) will sprout from wise women.

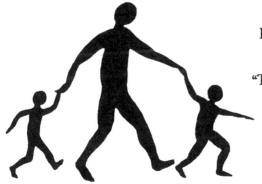

Take charge.
In peace, Patch Adams
3 August 2001

"Twenty years later, and
we're still weird."
Patch Adams
Camp Winnarainbow
28 June 2019

☉ I See the Wise Woman

Flowing deep in our psyches, healing impulses, like mythic springs, seep through our dreams and emerge into waking. The old wisdom bubbles to the surface. We vibrate with an ancestral beat. Old rivers flow in us. Mother to daughter, mother to son, spiraling down through the generations. In our dreams the Ancient Grandmothers make themselves known. They whisper to us. They reawaken the Wise Wo/man within each of us.

I see the wise woman. She carries a blanket of compassion. She wears robes of wisdom. Around her throat flutters a veil of shifting shapes. From her shoulders, a mantle of power flows. A story band encircles her forehead. She stitches a quilt; she spins fibers into yarn; she knits; she sews; she weaves. She ties the threads of our lives together. She forms a web of spiraling threads, intertwining our lives.

I see the wise woman at her loom. It is warped with days of light and nights of dark. White threads, black threads receive the flying shuttle. A shuttle filled with threads of many colors. Threads the colors of the earth, the common ground; threads the colors of the people of the earth. Some threads are short, some are long; each thread is different, each perfect and splendid.

The threads are alive with sound and color. The threads are mutable; they change at a touch. The threads are crystal antennae; they respond to our thoughts. And intertwined with each thread is a blood-red thread. A thread of such sensitivity, it seems invisible. A thread of such vitality, it can never be hidden. As our blood flows over and under the days and nights of our lives and binds each moment to the whole, so the red thread of the wise woman binds us in the tapestried, cosmic web and spirals lovingly around us in life and death.

I see the wise woman. And she sees me.

I see the wise woman. She is old and walks with the aid of a beautifully carved stick. She's the ancient grandmother of us all. She's the one who brought me here. I have been following her traces for years, finding here and there a thread from her clothes, many of them still strong and vibrant, especially among aboriginal women, earth-based women, women of earth colors, women of the mother cultures. The ancient wise woman speaks to me through each thread, each woman, each color, each glance. She speaks in song, in story, in dance.

The wise old woman winks at me; the cunning old woman spreads her arms as if to embrace me. I hear her say:

"These are the ways of our ancient grandmothers, the ancient ones who still live. We are one with all life in an ever-changing spiral. Every pain, every plant, every stone, every feeling, every problem is cherished as a teacher: not a teacher who grades, but a teacher who guides. We love the night for its darkness and the day for its light. We treasure each uniqueness. This is the Wise Woman way the world 'round.

"These are the ways of our ancient grandmothers, the ancient ones who still live. We eat with compassion, knowing we will be food for others. We view dying as a portal just as birth is. We celebrate comings and goings; they are the turnings of the spiral. This is the Wise Woman way the world 'round.

"These are the ways of our ancient grandmothers, the ancient ones who still live. We spin the invisible web which weaves us all together. We invite you to weave the threads of your own life back into the cloak of the Ancient Ones. We urge you to reweave yourselves with the sacred threads of nature, to remember your kinship with all. This is the Wise Woman way the world 'round."

🜨 *Note:* Woman (wo-man) includes all genders; it is inclusive. She (s-he)and Goddess (God-dess) also include all genders. They are the inclusive terms used throughout this book.

6 Steps @ 7 Medicines
DO NO HARM

Step 0: Do Nothing   Serenity Medicine
No harm ever.
No person, substance, or energy touches me.

Step 1: Collect Information   Story Medicine
Harm very rare; easily healed.
My mind is in contact; not my body.

Step 2: Engage the Energy   Mind Medicine
Harm rare; usually easily healed.
My mind and energy are in contact. Hands rest on my
clothed body or move slowly in sensitive, gentle ways.

Step 3: Nourish and Tonify   Lifestyle Medicine
Harm possible; usually easily healed; death rare.
My body, energy field, and mind are contacted by other
people, energies, and substances.

THE GREAT DIVIDE 🌸 THE GAP

Step 4: Stimulate/Sedate   Alternative Medicine
Addiction and side effects possible; harm easily healed.
My body, energy field, and mind experience deep and
sometimes painful contact that does not draw blood.

Step 5: Use Drugs   Pharmaceutical Medicine
Addiction likely; side effects very likely; death possible.
My body, energy field, and mind are altered by concen-
trated or synthetic poisons in appropriate doses.

Step 6: Break and Enter   Deep Medicine
Harm, side effects inevitable; injury, disability, death possible.
My body, energy field, mind, and spirit are broken into;
there is often blood or body fluids.

Use the Seven Medicines Now

You can start using the Seven Medicines right now.

If you have a new health challenge, read about Serenity Medicine, Step 0, choose a way to engage it, set a time limit, and see what happens. Go on to further Medicines, or add on further Steps as needed, until you are enjoying abundant health.

If you have a health challenge you are already dealing with, read about the Medicines that include the substances and techniques you are using. If it is one of the last three Medicines, that is, Steps 4, 5, or 6, perhaps it is time to add, or return to, the first four Medicines: Steps 0, 1, 2, and 3.

If you are healthy right now, and curious as to what abundant health would be like, browse the first four Medicines, and use what you will to improve your health and prevent problems. Then, browse the last three Medicines, and consider your relationship to stimulants and sedatives, drugs, and screening tests.

The Seven Medicines, also known as the Six Steps of Healing, is an ordering system designed to help us decide – in any specific instance and for each unique individual – which healing methods and which remedies will give the best outcome with the least harm.

The Seven Medicines/Six Steps system gives us a simple, safe way to choose wisely from all the health-care options available, from ancient wisdom to cutting-edge science, from hands-on healing to DNA diagnosis, and everything in between.

Like a well-organized herb cupboard or a good index to a favorite book, the Seven Medicines provide a framework for engaging different remedies and procedures while maximizing health.

Use the Seven Medicines in order, one at a time, or use them all at once. It depends on you, on what's happening.

For inspiration, go to page 281, where you'll find stories of those who used the Seven Medicines' complementary, integrated approach to their health challenges.

Safety and the Seven Medicines
First Do No Harm

The first four Medicines – Steps 0, 1, 2, and 3 – always improve health, even when they do not cure. The last three Medicines – Steps 4, 5, and 6 – always harm health, even when they do cure.

The first four Medicines require active daily attention and action. They build health and increase personal power for that very reason: they demand that we act consistently to create health, that we educate ourselves, and pay attention to ourselves.

The effects of these Medicines may be slow to appear, but they are long-lasting. They create little or no side effects. They steadily improve mental and physical functioning, while increasing our innate ability to heal and to stay healthy.

Serenity Medicine, Story Medicine, Mind Medicine, and Lifestyle Medicine are true preventative medicines. As such, they are most effective when used daily. They are generally safe to combine with remedies from Steps 4, 5, and 6 when addressing a problem.

The last three Medicines encourage passivity. When we cross from preventative medicine to urgent care, we seek a wise guide. Who may encourage, or actually tell us, to do what s/he says to do, without question or comment.

Relinquishing control of our own health isn't healthy. Caution and firm time limits protect us when we choose Alternative Medicine, Pharmaceutical Medicine, and Deep Medicine.

The effects of the last three Medicines can be dramatic and swift, incluiding unintended side effects that can threaten our well being, deteriorating and disabling us mentally and physically.

Trust your sense of what's right for *your* body and *your* feelings.

Play Safely

Pay attention to yourself.
Act sooner rather than later.
Set time limits.
Use the Medicines in order.

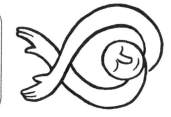

Complementary Integrated Medicine Revolution

The beginning of the twenty-first century is a fantastic time to be alive and well. It's a great time to be sick, too. With a little effort, one can access and make use of healing practices and substances from all over the world. The best of modern medicine and the best of ancient wisdom is available to any seeker.

Alternative medicine and standard care are no longer at war. Herbalists, naturopaths, acupuncturists, massage therapists – to name a few – have thriving practices and interface with their peers in the medical establishment. Alternative/complementary therapies are (sometimes) paid for by (some) insurers.

As good as this is, much more is needed. Many oncologists know that patients undergoing chemotherapy benefit from dietary and herbal support, and that herbs, massage and acupuncture effectively allay symptoms. Many cardiologists know that herbal medicine and lifestyle medicine are as effective in moderating blood pressure as drugs. Many healers understand the placebo effect. But few, even those in the most progressive centers, suggest or mention anything other than insurance-approved standard treatments.

Alternative/complementary medicines may be offered after Step 6 treatments in an attempt to heal the damage caused by chemo/radiation, surgery, and drugs. But medicines from the first four Steps are protective and effective when integrated with Steps 4, 5, and 6 – meditation and medication, herbs and drugs, radiation and acupuncture – into a kaleidoscope of expertise.

Seven Medicines is a map. Your abundant health is the destination. Your curiosity is my ally. Engage the first four Medicines as proactive health care for optimum health/wholeness/holiness. Integrate them with the last three Medicines to deal with traumatic injury, a chronic problem, a cancer diagnosis, or an acute illness, and be amazed at how abundantly well you feel.

It's a revolution in health care, and it starts with you.

The Three Traditions of Healing

The Seven Medicines help us stay abundantly well and restore health with the least harm. They can be used without knowledge of the three traditions of healing. But understanding the three traditions helps you individualize your healing journey.

We are all mixtures of all three traditions. Knowing your own predominant view, and the view of those you seek help from, will help you get the very best care on your own terms. And help you understand any treatments you may choose.

The three primary ways to envision health and healing are the Scientific way, the Heroic way, and the Wise Woman way. The Scientific tradition measures and fixes. The Heroic tradition cleanses and balances. The Wise Woman tradition nourishes the wholeness of the unique individual.

Scientific doctors are trained to use pharmaceuticals, surgery, chemo/radiation, and invasive tests. Heroic practitioners are trained in the use of supplements and cleanses. Wise Woman healers nourish wholeness in all circumstances, helping you embody self-love and self acceptance. (Wo/man includes all genders.)

Get Fixed Fast   *Be afraid*

Steps 5 and 6 predominate in the Scientific tradition. Drugs, surgical interventions, chemo/radiation, and tests are the primary tools of healing. We are measured so we can be fixed. Health has no definition in this tradition; it is merely the absence of disease. The emotion of the Scientific tradition is fear.

Health care in the Scientific tradition is a high-tech war on bacteria, viruses, disease, cancer, pain. Fearing for our lives, we often accept injury to our health as the price of staying alive. Its symbol is the measurable, unchanging line.

Science is reductionistic. Things are reduced – from cell to gene, from the one hundred factors of vitamin C to ascorbic acid, from the crude plant to a single, active constituent that can be synthesized. This approach offers a good representation of reality and does a fairly good job of distinguishing fact from fancy.

But living things, humans and plants, are complex, messy, and highly interactive. When the part is seen as the same as the whole, the hundreds of synergistic, holographically interwoven constituents in a plant are reduced to an active principle. Only part of the plant is used, only part of us is treated. We are separated into parts and those parts are fixed. No change, no growth, less aliveness.

Most MDs practice in the Scientific tradition. Some MDs – notably Bernie Siegel, Larry Dossey, Patch Adams, and Elisabeth Kübler-Ross – manifest the Wise Woman way. Some MDs – such as renegades who do unorthodox treatments, functional medicine doctors, and others who prey on their patients' weaknesses – clearly represent the Heroic tradition.

To nourish abundant wellness in the Scientific tradition, integrate the Seven Medicines, especially Alternative Medicine and Lifestyle Medicine, with all treatments.

Cleanse Away Toxins   *Be guilty*

Steps 3, 4, and 5 sustain the Heroic tradition. The primary tools of healing are *cleanses* – including chelations, colonics, fasts, purges, laxatives, cathartics, emetics, lancets, and leeches; *supplements* – including herbs, vitamins, minerals, CoQ10, SAMe, enzymes, and freeze-dried glands; *manipulations* – including adjustments, massage, and hydrotherapy.

In the Heroic tradition, health arises from, and results in, purity and balance; disease is caused by imbalances and toxins. The emotion of the Heroic tradition is shame, blame and guilt. Its symbol is the circle, or three circles, representing body, mind, and spirit.

Health care in the Heroic tradition is an all-out war on "bad" things: environmental chemicals, meat, germs, milk, unclean foods, gluten, impure thoughts, sweets. Since the problem is our own fault, we easily accept harsh treatments and difficult restrictions in a desperate attempt to overcome our problem/sinfulness and regain health.

In the Heroic tradition, the whole is the sum of its parts: body, mind, and spirit. But any view that separates us into parts breaks our wholeness and rends our unity.

The Heroic tradition predates the Scientific by thousands of years. It postulates that four *humors* cause disease when they are imbalanced or toxic. (More on pages 254-258.)

In the Scientific tradition, things happen to us. In the Heroic tradition, our problems are our own fault. We were negative. We were bad. We ate the wrong food. To be well, we must be absolved, punished, and purified. *No pain, no gain.*

Many naturopathic doctors, acupuncturists, chiropractors, massage therapists, aromatherapists, and herbalists practice and think in the Heroic tradition. Naturopaths trained in Australia and herbalists taught by my apprentices are likely to practice in the Wise Woman tradition.

Using the Seven Medicines can protect you from the harms inherent in cleansing and balancing, shame and guilt.

Nourish Wholeness   *Love yourself*

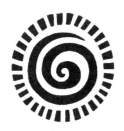

Steps 0, 1, 2, and 3 are used to create abundant health in the Wise Woman tradition. If needed, Steps 4 through 6 are integrated with the first four steps. Nourishing herbal infusions, compassionate touch, deep listening, and simple ceremony are the primary tools of healing.

Health is not the absence of disease but flexibility and resilience in the throes of life's inevitable traumas. Sturdiness and wholeness are nourished. The emotion of the Wise Woman tradition is delighted curiosity and loving kindness. Its symbol is the ever-changing, ever-moving spiral.

Life is a spiral, not a circle, not a line. It is ever changing, chaotic, and exactly as it ought to be. There are no mistakes. No blame, shame or guilt. No guarantees.

Health care in the Wise Woman tradition starts with complete acceptance of whatever we are experiencing. The focus is on the person, not the problem. Healer and patient work together to gather missing pieces, nourish the neglected shadow, integrate what is denied.

No matter how much care we take to eat organically and fasten our seatbelt, we may nonetheless find ourselves dancing with cancer or healing from a serious accident. Since there are no mistakes and no guarantees in this way of thinking, trauma and difficulties become doorways of transformation, not failures of our bodies or our selves. Disease and injury are not problems to be fixed, not imbalances to be righted, and not a result of toxins which we must purge. They are opportunities to nourish ourselves and become more.

In the Wise Woman tradition, the whole is greater than the sum of its parts. The relationships among the parts are as important as the parts; the trees of the forest depend on hidden mycelial nourishment. Substance, thought, feeling, and spirit are inseparably intertwined in dynamic disequilibrium in all living things.

The Wise Woman tradition is the world's oldest healing tradition. We see its spiral in the most ancient human sites. Its message of healing through loving kindness, nourishing body and soul, has found fertile ground and thrives in many diverse environments.

The Wise Woman way is validated by modern science, especially quantum physics. There are Wise Woman MDs like Kara Long, Tieraona Low Dog, and Aviva Romm. There are Wise Woman herbalists galore. There are Wise Woman midwives, osteopaths, therapists, acupuncturists, healers of all sorts. The wise woman is all around you, and inside you too.

> You are inherently whole.
> I am inherently whole.
> We inherently seek greater wholeness.
>
> You are naturally perfect just as you are.
> I am naturally perfect just as I am.
> We naturally desire greater perfection.

An Orchard at the Bottom of A Hill

Maurice Manning

Why don't you try just being quiet?
If you can find some silence, maybe
you can listen to it. How it works
is interesting. I really can't
explain it, but you know it when
it's happening. You realize
you're marveling at apple blossoms
and how they're clustered on the tree
and you see the bees meticulously
attending evey blossom there,
and you think the tree is kind of sighing.
Such careful beauty in the making.
And then you think, it's really quiet,
but I am not alone in this world.
That's how you know it's happening,
there's something solemn and wonderful
in the quiet, a slow and steady ease.
Whether the tree is actually sighing
is beside the point. It's better to wonder,
you needn't be precise with quiet,
it just becomes another thing.
It isn't a science, it's an art,
like love, or a dog who's pretty good,
asleep in the grass beneath the tree.

Step Zero

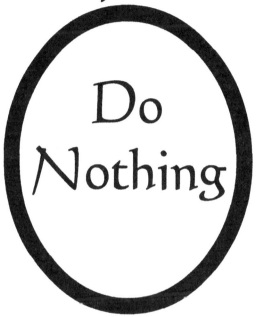

Do
Nothing

Serenity Medicine

"*To know nothing is the first condition of all knowledge.*"

Socrates

Do Nothing
Watchful Waiting

- Be
- Be silent
- Be still
- Be alone
- Relax
- Meditate
- Go with the flow
- Know nothing
- Sleep
- Surrender
- Float
- Rest
- Be serene
- Be foolish
- Retire
- Pull the plug
- Procrastinate
- Let go of time
- Observe it all
- Be content
- Daydream
- Settle down
- Allow wholeness
- Accept yourself completely
- Let the dust settle
- Hang out in a hammock
- Resign from responsibility
- Return to the cosmic egg

"On those special nights, I could absorb the long hours of nothingness in the half-light of the moon, where there was no sadness or boredom, and where I was nourished by silence. . . . "
Oria Douglas-Hamilton, *Among the Elephants*

Grandmother Growth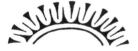

It is dusk; a stream gurgles. You feel the loving presence of your guardian angel, your spirit guide, your inner wisdom. You feel as if an unknown part of you has been triggered, a part that has been waiting for this moment. Words bloom in your mind.

"Right now I am free. Right now my breathing is steady and smooth. Right now I let go. Right now I surrender to the flow. Right now I exhale completely. Right now I rest in the emptiness, in the Void, in the Cosmic Egg of existence. Right now I float in the womb of the Great Mother. Right now I am spacious. Right now I am empty. Right now I am amazingly alive. Right now I am perfect. Right now I am whole/healthy/holy."

Benefits of Serenity Medicine

o Enhanced immunity   o Longer, healthier life
o Relief from chronic pain   o Better sleep
o More energy, creativity, fun   o Healthier hormones
o Less depression/anxiety   o Better digestion
o Fewer headaches/migraines   o Less dementia
o Increased birth weight   o Better breathing
o Decreased risk of cardiovascular diseases

Serenity Medicine is first. Whether the problem is acute or chronic, we begin at Step 0. Perhaps we will be spontaneously healed, perhaps we will need to add further Steps. We begin here.

We cultivate contentment. Seek inner silence. Return to fundamental consciousness. Spiral into the boundless cosmic womb. Allow the flow of the mysterious movement. Take time out.

Step 0 causes no harm. It is free. It requires no equipment, no physical presence, no outside touch.

We learn Serenity Medicine from others; we practice it alone. The more it is practiced, the greater the rewards.

Serenity Medicine engages complex biochemical and physical shifts that change the brain and body. Step 0 triggers the body's own self-repair mechanisms. It revitalizes the pluripotent stem cells in the marrow of our bones. Physicist David Bohm says there is a field of unbroken wholeness from which physical reality emerges. Serenity Medicine connects us to that wholeness.

"The more we learn about subatomic particles . . . the more the universe seems to be made of nothing at all. "   Robert Kunzig, *Discover*

"After two months [of practicing relaxation methods], the genes that fight inflammation, kill diseased cells and protect the body from cancer all began to switch on. [They] were not active in the control group."
Dr Herbert Benson, Harvard Medical School

"Some people experience a little improvement, others a lot, and there are a few whose lives are totally turned around."   Joan Borysenko,
relaxation program director, Boston's Beth Israel Medical Center

How to Do Nothing

Turn off outside input. Slow down. Deepen. Don't think. Go with the flow. Be insecure. Allow chaos. Be confused. Stop struggling. Relinquish desire. Abandon control. Stop feeling obliged. Trust. Drop out. Retreat. Enter the silence. Sink into the deep and nourishing dark. Leap off the edge. Surrender. Become the formless void. Be innocent. Be spacious. Be empty. Be present.

Doing Nothing is watchful waiting. It is not avoidance, where we hope that the problem will disappear if we refuse to face it, and we must continuously distract ourselves from the thing we are determined not to think about. Doing Nothing embraces the problem and faces it without delusion, strife, repulsion, or urgency.

". . . reaching out for the unlimited in which to lose herself."
Kate Chopin, *The Awakening*

We don't know, and we don't need to know. "I don't know" makes space for healing intelligence which comes without words, which exists outside of linear time.

"Having been reduced to nothing, nothing may then express itself. The expression of nothingness is love . . . without a source, without an object."
Steven Harrison, *Doing Nothing*

Step 0 gives us permission to live to our fullest potential, without apology. Step 0 helps us be still enough to hear the holy whisper, the invitation to acknowledge our wholeness and holiness, to give up our limits, lacks, and excuses, to live a life that is richer, brighter, fuller and more mysterious.

"The most valuable thing we can do for the psyche, occasionally, is to let it rest, wander, live in the changing light of a room, not try to be or to do anything whatever." May Sarton, *Journal of a Solitude*

Tranquility gives up the fight without giving in. Serenity Medicine connects us to the calm, undisturbed, eternal Self. We understand that we are already perfect, already healthy/whole/holy.

There is Nothing to do.

Relaxation

Relaxation is an essential Serenity Medicine. We could even say it is the goal of Serenity Medicine.

Relaxation is not just taking a nap, or chilling out. Relaxation leads to and builds on the "relaxation response" – a feeling of increased well-being. Breathing slows, blood pressure drops, heart rate calms, muscle tension relaxes, and cortisol levels decrease.

Much research has been done on the health benefits of relaxation. The results are often confusing, since techniques from Step 0 (progressive relaxation, autogenic training, biofeedback-assisted relaxation, meditation, mindfulness, and deep breathing) and Step 2 (prayer, guided imagery, and self-hypnosis) and Step 3 (yoga, Tai chi, and Qi Gong) are all lumped together in many studies.

Nonetheless, it is certain that the effects of a relaxation practice linger for months, even without further practice. And that they are cumulative. Those who practice the most, get the most.

Relaxation techniques
o   Counter anxiety associated with medical procedures
o   Offer a way to tap our inner capacity to heal
o   Lower cholesterol levels
o   Reduce insomnia
o   Lower blood pressure and keep it low for years afterward
o   Ease labor pain; ease chronic pain in children/adolescents
o   Stop chemotherapy-induced nausea
o   Strengthen the immune system
o   Widen restricted respiratory passages in asthmatics
o   Reduce the need for insulin in some diabetics
o   Ease TMJD (temporomandibular joint dysfunction)
o   Increase levels of antibodies and natural killer (NK) cells
o   Counter social anxiety disorder
o   Reduce the frequency and severity of chronic headaches

Serenity Medicine helps those dealing with post traumatic stress, attention deficits, hyperactivity, eating disorders, psoriasis, and those who wish to stop using alcohol, tobacco, or drugs.

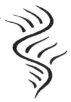 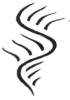

Serenity Medicine
to Remove Trauma

For relieving both acute and chronic trauma. A woman injured in a car accident 25 years previously found it relieved her chronic pain. Someone who fell off a cliff remembered to do this and walked away without a bruise. Repeat as often as desired.

Sit comfortably, with your back supported and upright. Relax more and more with each breath. Be at ease. Sink. Let go of your belly, your jaw, your throat. Relax more and more deeply with each breath. Be embraced.

Trust the breath. It is breathing you. Relinquish control. Do nothing. Be vast. Be spacious.

Allow your mind to be open and soft. Recall the incident that traumatized you. Focus on the impact. Remember the contact. The hard part.

Then, say: "I am made of atoms. Everything is made of atoms. Atoms are mostly empty space. Emptiness impacted emptiness. Nothing hit nothing. Spaciousness invaded spaciousness. I am untouched.

"I am spacious. I am serene. I am empty. I am spaciousness breathing spaciousness. I am breath arising from nothing, and returning to nothing. I am the vast open space of Nothing."

Breath arises and passes away. Thoughts arise and pass away. Sensations arise and pass away. Emotions arise and pass away. Life itself arises and passes away. Breathing in and breathing out. Arising and passing away. Arising out of emptiness and passing into emptiness. Alive with emptiness.

When you are ready, stretch, yawn, and sigh. Open your eyes. Say your name out loud. Reenter the world.

"Seeing nothing is the supreme insight."　　　Tilopa, Buddhist monk

Meditation/relaxation:
- o Reduces multiple dimensions of psychological stress, according to US Agency for Healthcare Research and Quality
- o Increases volume of grey matter in the happiness area of the brain (right precuneus)
- o Effectively treats obsessive-compulsive disorders
- o Increases resilience after emotional stress
- o Increases calmness; reduces anxiety
- o Creates a more coherent sense of self and identity
- o Improves emotional regulation
- o Helps decrease avoidance/suppression of emotions
- o Decreases over-arousal and heightened emotional reactivity in response to events
- o Can reduce or replace cognitive distortions, psychoses, substance abuse, and self-harm
- o Improves objectivity in emotional/morally difficult situations
- o Increases levels of feel-good chemicals, such as serotonin

♥ A meta-analysis of 30 randomized, controlled trials found high quality evidence for significant relief of depressive symptoms.

♥ At least 47 well-designed, reliable studies show meditation is as effective as medication in treating some forms of anxiety and depression. [Johns Hopkins, *JAMA*, 2014]

Serenity Medicines help prevent cognitive decline by:
- o Increasing grey matter in the hippocampus and parietal lobe, which improves attention span
- o Increasing memory and visual recall (sustained for six months)
- o Protecting against age-related brain atrophy
- o Significantly improving executive functioning (sustained for six months)
- o Increasing expressions of compassion
- o Increasing speed of learning; supporting memory
- o Increasing cognitive flexibility
- o Improving response times
- o Increasing verbal fluency
- o Promoting mitotic cell longevity
- o Increasing hormones that protect telomeres
- o Increasing production of human growth hormone (HGH)

Serenity Medicine is anti-inflammatory.
o   It relieves IBS (Irritable Bowel Syndrome) symptoms.
o   It eases flare-ups in those with ulcerative colitis.
o   It reduces arthritis and joint pain.

Serenity Medicine increases healthy immunity.
o   It boosts natural killer cell formation as we age.
o   It gives greater resistance to tumor formation.
o   It results in fewer viral infections.
o   It reduces the risk of cancer recurrence.

Serenity Medicine reduces pain.
o   Meditation and relaxation activate the anterior cingulate cortex and the ventromedial prefrontal cortex, giving rise to analgesic effects and a greater ability to tolerate pain.
o   Techniques such as conscious breathing and mantra meditation also improve pain tolerance. So does getting more sleep.

Serenity Medicine reduces risk of stroke/heart attack.
o   After reviewing 400 studies, the American Heart Association concluded meditation has "possible benefit on CVD risk reduction."
o   Research also suggests that relaxation may help those with chronic depression, fibromyalgia, nightmares, rheumatoid arthritis, tinnitus, epilepsy, and infertility.

When you experience Serenity Medicine are you . . .

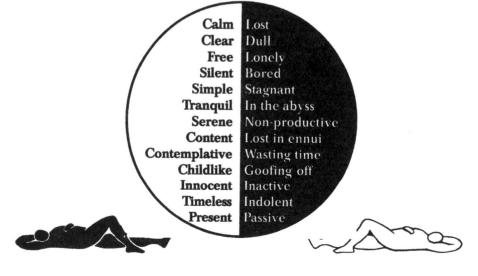

Calm	Lost
Clear	Dull
Free	Lonely
Silent	Bored
Simple	Stagnant
Tranquil	In the abyss
Serene	Non-productive
Content	Lost in ennui
Contemplative	Wasting time
Childlike	Goofing off
Innocent	Inactive
Timeless	Indolent
Present	Passive

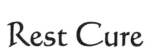

Rest Cure

The rest cure has been valued throughout medical history. Only recently – since industrialization enticed us to act like machines which never rest, and modern drugs gave us the means to carry on without rest – has respect for the healing power of rest been lost (except for induced coma in trauma care).

A rest cure is time off. Rest cures of many months were the norm a hundred years ago. Not today. Today we practice *Shinrin Yoku* (page 71), step into a float pod, or weave short rest stops into our busy lives.

William Osler, father of American medicine, was a proponent of the rest cure. He called it *"therapeutic nihilism."* Osler refused to use the revered treatments of his day (1884) – bloodletting, purgatives, and cathartics – or any unproven treatments, for that matter. Pure water, good food, clean sheets, and sunlit rooms were his sole treatments. The responses of his patients were usually rewarding and occasionally miraculous.

My mentor Elisabeth Kübler-Ross taught me to make use of every opportunity for rest, no matter how brief: waiting at a long traffic light, standing in line at the supermarket, while a file is downloading. I had complained that she didn't give us enough time to sleep. She replied that it was useless for me to sleep since I didn't know how to rest.

With her help, I learned to rest numerous times every day, as well as for long periods when I can. A brief rest promotes deeper, better sleep and sharper mental focus when it is time to work.

Quick Rest Stop: With closed eyes, slowly count backwards to zero. 10 - 9 - 8 - 7 - 6 - 5 - 4 - 3 - 2 - 1 - 0. Invite the relaxation response. Slowly count up from zero to ten. Open your eyes.

A **float pod** allows you to float in rich darkness and absolute silence on water that makes you super bouyant. It is a modern way to experience the traditional shamanic initiation of being buried alive, the ultimate rest.

"Idleness is only a coarse name for my infinite capacity for living in the present."
Cyril Connolly

Is It Safe to Do Nothing?

Serenity Medicine is a splendid way to maintain abundant health. But the idea of doing Nothing when faced with a serious injury or life-threatening illness seems absurd at best, fraught with harm at worst. Surely immediate action is better.

It isn't. Do Nothing is a healthy first response to all challenges. Watchful waiting, not fear-based reaction.

A First Responder told me: "When I arrive at a scene, I close my eyes and sink into the ground. When I open my eyes, I know where I need to go. How do I know? I don't. Nothing knows."

When I fell at the waterfall and hurt my wrist, I asked everyone to look for my lost glasses. Meanwhile, I sank into the river, allowing myself to be spacious, open, empty. They didn't find my glasses, but I had time to find myself and my strength, and understood how to proceed with my healing.

Many injuries and diseases are self-correcting. Our bodies want to be well, after all. Watchful waiting is a medically acceptable way to deal with prostate cancer and other problems. Oncologists I interviewed told me that it is almost always safe to wait 2-4 weeks before choosing treatment for cancer.

What distinguishes Serenity Medicine from denial (Stupidly-Burying-Your-Head-in-the-Sand Medicine) is a **time limit**. To do nothing for a reasonable amount of time can resolve problems, improve overall health even if the problem remains, and positively influence the eventual outcome. Denying a problem can make it more difficult to treat. Ignoring a problem can prove fatal.

In most non-acute cases – without bleeding, fever, or acute, unaccountable pain – watchful waiting on your own for 2-6 weeks is reasonable. Watchful waiting for a longer time is best done partnered with a skilled health care professional.

According to Dr. Kurt Kroenke, professor of medicine at Indiana University, more than 30 percent of unexplainable symptoms disappear forever – without treatment – within **two weeks**. And 47 percent of unexplainable symptoms are lessened – again without treatment – in two weeks. [*People's Medical Society, Aug 1998*]

Sleep

"Sleep is the single most effective thing you can do to reset your brain and body for health."   Matthew Walker, neuroscientist

Sleep is Step 0. Deep sleep brings deep healing. The sleep of induced coma helps heal those with severe trauma.

Sleeping and breathing are Step 0 remedies that we already do. Paying attention to them improves health. For most adults, most of the time, sleeping about 6-8 hours out of 24 will:

o Increase longevity
o Counter the effects of stress; decrease pain
o Increase physical strength, speed, and endurance
o Increase emotional stability
o Decrease inflammation; decrease C-reactive protein
o Lower blood pressure; lower cholesterol
o Improve immunity; prevent colds and the flu. Those who sleep less than 7 hours a night are 3 times as likely to get sick.
o Support creativity
o Improve the ability to reason and sharpen focus
o Improve reaction time and decision making
o Improve the consolidation and organization of memories
o Prevent anxiety and depression
o Increase testosterone levels and sex drive
o Prevent accidents; 20 percent of auto crashes are sleep-related
o Help children; those who get less than 8 hours of sleep are more likely to be hyperactive, inattentive, and impulsive
o Influence healthy weight; less sleep means less leptin and greater hunger, especially for high-calorie foods

For Deeper, Healthier Sleep:

Turn off the lights, especially electronics, or wear a sleep mask.
Turn down the alcohol. Turn down the heat.
Turn off all sounds or wear ear plugs.
Turn down the caffeine.
Try a weighted blanket.

Do Nothing: The Birth of Rose Moon

This true story was told to me by a woman in southern Virginia.

I was about six months pregnant when I realized my baby hadn't moved for hours. The midwife confirmed my worst fear: "There's no heartbeat." We looked at each other and wondered, "What shall we do?"

First, we accepted the situation and our powerlessness to change it. We acknowledged our grief and despair, our rage and regret.

Then we began to collect information. A local obstetrician said the baby would rot after a month and poison me and that I should be hospitalized as soon as possible to remove the fetus.

But I wanted to wait and see if my body would go into labor. For three weeks I was patient. Then I gave in to fear and, with the midwife's help, took lots of ginger tea and blue cohosh tincture. Labor did begin, but my cervix wouldn't dilate, even after hours of herbs and contractions, so nothing happened.

Finally, I stopped taking the herbs. I found myself thinking: "Let me really enter the Silence of this. Let me actively seek to do Nothing and see what happens."

I got in bed and stayed in the silence, in the dark. My dead child came to me in a dream. She said: "My name is Rose Moon. Make a hole in the ground for me. Make a space in your heart for me. Wait for me."

When I related my dream to my husband and children, a miracle happened. Whereas before they had been unhappy and angry, each feeling alone with the loss and pain, now they had a goal. Now they worked together to make space for the new baby. They ceased wondering who, or what, was to blame.

Just by chance, a few weeks later, I met an old retired general practitioner and confided my condition to him.

"Yup," he said. "It's a real sorry thing to carry a dead fetus."

"How did you get them out; what did you do?"

"Just waited 'til they came out on their own. Sometimes took a while, too."

"Don't they rot and poison the mother?"

"Now, who's telling you that?" He nodded. "You just hang on. Don't have to do a thing. It'll all work out just fine. You'll see."

And so it did. On my due date two months later, my daughter Rose Moon was born, and buried, at home. And all I did was Nothing.

"Not doing, the wise soul doesn't do it wrong."   Lao Tzu

Conscious Breathing

My teachers of Tai chi, yoga, and voice tell me to focus on my breath, to exhale fully. "Empty!" they demand.

"The breath is not simply to calm yourself . . . or develop concentration; it nourishes awareness throughout." Larry Rosenberg, *Insight Meditation*

Better breathing = Better health

Conscious breathing counters stress, activates the parasympathetic (peaceful) nervous system, trains and strengthens the respiratory system, and improves concentration. Learn to breathe better by observing your breathing. Then play with breath frequency, rhythm, phase durations, and the nostril through which you breathe. Deepen the breath; bring it into the belly. Slow the breath; lengthen the exhale. Make the breath light and feathery. Make the breath strong and definite.

In yoga, conscious breathing is called *pranayama.* Alternate-nostril breath is the queen of pranayama. Science agrees: It strengthens the heart, lungs, and nerves, making it especially useful for those with chronic obstructive pulmonary disease (COPD).

Alternate-Nostril Breath: Sit comfortably. Settle down. Fold the first two fingers of your hand into the palm. Place the thumb on one side of your nose, ring finger and little finger on the other. Press with your thumb to close one nostril. Breathe in with the other. Press with your ring and little fingers to close that nostril. Hold. Then release the thumb and exhale. Inhale and press the nostril closed. Hold. Release the opposite nostril. Exhale. Inhale and press that nostril closed. Hold. Continue for three minutes.

At first, inhale (2-3-4), hold (2-3-4), and exhale (2-3-4) to a count of four. After you are comfortable with this pranayama, alter it by increasing the length of the exhale or by holding each segment longer.

Nothing works all the time.
Nothing solves all problems.
Nothing makes everyone happy.

Meditate

"Meditation, not medication."   Robert Schneider, MD

Meditation can be transcendental or mindful, sitting or walking, zen or buddhist, alone or in a group. A meditation practice benefits from, but does not require: a quiet location, a comfortable pose, and something to focus on. Whatever kind of meditation you do, tradition and current science – including the *Journal of Pain, JAMA,* and *Frontiers in Psychology* – concur:
Meditation practices enhance overall health and well-being.

Scientific studies show meditation can:
- o Decrease chronic neck pain better than exercise
- o Improve sleep quality
- o Counter and prevent depression
- o Significantly lower stress hormones
- o Calm inflammation
- o Slow brain aging

Neuro-imaging reveals that different meditation styles are associated with different brain activity. Transcendental Meditation (TM) involves the repetition of a word or phrase (mantra). Mindfulness meditation (MM) uses focused attention. Tai chi and Qi Gong are moving meditations. You don't need incense or lots of time to meditate; even five minutes a day can make a difference.

The National Center for Complementary and Integrative Health (NCCIH), a division of the National Institutes for Health (NIH), is funding studies to investigate meditation as a way to:
- o Relieve chronic pain in adolescents
- o Moderate fibromyalgia pain; relieve headaches
- o Mitigate stress due to multiple sclerosis
- o Help those with post traumatic stress (PTSD)
- o Reduce hypertension

"Nothing, in its various guises, has been a subject of enduring fascination for millennia. Philosophers struggled to grasp it, mystics dreamed they could imagine it; scientists strove to create it; astronomers to locate it. . . ."
John Barrow, *The Book of Nothing*

Be Silent

". . . silence is to the spirit what sleep is to the body. . . ." William Penn

Step 0 is silent. Noise is a stressor linked to heart disease, high blood pressure, low birth weight, gastrointestinal disorders, headaches, fatigue, and insomnia. Enter into the silence.

"Everything that happens in our bodies happens in complete silence. The principle of healing is to invoke silence – going into the silence."
Mother Serena

Silence helps us become one with the sacred space where abundant health thrives. Let go of words and listen to your breath. Sit as silently as a hawk. Be still. Be in your body.

". . . the endless message forming itself from silence." Rainer Maria Rilke

Silence softens us, opens us in subtle ways, and increases our receptivity to new possibilities. When we step away from words, our animal nature comes closer, feelings rise, sensations abound, memories tickle us.

"Silence illuminates our souls. . . ." Khalil Gibran

"The Seneca believe that during silent communication the physical body undergoes stages of healing and upliftment." Twylah Nitsch, *Wolf Clan elder*

Silence is pre-verbal, pre-linguistic. It is the world of the primitive, ancient, essential Self who knows how to survive and thrive.

"Feminine silence . . . [is] ancient, deep and fraught with knowledge."
Stephanie Demetrakopoulos

"Practice silence and you will acquire silent knowledge. [It] is far more precise and far more accurate and far more powerful than anything that is contained in the boundaries of rational thought." Deepak Chopra

The poet Emily Dickinson speaks of an "appetite for silence." The British theologian, Robert Merrill Bartlett, invites us into "the Great Empire of Silence."

"Silence is for me a font of healing." Carl G. Jung

Seek silence. Quiet your mind. Set aside your fear. Fall into the well of nothingness. Experience the deep silence of the innermost cave of your being.

"[They] were trained to listen intently to nothing because the secrets lie in the spaces between the sounds . . . [to] listen when all is quiet and look when there is nothing to see." Lyall Watson, *Gifts of Unknown Things*

Know Nothing, Be Nothing

"L'essentiel est invisible pour les yeux." Antoine de Saint-Exupéry ["What is essential is invisible to the eyes."]

When we cannot envision the next step. When we are filled with confusion. When our very existence feels threatened. That is the time to be Nothing.

Whether we remain surrounded by activity or find time for retreat is immaterial. Nothing is a state of mind. Nothing requires us to be childlike, involved, trusting. We need not stop what we are doing; we need only to stop trying to do it right.

The gesture that means "I don't know" turns open palms to the sky. When we know nothing we open our hands; neither clinging nor resisting. Empty. Serene. Ready to improvise. Ready to heal.

Nothing is refined and charged, brilliant and full, a fertile, wide space of silence and awareness. Not knowing is Wu Ji – "beginner's mind."

A beginner knows nothing, which leads to Nothing. A beginner is open, receptive, free of preconception. In beginner's mind we don't know the right answer, or if there is a right answer, or even if there is a question.

"Remain as empty as possible, so God can fill you up." Mother Teresa

"I don't know.
I don't know.
Nothing, nothing,
Nothing do I know.
Nothing do I know.
Good, good."

Russian folksong

In the silence, in the stillness, in the dark, alone, I face the terror of surrender, of annihilation. Knowing seems safe. Not knowing seems risky. Who am I if I am Nothing? What remains if I am devoured by Nothing?

I am blameless. Perfect. Whole.

In the presence of Nothing there are no excuses, limits, lacks, or reasons. I am, just as I am, and just as I am is perfect in this moment. My problems are vital pieces of my wholeness seeking reintegration, not demons to be vanquished and overcome.

Nothing is everything, and thus it is larger than my problem. Nothing invites me to give up needing a solution right now, and let go, find zero and become accepting, available, playful.

"I wish there was a way to make 'I don't know' a positive thing, which it isn't in our society. We need to 'know'... and we substitute that quest for the actual experience... in all its complexity."   Keith Jarrett, jazz artist

"I did nothing, for there was nothing I could do. And doing that nothing, I saw at last how much I'd done, and hadn't done, and what the doing of it drained out of me...."   Drusilla Modjeska, *The Orchard*

The Do-Nothing Workout

Don't run or do yoga or go to the gym every day. "If you go hard every day, you'll never do your best," say professional coaches. Scott Trappe, director of the Human Performance Lab at Ball State University concurs: Without rest "you won't achieve your potential." Fitness experts advise a rest of a minute or two between sets of reps for maximum effect. Rest is essential in yoga.

"To sustain emptiness is to create enormous internal strength and wisdom...."   Chungliang Al Huang, Tai chi quan master/teacher

"Have you noticed that it's the little quiet moments in the midst of life that seem to give the rest extra-special meaning?"   Mr. (Fred) Rogers

Release LinearTime

Linear time is created by people. Nature, ourselves included, lives in cyclical patterns, not measured time. Release time and you discover the timeless present of health/wholeness/holiness.

Physicist Stephen Hawking maintains that time is an illusion. We are in a permanent Now. Everything already exists, contained within the "holographic potentiality of zero-point energy stored within a zero-point field." In Step Zero we access this permanent Now and allow it to create abundant health in our lives.

Releasing linear time is one of those simple, safe remedies that old wives, shamans, and healers of all sorts have used since time out of mind. You can do it too, easily and successfully.

Get rid of all clocks for a day, or even the entire weekend.

Listen to your rhythms, your cycles of sleep and wake, hunger and satisfaction. Reestablish your connections with the sun and the moon and the earth. Retime yourself to the pulse of the universe.

Let go of being up to the minute. Stop racing the clock, beating the deadline, counting the seconds. Just be, in timeless reverie.

Campers deprived of artifical light sleep two hours longer than normal and sleep better for weeks afterward. No time to camp? Take a walk in the sun; sleep in the dark. Sunlight is a powerful trigger to "feel-good, sleep-well" brain hormones.

No matter how pressed for time we feel, there is time for a breath, time to center, time to find zero.

The Sabbath is a "palace in time" set outside of time, a regular time of timelessness. My apprentices get a moon-day when they bleed, a timeless day with no responsibilities.

Lie down and listen to the crabgrass grow,
The faucet leak, and learn to leave them so.
Yourself, be still –
There is no living when you're nagging time
And stunting every second with your will.

Marya Mannes

Rushing to my train in Holland, I fidget tensely: my train leaves in two minutes and a dozen traffic lights block our approach to the station. My driver, noticing my distress, smiles and says "You have 120 seconds until the train leaves." I allow myself to know nothing. I release linear time. We arrive at the station. I find my track and board the train. It leaves, on time.

"Sometimes, on a summer morning, . . . I sat in my sunny doorway from sunrise 'til noon, rapt in a revery, . . . in undisturbed solitude and stillness . . . until by the sun falling in at my west window . . . I was reminded of the lapse of time."   Henry David Thoreau

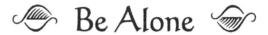

Be Alone

". . . being alone, constructively alone, is a prerequisite for every phase of the creative [healing] process."   Barbara Powell, *Alone, Alive & Well*

Whether on the mountaintop or on a city street, solitude is an important way to nourish abundant health/wholeness.

"If a woman is to know herself, then periods of solitude should be courted, planned, and embraced."   Mary Kay Blakely, *The Wonders of Solitude*

"Solitude is good after you're full . . . [not] if your spirit is empty. . . . "
                                        Isaac Bashevis Singer

By yourself, alone, the cables, strands, and strings of tension can be loosened. The mind can be allowed to relinquish the need to control. The heart can break open.

"There is nothing either/or about being alone, because it is not a role. It is not a reduced way of life. It is . . . the discovery of our whole selves."
                                        Phyllis Hobe, *Never Alone*

". . . certain experiences and truths are so alien to ordinary conscious-ness that [one] must withdraw in order to experience them."
                            Carol Christ, *Why Women Need the Goddess*

We all need time alone now and then, more after a major loss. Some menopausal women need several years of solitude during their Change, others find the occasional solitary retreat better than a sharp retort. Let your solitude be full of you, an independent being. Let your personal priorities become clear.

". . . if one says: I cannot come because that is my hour to be alone, one is considered rude, egotistical or strange. But women need solitude in order to find again the true essence of themselves. . . ." Anne Morrow Lindbergh

A clear signal helps when courting solitude: sit in a special place, wear a certain scarf, close the door, go for a walk.

"A moment without weight or duration, a moment outside the moment . . ."
Octavio Paz (trans. by Eliot Weinberger)

In solitude you can give in to grief, give in to exhaustion, give in to failure. In solitude you can allow confusion and let go of control. In solitude, in Nature, it is clear that the spiral of life always offers us greater, deeper, richer, more spontaneous wholeness/holiness/health. In solitude, Do Nothing. Offer yourself to emptiness. Release desire, attachment, and expectation. Allow yourself the freedom to envision health differently. Make yourself available for a miracle.

Many conditions improve when rest allows the body's own natural healing powers to work.

". . . the finite becomes conscious of the infinite residing in it."
D. Suzuki

" The diagnosis: metastatic cancer, so far advanced that treatment was useless. I had two weeks of life left.
"I was frightened. I was sad. I was angry. Who were they to tell me when to die? I'd show them: I'd die sooner!
"I went home, unplugged the phone, pulled the shades down, turned off the lights, threw away the clock, got into bed, pulled the covers over my head, and went to sleep, hoping never to wake up.
"I did wake up, but I refused to get up. I lay in the dark for days. I couldn't tell if I was asleep or awake. I did not speak, I did not eat, I did not read or watch TV. I did Nothing.
"Time must have passed. I felt restless. I felt hungry. I got up. That was five years ago. " Sophia, age 55, CPA

Fast

There are water fasts, juice fasts, brown rice fasts, grapefruit fasts, and fasts from specific foods, like meat. Not eating is a Step 0 technique that can improve health or injure it. Severe fasting is anorexia. Since the brain must eat constantly, it is rarely healthy to go without solid food for more than twelve hours.

Intermittent, rather than continuous fasts, are healthiest. That means 12 hours between dinner and breakfast, or alternating days of 500 and 2000 calories, or alternating two weeks of full calories and two weeks of reduced calories. I now see my aversion to eating breakfast too early as a healthy desire to be foodless for 12 hours.

o Medically supervised fasting eliminated the need for insulin in some type-2 diabetics. [*British Med Journal Case Reports*, 2018]

o Rats fed every other day live 83 percent longer than those fed daily.

o Intermittent fasting reduced Alzheimer's symptoms in nine out of ten patients. [www.aging-us.com/article/100690]

o Fasting protects against stroke damage; slows cognitive decline.

o Intermittent fasting is a mild stress that stimulates cellular defenses against molecular damage.

o Occasional fasting increases the number of special proteins that prevent mistakes in the assembly of cellular molecules.

o Fasting mice have higher levels of brain-derived neurotrophic factor, a protein that prevents stressed neurons from dying.

o Fasting increases a cell's ability to rid itself of damage.

o A rapid, significant alleviation of symptoms occurred in over-weight asthmatics who fasted every other day for two months.

o Fasting may protect against neurodegenerative diseases like Parkinson's and Huntington's.

o Fasting may improve the effectiveness of chemotherapies.

But:

o A 2011 study found long-term intermittent fasting increased tissue levels of glucose and damaging oxidizing compounds.

o A 2010 study found rats who periodically fasted developed stiff heart tissue, which impeded pumping ability.

Step 0: Serenity Medicine
References and Resources

"Inside the proton lies the deep, unsettling truth. Stuff is made of nothing. . . ."   Robert Kunzig, physicist

Barrow, John D. *The Book of Nothing: Vacuums, Voids, and the Latest Ideas about the Origins of the Universe.* Pantheon Books, 2000.

Benson, Herbert MD. *The Relaxation Response.* Morrow, 2000.

Connelly, Dianne. *All Sickness is Homesickness.* CTA, 1986.

Genz, Henning. *Nothingness: Science of Empty Space.* Perseus, 1999.

Gross, Amy. "The Art of Doing Nothing." *Tricycle,* 1998.

Hampl, Patricia. *The Art of the Wasted Day.* Viking, 2018.

Harrison, Steven. *Doing Nothing.* Tarcher, 1998.

Hodgkinson, Tom and Matthew De Abaitua, eds. *The Idler's Companion: An Anthology of Lazy Literature.* Ecco, 1997.

Holland, Barbara. *Endangered Pleasures: In Defense of Naps.* Little, Brown & Co, 1995.

Huber, Cheri. *When You're Falling, Dive: The Power of Acceptance.* Keep It Simple Books, 2003.

Japenga, Ann. "The Siesta Cure." *Utne Reader.* Feb 2004.

Kaplan, Robert. *The Nothing That Is: A Natural History of Zero.* Oxford University Press, 1999.

Keizer, Garret. "Sound and Fury." *Harper's Magazine,* March 2001.

Lao Tzu. *Tao Te Ching,* trans. Ursula K. Le Guin. Shambhala, 1977.

Levine, Stephen. *A Gradual Awakening.* Anchor, 1979.

Lindbergh, Anne Morrow. *Gift From the Sea.* Pantheon Books, 1955.

Nitsch, Twylah; Yehwehnode. *Entering Into the Silence, the Seneca Way.* Seneca Indian Historical Society, 1976.

Paz, Octavio. "Repose, Reconciliation," trans. Eliot Weinberger. 1998.

Park, Alice. "The Sleep Cure." *Time.* Feb 2017.

Rosenberg, Larry. *Breath by Breath.* Shambhala, 1998.

Russell, Bertrand. *In Praise of Idleness.* Routledge, 1932.

Salwak, David. *The Wonders of Solitude.* New World, 1998.

Siegel, Bernie MD. "I Want to Be a Nobody . . . and Have Nothing to Offer You." *Massage Therapy Journal.* Spring 1998.

Smith, Robert L. *A Quaker Book of Wisdom: Life Lessons in Simplicity, Service, and Common Sense.* William Morrow, 1998.

Tarrant, John. "Not Doing." *Personal Transformation.* Summer 1999.
Vienne, Veronique. *The Art of Doing Nothing: Simple Ways to Make Time for Yourself.* Clarkson Potter, 1998.
Wolinsky, Stephen, PhD. *The Book of Serenity.* Quantum Press, 2010. stephenhwolinskyphdlibrary.com/downloads

> "*To do nothing at all is the most difficult thing in the world.*"
>
> Oscar Wilde

Serenity. Go to these websites and type in "relaxation therapy."
- www.cochranelibrary.com [43 meta-studies]
- www.nccih.nih.gov [several dozen studies]
- www.ncbi.nlm.nih.gov/pubmed ["A randomized controlled study of mindfulness meditation versus relaxation therapy."]

> "*I loaf and invite my soul.*"
>
> Walt Whitman

Meditation
- https://nccih.nih.gov/health/meditation
- www.wildmind.org/resources
- http://marc.ucla.edu/mindful-meditations
- www.freemindfulness.org/download
- www.insighttimer.com
- www.plumvillage.org

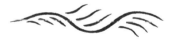

Fasting
- https://www.jwatch.org/fw114657/2018/10/10/therapeutic-fasting-could-be-alternative-insulin-some
- www.scientificamerican.com/article/does-intermittent-fasting-work

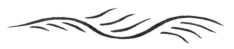

> *Form is emptiness, emptiness is form.*
> *Form does not differ from emptiness.*
> *Emptiness does not differ from form.*
>
> The Heart Sutra

> *You must have been warned against Letting the golden hours slip by.*
> *Yes, but some of them are golden Only because we let them slip.*
>
> J. M. Barrie

The Truth Is . . .

"The truth is that doctors *have no idea* how you feel and will never know how you feel because the doctor does not live inside your body – you do.

"The truth is that to get the correct healthcare for you, you have to understand how you feel and express it in everyday language without fear of being judged.

"The truth is you have no real choice but to seek a doctor who listens to you and is going to protect you with sound advice that resonates with you. That doctor must be committed to *you* and work only for *you.* To truly represent you, the doctor cannot have other masters – not malpractice fears, pressure from drug companies, insurance companies, equipment companies, or any other 'invisible presence' in the examination room.

"The truth is that if you don't feel right about a doctor's advice, but accept it out of fear, you are risking your health and potentially your life.

"The truth is that not every doctor is right for you. The doctor-patient relationship isn't different from any other human relationship. If it's a good fit, stay with it. If it's not right and you choose to stay, it might kill you.

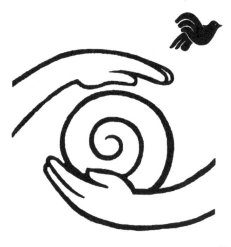

"The truth is that every word a doctor speaks to a patient has tremendous impact. In medical school, there is no training in sensitivity or how to speak to a patient. If your doctor is not impeccable with his [her] words and care, no matter how adept [s]he is in his [her] field, this deficiency may be devastating to your life and health."

Erika Schwartz MD, June 2015
Don't Let Your Doctor Kill You
with permission from Post Hill Press

Step One

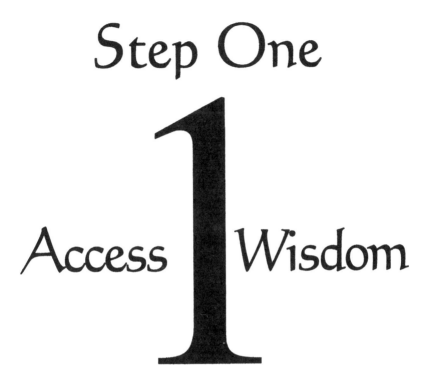

Access **1** Wisdom

Story Medicine

"Keep some room in your heart for the unimaginable."
Mary Oliver, poet, Pulitzer Prize winner

Gather Information, Access Wisdom

o Read	o Write
o Discuss	o Dream
o Listen	o Draw
o Question	o Invite guidance
o Study	o Try hypnosis, self-hypnosis
o Ask your circle of friends	o Cast an oracle
o Become your own expert	o Visit the Wise Healer Within
o Tell your story	o Listen to your intuition
o Name your problem	o Consult a medical intuitive
o Consult a healer	o Go to a medical astrologer
o Get a hands-off diagnosis	o Ask a pendulum
o Get a second opinion	o Get a reading
o Consult a specialist	o Consult a shaman
o Join a support group	o Open your mind

"She looks within herself and acts according to her intuition and the situation. Her acts are deliberate, but without deliberation. Her perspective is that of a person who knows rationality but understands she is dealing with irrational forces."   Stephanie Demetrakopoulos

Set aside half an hour each day for the next four days to write down any and all thoughts, feelings, and memories about a traumatic or important issue from your past, your present, or a desired future. Give your self permission to explore all your emotions. Decide on a topic before you begin. It is fine to write about the same topic on all four days, or to choose different ones. You will not be graded on grammar or spelling or anything else. In fact, you never have to show it to anyone at all.

As long as you write for 20 minutes with only brief pauses, you have succeeded. (Give yourself ten minutes afterwards to return to normal life.) Soft, instrumental music may be helpful. A safe, private place is essential. Do not write just before bedtime.

Benefits of Story Medicine

Wise use of Story Medicine can promote
o   Increased self worth
o   Decreased anxiety
o   Strengthening of overall health
o   Improvement in mood
o   More satisfaction with life
o   Greater creative energy
o   Sharper memory

Story Medicine is the stories we tell ourselves, the stories our culture tells us, the stories we believe, the stories we trust. Change the story and you change how you perceive, and relate to, your problems. Change your story and you change your life.

Story Medicine gathers information and accesses wisdom. We move from Serenity Medicine, where we are alone, in our own minds, to Story Medicine, where we share stories with others.

Story Medicine is universal and individual, mythic and specific. Story medicine spins meaning into the fabric of our lives, and anchors us through time. Story medicine gives voice to our mysterious, sacred, inner knowing.

If Serenity Medicine doesn't resolve our problem within the time allotted, we add on or we move on to Story Medicine. We seek the story of our problem. We want to know what is wrong. We want a diagnosis. We want to hear a trusted other assure us all is well. Or, if it isn't, to help us figure out what we can do to regain health. We want a story, and we want someone to hear our story, to listen to us.

Story Medicine is safest with non-invasive diagnostic techniques. Dangers lurk both in believing a story that delays needed treatment and in moving too quickly into Step 6, where diagnostics can kill.

Story Medicine is most helpful when we write our own story, when we question authority, when we demand answers. If our fear dominates, then any story, any protocol (standard or alternative) can disempower us and make it harder to hear, understand, and act on our inner wisdom.

Grandmother Growth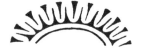

You breathe out and open your eyes, feeling wonderfully re-laxed, as though you have been held close, rocked, and cherished. The voice within you, the voice you think of as your inner Wise Woman, is vivid and clear, convincing and real.

"What do you know?" she questions you. "What do you need to know? Who will tell you? What is your story?"

You realize, with some surprise, that, in addition to hearing your imaginary Wise Woman, you can almost see her. She is in-distinct, but definitely there. More substantial than a shadow, wavering, like a mirage off a hot road.

Her eyes are the steadiest part of her, and you feel her gaze searching you, looking into you, awaiting your answer. She is all curiosity, all attention. You are aware of your breath.

"I want to know how to solve my problems," you tell her. "I want to know the right thing to do. I want to know the best way to do it. I want to be healthy. Can you help me?"

"Yes," she answers firmly. "I can help you investigate options, ask questions, lure intuition, and access wisdom. Tell me, what do your dreams say about your problems?"

"I don't know," you reply with a puzzled frown. "And it doesn't matter. I certainly wouldn't trust my dreams to tell me what to do about my problems. Isn't it better, and safer, to ask the experts?"

"Yes. Ask the experts. And ask yourself. Become, as the Mazatec shaman María Sabina would say, a woman who 'looks into the insides of things.' Become your own expert. Your inner vision is vaster than the experts' limited knowledge. Let it guide you. Let it tell you what questions to ask. Let it protect you.

"Listen to the experts, yes. And pay close attention to your dreams. Be open to the omens. Seek wise words and clear vision. Name what needs to be named. Be neither too skeptical nor too gullible. Create the story of health/wholeness/holiness that is best for you right now."

Her image fades away like drifting fog, but her voice remains in your memory, in your psyche, beckoning you. You breathe in, close your eyes and reach for her hand.

Diagnosis is a Story

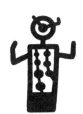

Story Medicine is diagnosis; diagnosis is a story. Step 1 is about choosing a story to guide us in our quest for health/wholeness/holiness.

And Step 1 is about sharing the story of our quest. When we have a problem, we want to know what is wrong with us. We want a story about it. We want to tell someone we trust about our problem. Sometimes the act of telling our story solves our problem. More often, it predicates our treatment.

A wise diagnostician will arrive at a "differential diagnosis" by listening, looking, feeling, intuiting, and reasoning. Many alternative/complementary/integrative health workers know and use non-invasive diagnostic techniques, keeping you safely in Step 1, away from the temptations of Step 6.

Seeker and healer alike, we are tempted to look deeper, know more, find out at any cost, flirt with danger. Step 6 high-tech diagnostics − such as biopsies, x-rays, MRIs, CT scans, exploratory surgery − invade, harm, poison, damage, maim, and even kill us.

These diagnostic tools provide useful, rational, science-based stories about our problems. But they are not the whole truth. Our DNA partakes of quantum reality, where truth is unquantifiable.

Insofar as we accept science as truth, and view intuition as mere story, we miss half the information available to us, the wisdom half. For the richest story, we need both halves.

Diagnosis, the story of our problem, affects our health in powerful ways. Accepting the stories of our doctors and our culture without question can cure our problems, but, far too often, the cure ruins our health and leaves us in chronic pain or in need of daily drugs or in deep emotional distress. For abundant health, we often need to question the popular story/diagnosis/protocol.

Each person, each problem, and each situation is unique; there is a unique story that nourishes the health/wholeness/holiness of that person, with that problem, in that situation.

"Doctors are, and always have been, the health care alternative of last resort. The real 'primary care practitioners' are non-physicians, the millions of people who practice informed self-care."   Anne Simons MD

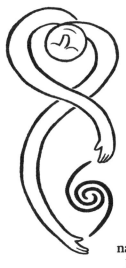

Access Wisdom

Access wisdom from your body. Access wisdom with your feelings. Access wisdom via intuition. Access wisdom in dreamtime. Access wisdom using altered states of consciousness. Access the wisdom of your inner artist. Trust the ancient wisdom in your bones, in your blood, in your DNA. Access wisdom with an oracle. Access wisdom with portents. Access wisdom through clairvoyants, intuitives, and medical astrologers. Access wisdom by listening to your guides. Let divination be part of your diagnosis.

Like Isis, who gathered the dismembered parts of her beloved, gather all the parts of your story. Wholeness/health/holiness is complex, chaotic, and contradictory. Allow yourself to accept your contradictions, your chaos, and your complexity.

Mind is uneasy with Psyche. Order abhors chaos. Orthodoxy distrusts unmeasurable, individual, unique wisdom, and warns us (rightly) against superstition, wishful thinking, and false hope.

As foolish as it would be to ignore information and decide from wisdom alone, it is more foolish, I believe, to decide only from information, ignoring wisdom.

Be open. Be skeptical. Create health/wholeness/holiness with both sides of the brain: medical facts and intuitive truths.

Non-invasive Diagnosis

o Pulse diagnosis	o Look
o Tongue diagnosis	o Listen
o Facial diagnosis	o Touch
o Tibetan urine diagnosis	o Smell
o Hara/belly diagnosis	o Ask pointed questions
o Psychic diagnosis	o Divine
o Auric diagnosis	o Intuit

Gather Information

"We can be knowledgeable with other [wo]men's knowledge, but we cannot be wise with other [wo]men's wisdom."   Michel de Montaigne

Gather information from large, controlled studies and meta-studies. Gather information from respected, peer-reviewed sources. Gather information from cutting-edge research. Gather information from those who have been there, done that.

Read widely. Listen closely. Question everything, even your own assumptions. Gather information from those studying the problem. Gather information from those personally dealing with the problem. Gather details. Compare, contrast.

Gather figures; gather facts. Gather information – it may seem odd – with hands-off diagnosis. Gather information – but be aware of the risks – with high-tech diagnosis.

Caution: Step 6 diagnostics can endanger your health.

A prevalent story in modern medicine is that diagnosis – and even good health – requires high-tech tests. This puts the patient at risk. (Specifics start on page 223.) Useful, yes. Necessary, no.

Non-invasive diagnosis is Step 1 because it does no harm. Non-invasive diagnosis is reliable, though not the "standard of care." If you are told you need a high-tech test, you will be healthier if you say: "I need time to consider my options."

"Each [diagnostic] sign means nothing by itself . . . only in its relationship to other signs."   Ted Kaptchuk

In Step 1 contact is minimal and gentle.

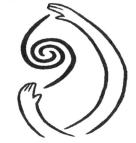

"My doctor insisted I have an MRI. I went into anaphylactic shock when they injected the contrast dye. Now I'm allergic to everything. The results of the MRI? Inconclusive!"   Abigail, chef, 47

Applied Kinesiology? Weak

"Muscle testing" has limited applications. It is easy to demonstrate that the patient responds more strongly to what the practitioner thinks than to anything else. Most AK practitioners are true believers. So were phrenologists.

Iridology? Unsound

The sticky elastic fibers covering the iris congeal into a permanent, unchangeable pattern before birth. The iris is not diagnostic, nor can it record any event occurring after birth.

Your iris is more unique than your fingerprints or your DNA, and more difficult to change.

Super-secure computers rely on iris IDs, not passwords.

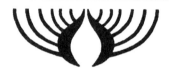

My body is innately wise.

Differential Diagnosis from the Skin
Healthy skin is smooth, warm, even, continuous, and "rosy."
Look at texture, temperature, color, flexibility, moisture

Ashy: cancer, TB, severe anemia, nephritis
Bronzing: poisoning, Addison's disease, pellagra
"Liver spots:" age, thyroid/goiter, liver cancer, irritants
Cherry red: carbon monoxide poisoning
Cold: thrombosis, poor circulation, diet lacking in heme
Cyanotic (blue): asthma, goiter, TB, ovarian tumor
Cyanosis with pallor: typhoid, silver poisoning
Dry, abnormally: thyroid deficiency, diabetes
Edema: anemia, cardiac/renal diseases
Hot and dry: fever, excess salt, extreme excitation
Moist (often): Graves' disease, malaria, pneumonia, TB
Pale: malnutrition, dropsy
Pallor: internal hemorrhage, shock; leukemia; TB; lead, mercury, or arsenic poisoning; syphilis, malaria
Purplish: asthma, typhus
Red: sunburn, irritation, alcoholism, allergies
Sallow: syphilis, constipation, anemia, gallbladder or liver disease
Yellow: jaundice, liver disease, excessive carrot juice consumption

Safe, effective, no-tech, Step 1 ways of creating a diagnostic story have been used in China, Tibet, and India for centuries. These techniques, thanks to the Internet and the jet plane, are now readily accessible to us all.

The face, tongue, and skin reveal, to the practiced eye, a wealth of diagnostic information. Palpating the feet, feeling the pulses, touching the belly reveals, to those who have training and experience, as much as Step 6 invasive tests. Healers from China say seventy percent of a person's health problems are revealed in their face.

Non-invasive diagnosis is also done by psychics and shamans with the aid of psychoactive plants. (If you take a mind-altering plant, that is Step 6.) This type of diagnosis addresses physical, emotional, and spiritual problems.

Some non-invasive diagnostic techniques are shams. Some psychics aren't psychic. Wisdom is discerning. You don't have to believe the first story you are told about your problem. Or the fifth story. And you don't have to rush, either.

The next time you have a health problem, take the time to seek out non-invasive diagnosis (resources, page 42), look for an alternative diagnosis, and become your own expert.

Scientific Tradition

Step 1 Diagnosis > *low risk* <	Step 6 Diagnosis > *high risk* <
visual examination	mammogram
urinalysis	x-rays (exposure accumulates)
swab/culture	MRI scan; PET scan
thermogram	CT/CAT scan
answering/being heard	lumbar puncture
stool sample/FIT	colonoscopy
eye exam	exploratory surgery
hearing exam	biopsy, colposcopy
EEG	endoscopic exam
ECG	angiogram
blood pressure test	laparoscopic exam
memory test	cystoscopic exam
blood draw	injection of contrast dyes

Get A Second Opinion

Our pains and our problems lead us to look for a diagnosis, and that leads to a treatment. If the treatment will improve (or not injure) your health – that is, Steps 0, 1, 2, 3, and possibly 4 – then it is safe to proceed.

If your diagnosis is linked to a treatment that will injure you – drugs, chemotherapy, radiation, surgery, cleanses (colon or liver) – it is critical to get a second opinion before proceeding.

Protect your health before agreeing to any treatment in Steps 5 or 6 by setting up another appointment with a different practitioner. A second opinion reminds us that we are not dealing with "Mommy/Daddy/Doctor/God" whose word is law. All practitioners are people, and people, even the best people, can get it wrong, can make mistakes. Get a solid second opinion.

A second opinion gives us the most information when it is outside the box. When looking for a second opinion, seek a different worldview, a different paradigm of healing, and you will find a different diagnosis, a different opinion, a different way of healing. (Most health insurance does not yet see the wisdom in supporting a wide variety of Medicines and most likely will not reimburse you for seeking a second opinion. Nonetheless, you are worth it.)

What would someone trained in Traditional Chinese Medicine have to say about your pain or your problem? What would a shamanic healer suggest? What would a medical specialist do?

The most useful second opinions come from those who have different training and a different worldview than the practitioner who is suggesting a treatment. If a surgeon says you require surgery, what would a physical therapist say? What would an acupuncturist suggest? You are worth the time and effort it takes to get a different opinion.

And it is well worth the extra expense to get a second opinion on lab tests, especially biopsies. Find a specialist. Those who have spent the most time dealing with your problem are the ones who are most likely to be of real assistance to you.

Become Your Own Expert

You don't always have to ask someone else for a diagnosis. Becoming an expert on your own health may sound like a lot of work, but it's easier than it seems, and tremendously empowering. When you're your own expert, you are the teller of your own story, the author of your own script, the creator, not the victim.

Become an expert on your own health by learning about your body and your risk factors. Then, become an expert by taking responsibility for your health, one day, and one problem at a time.

Tend yourself well. Collect and create remedies for your most common problems. Explore alternative and complementary ways of helping yourself when faced with chronic problems or trauma.

Learning about your body and your health doesn't make you an expert on all bodies. It does give you a basis for setting reasonable time limits as you explore possible ways of helping yourself. And it gives you the knowledge and wisdom to choose the safest diagnostics and the best help, when needed.

Health-care professionals have to know about many problems, many bodies. You only have to know about your own.

Become your own expert by reading articles and studies that pertain to your specific problem. Become your own expert by consulting old books, written before Step 6 became the norm. Become your own expert by collecting information about your family's health so you can forestall future problems. (Diabetes runs in some families, as does heart disease and some cancers.)

Become your own expert without reading a word. Seek out those who have studied your problem and listen to them. Seek out those who have had your problem and ask for their advice. I have learned more about my options from those who have "been there" than from any other source.

Become your own expert by realizing that there are many ways to deal well with any specific problem. Become your own expert by realizing that your way may be different from accepted norms.

How can you find knowledgeable people? Call a friend. Any two living people are, according to numbers theory, only "six degees of separation" apart. [*Sci News,* 22 Aug 98] That means you'll find the knowledge or person you need in six calls or less.

Many times I have called seasoned, educated professional friends and asked, "What would you do if this were happening?" More often than not, what they recommend can be done right at home, without a diagnosis. Whom can you call upon to help you when there's a problem?

"The universe is not only queerer than we suppose, but queerer than we can suppose."
                                              J. B. S. Haldane, biologist

Diagnosis the Wise Woman Way

A diagnosis helps us treat problems. But the Wise Woman tradition treats people, not problems, so a diagnosis is not always necessary. Nourishing health and wholeness can be independent of a diagnosis when there is nothing to fix, balance, or cleanse.

The Wise Woman tradition, still widely used in Eastern medical models, like the Buddhist Bon tradition, looks at the *relationship* between things and adjusts that. The more familiar Western model looks at *things* and treats them with little or no regard for their connections. Wholeness/health/holiness is a relationship, a process, not a task to complete.

A diagnosis allows us to focus on the problem and forget the person. A diagnosis allows us to believe that eliminating the problem is enough to make the person healthy. The Wise Woman tradition insists that the problem and the person are one, and that problems are allies of wholeness. Problems which are fixed often return. What is cleaned gets dirty. Nourishing all parts of ourselves creates abundant health.

Herbs aren't for problems, they are for people. When someone asks: "What herb is good for a headache?" I reply: "I don't know of any herb good *for* a headache, but some are good for *you* if you have a headache."

Nourishing wholeness is complex. We resist loving the unloved parts of ourselves. We deny that they even exist. It is easier to treat a diagnosis than it is to be whole. It is easier to treat a problem than to embrace ourselves as we are, right now.

It is tempting to seek information and settle for guilt. When we blame and shame ourselves, we slow down or stop healing.

A diagnosis allows us to say "why" we have the problem. But the wise woman doesn't ask "why?" Asking "why?" is asking for a reason, a cause, a something or a someone to blame. Asking "why?" is a way to escape the reality of what is happening. Asking "why?" (and changing what's wrong) takes so much time, there's none left for asking what's *right* with the problem.

When my problem is caused by something outside myself, my cure is outside myself. When my problem is my fault, my cure must be administered by someone else. When my problem is my ally of wholeness, I can claim my power and accept the gifts of my problem. I am free to nourish and love my problem.

Getting well is a fight. Getting whole is an expansion.

Abundant health is wholeness. Wholeness is all of me. There are no enemies. The Wise Woman asks: "What story is this problem telling? What piece of wholeness does it hold? How is this problem an ally of wholeness? What is asking for recognition, care, love, and kindness? How can I nourish what I dislike?"

"If healing is about being whole, then every expression of being wants acknowledgment, including the things I don't like."
Dianne M. Connelly, acupuncturist, author

A **time limit** helps ensure that gathering information doesn't become avoidance. "I can't decide until I have all the information." *You won't ever have all the information.* "I don't want to make the wrong decision." *There are no wrong decisions.* "What if I change my mind?" *You can't change your mind until you have made a decision.* "How can I be certain I'm doing the best thing?" *There are no guarantees.* "Who's telling the truth?" *Everyone has a piece of truth.* Access your inner wisdom and feel into the whole picture. *Listen to the whisper of your deepest desire.*

Problems can be resolved without a diagnosis.

Mind-Opening Diagnosis

"These plants [are] called 'doctores'... if ingested under certain conditions, they ... 'teach' the shaman."   T. McKenna, psychonaut

Mind-opening, mind-altering plants help healers access the deep story of the problem. Throughout the world these "power plants" are considered "the surest diagnostic tool," "repositories of holy wisdom," and "gateways to the truth."

"The medicos or curacas take an aqueous maceration of the leaves ... [and] they see the solution of difficult cases of ... diagnosis."
J. F. Theikuhl, 1957

Richard Evans Schultes and Terence McKenna, respected professors and pioneers of reclaiming power plants, have long advocated that traditional uses of these plants have a place in modern medicine; diagnosis is most interesting in this regard.

"Forthewith ... he toke [sic] certain leaves of the Tabaco and caste them into the fire and did receive the smoke ... he fell doune uppon the grounde as a dedde manne ... and when the hearbe had doen his woorke he did revive and awake and gave theim their answeres according to the visions and illusions which he sawe ...."
Nicolas Monardes (1493-1588), Spanish physician, botanist

As with any diagnostic tool, training and practice increase the reliability of the results. Not every shaman uses mind-altering plants as a means of diagnosis. María Sabina did. She saw the cause and the cure of problems by reading the "Book of Life" with the help of her friends, the "little people" (psilocybin mushrooms).

"Wisdom is Language. Language makes the dying return to life. The sick recover their health when they hear the words...."   María Sabina, shaman [speaking of the words she chants after eating psilocybin]

Power plants remind us: There is no place to hide; no one and nothing is to blame; chaos is a natural state of being; no action guarantees any outcome; and no one knows the right answer.

Tell Your Story Medicine

Even brief autobiographical storytelling improves mental and physical health and resilience, both immediately and for many months afterward.

"A drug intervention reporting effects similar to those found for expressive writing would be regarded as a major medical advance."
J. M. Smythe MD, *How Expressive Writing Promotes Health*

Expressive writing has been shown to:
o   Increase physical and mental performance
o   Improve lung function significantly, esp. in asthmatics
o   Reduce blood pressure
o   Sharpen memory
o   Improve immune system function, esp. in HIV patients
o   Increase liver functioning
o   Decrease anxiety and depression, esp. social anxiety
o   Lessen joint stiffness in rheumatoid arthritis
o   Reduce the intensity of chronic pelvic pain
o   Hasten the onset of sleep
o   Relieve PTSD symptoms
o   Improve recovery post-operatively
o   Support self-worth
o   Increase well-being and sense of personal power
o   Decrease hospital admission rates for chronic diseases
o   Raise grade point average for students
o   Reduce visits to health-care providers
o   Improve lifestyle: better diet and more exercise
o   Shorten the grieving period and make it more bearable

"Humanity has but one product, and that is fiction."   Annie Dillard

If diagnosis is finding a story, telling our story is the healing. When we tell our story, whether by writing or actually speaking, we empower ourselves and we empower others. When we give ourselves permission to tell the truth, we find that shame, guilt, and fear loosen their hold on us, revealing our health/wholeness.

Telling our story helps us understand the ambiguous nature of experiences, and the multiple ways they can be viewed. Fiction is not the opposite of truth. Metaphors matter.

When we tell our story in any way, we are no longer the victim, we own ourselves. "I saw I could create any ending I wanted for my own story," said Elishiva, a fifteen-year old mom (as a result of being raped when she was fourteen).

"You cannot heal what you conceal."   African proverb

Support groups allow members to share their ongoing stories, improving both quality and length of life after diagnosis of a terminal or chronic condition. Chat rooms are the Internet equivalent, and are especially helpful for those who are homebound. Whether in person or online, do take care to choose a group that focuses on gratitude and love, emotions that even the worst diagnosis cannot vanquish.

"Dismiss whatever insults your own soul, and your very flesh shall be a great poem."   Walt Whitman, American poet

People who write about past problems show increased ability to resolve longstanding issues. People who read or tell their story out loud in front of others say the hope that someone might be inspired or helped by their story gives them a sense of validation and self-worth. Those who do not share reap the same benefits if they write out their story, even if no one else reads it.

"Besides learning to see, there is another art to be learned – not to see what is not."   Maria Mitchell, astronomer

Writing Therapy

In a study of folks with asthma and arthritis who were assigned to write for 20 minutes three days in a row, twice as many who wrote about a stressful life event improved compared to those who wrote about mundane topics. After four months the progression of disease slowed in the first group. "Anyone with a chronic disease who tries writing therapy has little to lose," says Harry Greene MD [*JAMA* 4/14/99]

Is Story Medicine Safe?

What if you know something is wrong but the medical profession denies your problem? What if skilled diagnostic help is unavailable? What if you refuse invasive diagnostic tests? Is it safe to continue without a definite diagnosis? Is it possible to diagnose yourself? Do you really need a diagnosis? It depends.

Most problems don't signify something terrible. It is usually safe to diagnose yourself, and proceed with treatment, if you set a time limit, become your own expert, and understand what the worst could be. A time limit compels you to seek help if your problem worsens. Becoming your own expert means you read and study and ultimately participate in your own diagnosis. And understanding the worst focuses your attention on what is important.

Sometimes we have to help ourselves without a diagnosis, stick to what we know when we are told we are imagining things, and create abundant health on our own. Slowly, if we insist that our symptoms deserve a story and a name, we will be rewarded with recognition: PMS/premenstrual syndrome, fibromyalgia, lupus.

A diagnosis gives us access to drugs, surgery, and high-tech treatments. A diagnosis opens the door to supplements, cleanses, and other dangers. A diagnosis is required for insurance payments. But a diagnosis does not create abundant health.

Ignorance is Bliss

"When I received my prostate cancer diagnosis, you gave me things to read. When I decided to have the radioactive implants, you offered information about that.

"I didn't want to read anything, or to understand my treatment options. I really didn't want to know what was happening or what they were doing to me.

"I remained blissfully ignorant."

Evan, 68, actor

Get it in writing. A meta-study found most people forget 80 percent of the medical information offered them, and half of what they do recall is incorrect. **Make a recording.**

Step 1: Story Medicine References and Resources

Diagnosis

Beinfield, Harriet and Efrem Korngold. *Between Heaven And Earth: A Guide to Chinese Medicine.* Ballantine, 1991.

Benjamin, Ben. *Listen to Your Pain.* Penguin, 1984.

Kaptchuk, Ted. *The Web That Has No Weaver.* Congdon & Weed, 1982.

Kushi, Michio. *Your Face Never Lies.* Avery, 1983.

Lowell, Bruce MD. *Body Signals: Symptoms and What They Mean.* Harper Collins, 1995.

Ohashi. *Reading The Body (Oriental Diagnosis).* Penguin Arkana, 1991.

Welfeld, Renee. *Your Body's Wisdom.* Sourcebooks, 1997.

"The brain's resting-state circuitry – which is turned on when you stop focusing on a problem and just veg out – is very likely the best place to park a problem, for it employs the best, wisest, and most creative (though not necessarily fastest-working) mechanics."   Marcus Raichle MD, neuroscientist

Online Diagnostic Resources

- www.IsabelHealthCare.com

Tongue diagnosis

- http://eagleherbs.com/self-tests/tongue-diagnosis-38/

Pulse diagnosis

- www.greekmedicine.net/diagnosis/Pulse_Diagnosis.html
- www.ayurvedacollege.com/articles/students/pulse
- www.acupunctureandherbalmedicine.com/pulse-diagnosis/

Facial diagnosis

- http://mienshiang.com/musings-facts/the-ancient-art-of-face-reading

Tibetan urine diagnosis

- http://hps-online.com/hurinetibetean.htm
  (The urine sample is stirred with a stick in a white porcelain container; color, vapors, smell, bubbles, sediments, and film are noted.)

Be Your Own Expert/Books

Boston Women's Health Collective. *Our Bodies, Ourselves For the New Century.* Touchstone, 2011.

Burns, A. A., Ronnie Lovish, Jane Maxwell, Katharine Shapiro. *Where Women Have No Doctor: A Health Guide.* Hesperian, 1997.

Cohen, Elizabeth S. *The Empowered Patient: How to Get the Right Diagnosis, Buy the Cheapest Drugs, Beat Your Insurance Company, and Get the Best Medical Care Every Time.* Ballantine, 2010.

Federation of Feminist Women's Health Centers. *New View of a Woman's Body.* Simon & Schuster, 1981; *How to Stay Out of the Gynecologist's Office.* Women to Women, 1981.

Lanctôt, Guylaine MD. *The Medical Mafia, How to Get Out of It Alive and Take Back Your Own Health.* Here's the Key, 1995.

Lowell, Bruce. *Body Signals: When to Relax, When to be Concerned, and When to go to the Doctor Immediately.* Harper Collins, 1995.

Mayell, Mark and the editors of Natural Health Magazine. *The Natural Health First-Aid Guide.* Pocket Books, 1994.

Michelson, Leslie D. *The Patient's Playbook.* Vintage, 2016.

O'Sullivan, Suzanne. *Is It All in Your Head? True Stories of Imaginary Illness.* Other Press, 2017.

Pole, Nick. *Words That Touch: How to Ask Questions Your Body Can Answer.* Singing Dragon, 2017.

Simons, Anne MD, Bobbie Hasselbring, Michael Castleman. *Before You Call The Doctor.* Fawcett Columbine, 1992.

Smyth, Angela. *The Complete Home Healer. A Guide to Every Treatment Available for over 300 Health Problems.* HarperSF, 1994.

Werner, David. *Where There Is No Doctor.* Hesperian Foundation, 1992. www.hesperian.org

Be Your Own Expert/Internet
- www.ahna.org [American Holistic Nurses]
- www.ahrq.gov [Agency for Healthcare Research and Quality]
- www.alternative-therapies.com
- www.canhelp.com [Complementary medicine/cancer]
- www.hrsa.gov [Health Resources and Services Administration]
- www.labtestsonline.org
- www.liebertpub.com/overview/alternative-and-complementary-therapies/3/
- https://nccih.nih.gov/health/integrative-health

- www.health.gov/nhic/ [National Health Information Center]
- www.nwhn.org [National Women's Health Network]
- www.ourbodiesourselves.org [Our Bodies, Our Selves Self-Help]
- www.ncahf.org [National Council Against Health Fraud]
- www.planetree.org [Planetree Health Information]
- www.healthfinder.gov [Reliable orthodox health info sources]
- www.medscape.com [Medical news and education]
- www.nlm.nih.gov [World's largest medical database]
- www.wrf.org [World Research, all therapies]
- www.consumermedical.com

Mills, James et al. "Data Torturing." *NEJM.* Oct 1993.

"There's a world of difference between . . . data and the knowledge that people have in their bones. . . ."   Wendell Berry

Access Wisdom
Adair, Margo. *Working Inside Out.* Wingbow, 1984.
Auw, Audre. *Gentle Roads to Survival; Making Self-Healing Choices in Difficult Circumstances.* Aslan, 1991.
Blum, Ralph & S. Loughan. *The Healing Runes.* St. Martin's, 1995.
Demetrakopoulos, Stephanie. *Listening to Our Bodies.* Beacon Press, 1983.
Estrada, Alvaro. *María Sabina, Her Life and Chants.* Ross-Erikson, 1981.
Mariechild, Diane. *Mother Wit.* Crossing Press, 1981.
Markova, Dawna. *No Enemies Within.* Conari, 1994.
Masters, Robert. *Listening to the Body.* Delacourt, 1978.
McMurray, Madeline. *Illuminations.* Wingbow, 1988.
Mehl-Madrona, Lewis MD. *Narrative Medicine.* Bear & Co, 2007.
Mindell, Arnold. *Working On Yourself Alone.* Arkana, 1990.
Palmer, Helen (ed). *Inner Knowing: Insight and Intuition.* Tarcher, 1998.
Prendergast, John J. *In Touch: How to Tune in to the Inner Guidance of Your Body and Trust Yourself.* Sounds True, 2015.
Pennebaker, J. W. *Opening Up.* Guilford Press, 1997.
Roman, S. & D. Packer. *Opening to Channel.* HJ Kramer, 1987.

Story Medicine
Banayat, Melanie. *Stretch Your Brave, Hack Your Story: Break Through Chronic Disease with Storytelling.* Nourish Me Academy, 2015.
Dillard, Annie. *Living by Fiction.* Harper & Row, 1982.
Ditkoff, Mitch. *Storytelling at Work.* Ideas Champions, 2015.

Endicott, G. *Spinning Wheel: The Art of Mythmaking.* Attic Press, 1994.

Estés, Clarissa. *Women Who Run With the Wolves.* Ballantine, 1992.

Gates, Henry Louis and Maria Tatar, eds. *Annotated African American Folktales.* Liverwright, 2018.

Lepore & Smyth (eds). *The Writing Cure.* American Psychological Association, 2002.

Meade, Erica. *Moon in the Well: Wisdom Tales.* Open Court, 2001.

Perroe, Susan. *Therapeutic Storytelling.* Hawthorn Press, 2012.

Smythe, J. M. *J. of Consulting & Clinical Psychology,* 66, 174–184(1998).

Stone, Richard. *The Healing Art of Storytelling.* Hyperion, 1996.

Trevanian. *The Summer of Katya.* Ballantine, 1983.

"The health benefits of writing your life story." *Harvard Men's Health Watch.* May 2018.

"Intuition is arriving at accurate conclusions based on inadequate information."   Mona Lisa Schultz

- www.thesunmagazine.org [the *Sun* is stories]
- http://apt.rcpsych.org/content/11/5/338
- www.freerangestories.com
- www.psychologytoday.com/us/blog/brain-babble/201208/turning-trauma-story-the-benefits-journaling
- file:///C:/Users/Owner/Documents/sandelowski_telling stories.pdf
- www.hawthornpress.com/books/storytelling/therapeutic-storytelling/

"If you want to change the world, change the metaphor, change the story."   Bill Moyers

"Story is at the very crux of healing, at the heart of every ceremony and ritual. . . . "   Linda Hogan

"Research has been substituted for imagination; the True has fallen victim to the Actual."
      Trevanian, *The Summer of Katya*

"There are no mistakes, no coincidences; all events are blessings. . . . "   Elisabeth Kübler-Ross

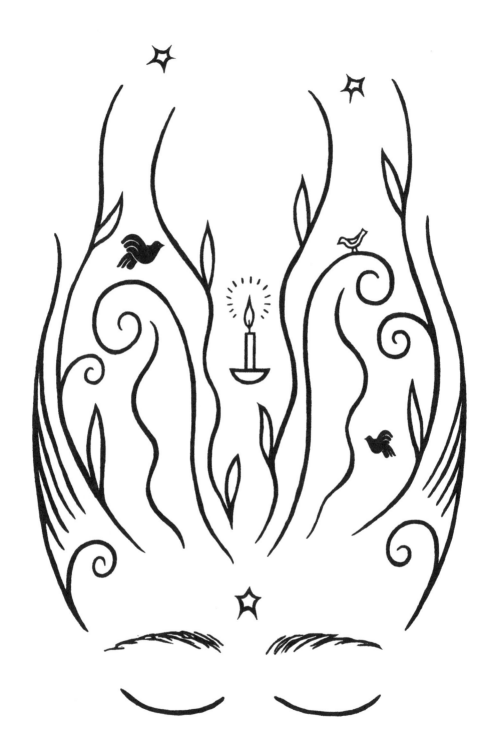

Step 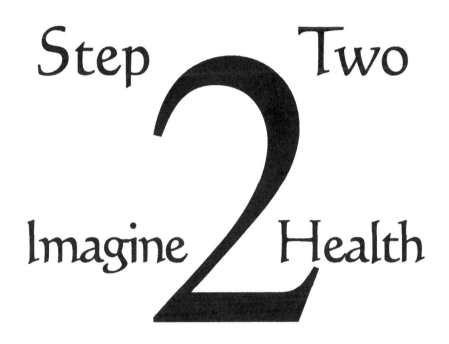 Two

Imagine 2 Health

Mind Medicine

"Natural forces are the healers of disease." Hippocrates (460-370 BCE)

Imagine Health

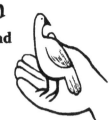

**Enter The Shaman's Playground
Embrace Your Unique Life
Symbolize Your Intention
Engage the Energy
Trust the Invisible**

Mind Medicine: Belief/Faith

o Prayer   o Abiding Hope   o Candle Magic
o Faith Healing   o Distant Healing   o Animal Allies
o Soul Retrieval   o Guides, Guardians o Miracles
o Amulets, Talismans o Rituals, Spells o Green Allies
o Unfathomable Certainties

Mind Medicine: Placebo

o Homeopathic Remedies   o Bach Flower Essences
o Gemstone Elixirs   o Willard Wonder Water
o Tissue Salts   o Acupuncture

Mind Medicine: Intention

o Word Medicine   o Affirmation   o Visualization
o Past-life Regression o Trance   o Hypnosis
o Art Therapy   o Color Healing   o Mandalas

Mind Medicine: Energy/Vibration

o Shamanic Healing o Reiki   o Polarity Therapy
o Chakra Therapy   o Medicine Wheels   o Feng Shui
o Therapeutic Touch o Ley lines   o Nature Spirits
o Auric Healing   o Rosen Method   o Mudra
o Feldenkrais   o Qi Gong   o Mariel Work
o Crystal Healing   o Psychic Healing   o Mantra
o Network Chiropractic   o Zero Balancing
o BRETH work (Breath Release Energy Transformation Healing)

"There is a common thread among healers throughout the world that vibration underlies the way to intercept illness."   Pat Moffitt Cook

Benefits of Mind Medicine

o   Requires no diagnosis   o   Engages social support
o   Free or low cost   o   Symbolic, archetypal
o   Patient empowered   o   Holds space for miracles
o   High percentage of cures with few side effects

Mind Medicine is Step 2. Because it is based on belief, it is Faith Medicine. Because there is no mechanism of action, it is Placebo Medicine. Because it asks us what we are thinking, it is Intention Medicine. Because it engages invisible healing energies, it is Vibrational Medicine.

It is easy to get lost in Mind Medicine, for it is as various and vast as the human imagination. It is important to see it as one of the Seven Medicines; if Mind Medicine does not resolve the problem within our time limit, then we go on to Step 3, Lifestyle.

In all cultures and through all times, healers engage the energy with intention, belief, and direct contact with life force. Scientifically-trained medical professionals are often uncomfortable with, or deeply suspicious of, Mind Medicine. They may see it as quackery, superstition, or hype. They may ridicule, ignore, or fear it so much they support legislation against those who practice it.

Mind Medicine is the stuff of miracles. Engage with it.

"[Sound scientific evidence shows] our thoughts and beliefs control the destiny of our living bodies. At the cellular level, we possess an innate intelligence that is far more crucial to shaping our lives than even our genes."
Bruce Lipton, *The Biology of Belief*

"The human body is a linkage of oscillating solid and liquid crystals that form an overall energy pattern. . . . The bones have a solid crystal structure with piezoelectric properties."   Gabriel Cousens, MD

". . . the universe resembles incandescent threads stretched into infinity in every conceivable direction, luminous filaments that are conscious of themselves in ways impossible for the human mind to comprehend."
don Juan, as reported by Carlos Castaneda

Grandmother Growth

A shimmering luminescent mist pulses rhythmically and sets the air aglow. Every plant, every rock is shimmering with energy and light and throwing off tiny sparks. You feel it in your nerves; you breathe it in. It enters through your skin. It touches every cell. It settles deep in your bones. You laugh with delight as you see yourself glowing and shimmering.

Your senses sharpen and expand, flow together, overlay and interplay with each other. The breeze leaves a honeyed taste on your skin. You are filled with curiosity, wonder, and eagerness.

"Ah, you are here at last," says a delighted, resonant voice.

How long has the Wise Woman been beside you? Has she been with you all along? The glow that surrounds her sparkles musically and gives off a reassuring and familiar scent. Light seems to spill from her every pore and pop off the ends of her hair.

"Welcome to the shaman's playground. Welcome to the temple, the grove, the sacred ceremonial space. Feel the mysterious movement, the shape shifting, the permeable boundaries. Here stories come to life. Past and present dance with the future. Energy becomes matter. And anything you can imagine can come true. Just being here will alter your view of reality."

Her eyes twinkle. "And if you believe, who knows what will happen? Strange sights, amazing creatures, and fantastic places await us. Come! Follow me."

And she's gone . . . but for a swirling cinnamon-scented golden mist. Leaving you to wonder how to follow her.

"Close your eyes and click your heels," you find yourself thinking, "and imagine it is so!"

Could it really be as easy as that?

"True faith isn't believing outlandish things, but being perfectly open and free to see the sacred in the ordinary and the commonplace. To come at reality without prejudices or preordained views means, at times, that we can sense and experience something truly miraculous without rejecting it outright."

Stephen Kendrick, *Prayer Works*

Mind Medicine: Belief/Faith

People who use Faith Medicine
o   Have stronger immune systems
o   Are less anxious
o   Have more stable blood sugar
o   Have improved cardiovascular functioning
o   Have better outcomes from coronary disease
o   Deal with rheumatoid arthritis better
o   Are less likely to be depressed
o   Resist suicidal thoughts better
o   Recover from breast cancer more quickly
o   Are less likely to have a child with meningitis

"From a scientific perspective, faith healing is unexplained, incomprehensible, and should not work. Yet it does work."   Nigel Barber Ph.D.

Mind Medicine starts with belief, which cannot be measured or quantified. Belief resists scientific investigation.

Critics contend that faith has absolutely no part in medicine; its effectiveness has not been proven, and ethical and professional problems immediately arise when it is introduced.

Those who believe, those who have faith, are not swayed by scientific evidence or lack of it.

"We've been praying a long time, and we've seen prayer work, and we know it works."   Bob Barth, director, Spiritual Unity

After researching and writing about the power of prayer, Tom Knox found himself overwhelmingly convinced that faith prolongs life. One study found those who attended a religious service weekly lived seven years longer than those who never attended. Another study found that religious people, even if they don't go to a place of worship or congregate with others weekly, live longer than atheists do.

Dr. Koenig – director of Duke University's Center for Spirituality, Theology and Health – says prayer has a remarkable effect on patients with hearing and visual deficiencies.

How to Pray

Effective prayer follows this pattern, using your own words.

Release

I release my judgments, desires, fears, and hopes about . . .
I release my past problems and my future wishes for . . .
I release all images of . . .

Affirm

I affirm that I am a being of infinite love and abundant health.
I affirm that I am whole.
I affirm that I radiate infinite love, abundant health, and
     wholeness to everyone and everything, including myself.

Protect

Infinite love, abundant health, and wholeness protect me.
I am surrounded by infinite love, abundant health, and wholeness.
I know only infinite love, abundant health, and wholeness.

Express Gratitude

I am grateful for my life.
I am grateful for my problems.
I am grateful for my body.
I am grateful for everyone and everything in my life.

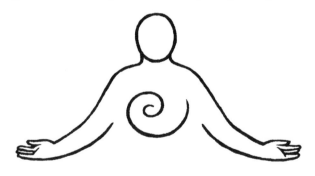

"Perhaps . . . it is not so much a matter of which road we select. Perhaps the real issue is us: our attitudes, our perceptions, what we see, smell, taste, and feel along the road, how well we listen, how we relate to the road, and what we choose to leave behind. . . ." John Perkins, minister

Eighty-five out of 125 studies (68 percent) investigating the effects of regular worship on health found those with faith lived longer. Over a five-year period, seniors who attended religious services were 36 percent less likely to die than non-attendees.

"The benefits of devout religious practice . . . are that people cope . . . with stress better . . . have more hope, they're more optimistic." Dr. Koenig

A study led by Karin Jensen found that when we see images that we associate with healing, "the mind automatically makes associations that can lead to actual positive health outcomes." [Proceedings of the National Academy of Sciences, Sept 2012]

Critics don't question these findings; they simply don't believe faith is responsible. Involvement in any social network correlates positively and consistently with better health and longer life. Companionship is probably more important to our health than faith is.

Consider a 2006 study of nearly two thousand people undergoing heart surgery. Those who knew they were being prayed for did worse than those who were prayed for and didn't know it. *Those who weren't prayed for at all did the best.* Prayer increased postsurgical complications like heart-rhythm disturbances, stroke, and heart attack. Another study that found recovering alcoholics who were prayed for fared far worse than those who weren't.

Most studies fail to distinguish between personal prayer and intercessory prayer. In the study above, for example, strangers interceded with prayer. To the scientific mind, all prayers are equal. To the magical mind, your own prayers are more powerful than any others and have a greater healing effect. The prayer we say ourselves is an affirmation of self love, and self love leads to abundant health.

". . . rituals and repetition resonate with and comfort people. These things that I do have been done by those before me and will continue to be done after I am gone, limiting my self-importance while at the same time connecting me with my community." Amy B. Gregory, minister

Subliminal (but not overt) messages make elders' perceptions about aging more positive, enhance their physical strength, and improve their balance. The "cascade of positive effects" persists for at least three weeks.

Embrace Your Unique Life

Mind Medicine is more than the power of positive thinking. Mind Medicine is the portal to the psyche, your personal storehouse of ancient survival wisdom. Traditional psychological therapy, where the therapist says little or nothing, merely asking about your dreams, your associations, your inner world, is clearly Mind Medicine. When we open that door, engage the energy, and ally with our problems, we almost always find "difficult" feelings.

Healers of all persuasions say physical symptoms are related to unexpressed feelings. Primal emotions are intense, uncivilized, raunchy, totally terrifying, and strong enough to help us create miraculous changes in health when listened to, accepted, loved.

Mind Medicine evokes deep healing because it draws our attention to our emotions as they live inside our body. One day, during a period of my life when I felt deeply betrayed, I experienced the actual physical effects of my bitterness and helplessness. After that, it was much easier to let those feelings go.

Wise women have listened to me, validated me, questioned me, and taught me how to embrace myself exactly as I am, right now. Pretending to be happy creates changes in my body that make me happy. When facing a challenge, I respond better thanks to the teachings of Eva Pierrakos (*Pathwork of Self-Realization*), Jean Houston (*The Possible Human*), and Judith Blackstone (*The Realization Process*). They help me invoke the no fault clause, remember I am co-creating my story, and acknowledge reality as it is.

" *When sorcerers talk about molding one's life situation they mean molding the awareness of being alive. Through molding this awareness, we can get enough energy to reach and sustain the energy body, and with it we can certainly mold the total direction and consequences of our lives.* "

don Juan, as reported by Carlos Castaneda

I believe that the Mind Medicine of reinhabiting the corpus and joining it with the psyche is a core practice for anyone wishing to gain or maintain abundant, optimum health.

Mind Medicine: Placebo

Placebo Medicine has been found to relieve (but not cure)

o Chronic pain	o Asthma
o Migraines	o Depression
o Anxiety	o Chronic fatigue
o IBS	o Parkinson's

o Cancer symptoms
o Cancer treatment side effects (fatigue, nausea, hot flashes, pain)
o Musculoskeletal, gastrointestinal, and urogenital disorders

Yes, a placebo is an inert substance, a sham treatment, a fake medical procedure. Yes, a placebo is wishful thinking and fervent hope. Yes, Placebo Medicine works. It works as well as drugs or surgery . . . for some people, for some problems.

Recent research from clinical science, psychology, anthropology, biology, social economics and neuroscience provides compelling evidence that Placebo Medicine is a "genuine biopsychosocial phenomenon that represents more than simply spontaneous remission, normal symptom fluctuations, and regression to the mean."

Placebo Medicine is distinct from "symptoms subsiding without treatment – the inevitable trajectory of most chronic ailments."

Neuroscientist Fabrizio Benedetti of Turin says Placebo Medicine creates direct and real physiological responses in heart rate, blood pressure, and chemical activity in the brain.

Placebos induce the brain to make pain-relieving neurotransmitters, some similiar to cannabis, some more like opium.

Placebos activate and increase the amount of endorphins and dopamine (related to emotions, pleasure, and rewards) produced in the brain, even in the brains of Parkinson's patients.

Placebos activate specific, quantifiable, relevant electrical and metabolic activity in the prefrontal cortex, anterior insula, rostral anterior cingulate cortex, and amygdala.

The placebo effect extends to real medications and actual treatments, too. A pain-relieving drug labeled as such worked 50 percent better than the same drug labeled "placebo."

Ted Kaptchuk, an acupuncturist and Associate Professor at Harvard Medical School, Program in Placebo Studies and the Therapeutic Encounter (PiPS) has shown that every part of our experience is important in Placebo Medicine:

- ✓ The size, shape, and color of the treatment
- ✓ The sounds, smells, and sights of the treatment venue
- ✓ The beliefs, experiences, and mood of the practitioner
- ✓ The amount of attention given to the patient
- ✓ Contextual and environmental cues
- ✓ Paraphernalia and settings
- ✓ Rituals, symbols, and interactions in the therapeutic encounter
- ✓ Emotional and cognitive engagement and clinical interactions:
  - empathic and intimate witnessing
  - touch, laying on of hands
  - nonjudgmental interaction with the patient's beliefs

"Sham treatment won't shrink tumors or cure viruses," Kaptchuk says. But disregarding placebos "ignores a huge chunk of healthcare."

Whatever protocol is used – alternative, orthodox, complementary, unproven – the *practitioner* has a significant effect on the outcome.

Forty-four percent of those told that a drug *causes* erectile dysfunction experienced ED after taking a placebo labeled as that drug.

Patients with irritable bowels (IBS) who receive fake acupuncture plus 20 minutes of focused personal attention, including light touch and affirmation about the treatment's success, have the greatest relief. Patients with IBS who *know* their pills are placebos still report twice as much symptom relief – or about as much improvement as the best IBS drugs provide – as the no-treatment group.

- o Yellow pills are more effective against depression symptoms.
- o Green pills counter anxiety best.
- o Blue pills are calming and sleep-inducing.
- o Red pills are energizing; they increase alertness.
- o White pills soothe digestive woes, especially ulcers.
- o Placebos with a "brand name" work better than those without.
- o Catchy names increase effectiveness.
- o Injections (and surgery) are more effective than pills.
- o Placebos taken four times a day are more effective than those taken twice a day.

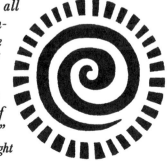

Placebo Medicine rarely changes the underlying pathology of a disease. Its effect is primarily on our relationship to our symptoms, our subjective sense of health. Placebo Medicine helps us heal the split between how we wish to be and how we really are.

The placebo effect is magnified when both the patient and the practitioner believe that the remedy will work. This is why the best scientific studies are "double-blinded" (neither patient nor practitioner knows what the patient is taking).

Ideally, a placebo costs little or nothing, and is easily accessible. Water and lactose – the substances most commonly used as placebos – certainly fulfill these requirements. (Little white homeopathic pills are lactose; flower essences are water.)

Placebo medicine is dangerous, according to Dr. Harriet Hall, retired family physician, because there can be a discrepancy between objective and subjective results. "If the patient's function is worse but a placebo makes them feel better, they might delay treatment until it is too late."

"Rituals and drugs use the very same biochemical pathways to influence the patient's brain."　　　　Fabrizio Benedetti, neuroscientist

Another downside to Placebo Medicine is called the Nocebo effect: the ability of an inert substance to harm. (*Nocebo* is Latin for "I shall harm." *Placebo* means "I shall please.") Nocebo effects are seen in the hippocampus. Up to a quarter of those getting placebos in drug trials experience nocebo effects, usually headaches, nausea, insomnia, pain, or fatigue.

One depressed person was almost successful in committing suicide by taking placebo pills he was given as part of a study.

"The Universal Energy Field permeates all space, animate and inanimate objects, and connects all objects to each other; it flows from one object to another. . . . It also follows the laws of harmonic inductance and sympathetic resonance . . . . [T]he field [is] highly organized in a series of geometric points, isolated pulsating points of light, spirals, webs of lines, sparks and clouds."
Barbara Ann Brennan, *Hands of Light*

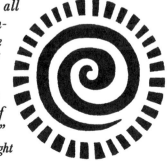

Homeopathy

Homeopathy is perhaps the most organized, written about, and practiced technique of Mind Medicine. Homeopathic remedies, because they contain nothing measurable by science, are placebos.

"Homeopathic 'remedies' enjoy a unique status in the health marketplace: They are the only category of quack products legally marketable as drugs." Stephen Barrett MD, Quackwatch

Allo- means opposite, while *homo-* means same. Allopaths counter disease by doing the *opposite*. Homeopaths by doing the *same*. "Like cures like" – the Law of Similars – is one of the foundations of homeopathy.

A homeopathic remedy begins as a Mother tincture. This is diluted by a factor of ten, then another factor of ten, and so on. Mother tinctures are not homeopathic remedies until they are diluted to the point where not a single atom of the plant material remains. (In a 30X dilution, the original substance has been diluted 1,000,000,000,000,000,000,000,000,000,000 times. In a 30C solution, the original molecule is dissolved in a minimum of 1,000,000,000,000,000,000,000,000,000,000,000,000,000,000,000, 000,000,000,000 molecules of water.)

According to the Law of Infinitesimals, dilution increases the energetic effect of the plant and makes the remedy more powerful. The less plant material, the better. Extreme dilutions allow homeopaths to use poisonous plants, deadly diseases, heavy metals, and even cancer strains as curative agents.

"[Homeopathy, created by Samuel Hahnemann (1755-1843), a German physician] has no coherent physical, biochemical, or anatomical theory, at least by modern standards. [It] originates from an historical event at the close of the eighteenth century and has not been definitively reevaluated or updated since." Richard Grossinger, *Planet Medicine*

Classical homeopaths treat people, not problems, with simples, not combinations. After a lengthy interview (a classic placebo effect technique), a remedy is chosen based on reported symptoms being carefully matched with symptoms observed by those who have "proven" the remedy by taking an overdose of the Mother tincture.

In 2015, the National Health and Research Council of Australia issued statements about homeopathic treatment. [*My comments*]:

o   No reliable scientific evidence has shown homeopathy to be effective against any health condition. [*Nor any that show harm when homeopathy is integrated with safe and effective treatments.*]

o   No good-quality, well-designed studies with enough participants have found homeopathy causes greater health improvements than [*any other*] placebo.

o   Those who use homeopathy may put their health at risk if they fail to take prescribed drugs, and/or reject or delay treatments for which there is good evidence for safety and effectiveness. [*Using the Seven Medicines encourages us to set time horizons, or due dates, when progress is reassessed and needed actions are taken.*]

"I was struck by the idea that not only can the symptoms of disease recapitulate old trauma, but that the very cures people select, both individually and collectively . . . can do the same thing." Julie Motz, medical intuitive

Bach Flower Essences

This specialized set of homeopathic remedies was created by the pediatrician Dr. Edward Bach, who deplored the blood-letting, purging, and catharsis used as treatments. Chicken pox was treated by bleeding the child and setting the dish of blood on the windowsill "so the contagion can be dispersed." His vision of gentle remedies made from tree flowers includes Rescue Remedy, one of the most cherished placebos in common use.

One set of Bach Flower Essences is meant to last for at least three generations, so it is a wise investment in placebo medicine.

Other homeopathic-type placebos, such as **flower essences, gem stone elixirs,** and **magic waters** of all sorts are generally not worth buying. Make your own. It engages your energy in a deeper way, bringing more profound healing. And it's easy too. (Recipe on page 312.)

". . . trials in irritable bowel syndrome, migraine, and attention deficit hyperactivity disorder suggest that placebos help even when people know they are taking them."   Jo Marchant, science journalist

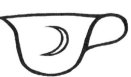

Mind Medicine: Intention
The Power of Positive Thought

". . . mental power exists for healing all types of physical and mental maladies. Release this power by developing such self-healing skills as meditation, visualization, and positive thinking."   Steven F. Brena MD

Imagine abundant health. Visualize abundant health. Affirm abundant health. Ask a hypnotist or an art therapist for help. Find someone who can lead you on a past-life regression or look at your Akashic Records.

The human imagination is one of the most profound and effective means of healing known. Imagination is sympathetic magic. You can create a new reality with visualization, affirmation, art, archetypes, guided meditation, shamanic trances, and mandalas.

Intention Medicine is as direct as an affirmation, as stirring as a visualization, as deep as a trance, as expressive as art, as centered as a mandala, and as esoteric as chromotherapy. Intention Medicine uses simple language and short declarative sentences. Intention Medicine chants mantras. Intention Medicine draws upon the subconscious in colorful, dramatic, symbolic ways. Intention Medicine creates healing images. Intention Medicine invites the psyche to take an active part in resolving problems. Intention Medicine awakens the Collective Consciousness, for abundant health/wholeness/holiness.

I clearly envision myself enjoying abundant health.

I created a visualization of the farm I wanted to live on. I spent time there every day. I saw myself driving up to a white house at the end of a dead-end road, feeding the horses, swimming in the pond, tending to gardens overflowing with flowers, herbs, and food. I talked about it as though it were mine. When a friend called and said I should to fly to New York immediately to interview for a caretaker position at a farm, I didn't hesitate. And that's how I came to run the farm of my dreams, complete with horses, a pond, and gardens for John and Yoko." Penny, 64, landscaper

"Those holding more negative age stereotypes earlier in life had signifi-cantly steeper hippocampal volume loss and greater accumulation of neu-rofibrillary tangles and amyloid plaques" [indicators of dementia and Alzheimer's].   Baltimore Longitudinal Study of Aging, 2017

We are what we believe. We are what we think. We are what we say. Every teacher I have ever valued has impressed this litany on me. This is the essence of Mind Medicine: the belief that my thoughts create my reality.

But how do I create a different reality if I don't like the one I am in? One way is through Art.

There are four primary expressive arts: Sound Arts, Movement Arts, Word Arts, and Image Arts. Sound and Movement Arts are part of Lifestyle Medicines; Word Arts are both Story and Mind Medicine; Image Arts are Mind Medicine.

When sounds, movement, words, scents, and bold images are brought together for healing, we have Ceremonial Medicine and Shamanic Healing

Word Art Intention Medicine gives rise to affirmations, stories, visualizations, trances, and hypnosis. Image Art Intention Medicine gives us color therapy and art therapy.

"I can't change what happened in my childhood, but I can use my story of protection, empowerment, and spiritual connection to weave a layer of healing energy. . . ."   Susan Wright, 56, author

Sound Arts: Listening to music, humming, ton-ing, chanting, singing, playing an instrument

Movement Arts: Observing motion, dancing, Tai chi, Qi Gong, martial arts including aikido and karate, yoga, computer games

Word Arts: Listening to someone tell a story or read aloud, reading aloud, reading to one-self, writing, hypnosis

Image Arts: Looking at/touching art, coloring, drawing, painting, sculpting, modeling, wood-, metal-, gem-crafts, mosaic, stained glass

Word Arts:
Affirmation, Visualization, Trance, Hypnosis

Affirmations

These short, declarative statements affirm in the present tense; they do not deny. Affirmations are meant to be repeated, often.

The words we think and say cause actual chemical changes in our brains, which can change our bodies. Our bodies physically express every thought we repeat and every image we dwell on.

I heal rapidly and well.

Thinking about something is not the same as doing it, but thought does precede action. Our habitual thoughts and unconscious inner dialogues create the body we inhabit as much as what we eat does.

Every single cell in my body is a healthy cell.
Unexpected delights are mine.
My greatest aspirations come to pass in miraculous ways.

Visualization

Imagining something triggers the visual cortex and changes the chemicals produced in the brain. Mandalas and thangkas are aids to visualization. Anything meaningful to you is an effective visualization. A color can be a visualization.

Our brains repeat scary, bad things that happen to us, over and over. That is good; it keeps us from doing it again. That is bad; it increases our chances of depression and anxiety. Visualization is the fastest way to divert the brain into the pathways of abundant health. When my mind conjures up life-threatening images from my past, I replace the horrific scenes with the color green. I look for green; fill my eyes with green; visualize green; repeat the word green, green, green. I am calmed. I am soothed.

A **Guided Meditation** is an assisted visualization. It is traditionally done in person, with a guide, who uses a drum or rattle in cadence with their spoken word to take you on an inner journey of discovery to meet your allies or to experience images like the Tree of Life or Grandmother Spider's Web.

Hundreds of excellent guided meditations are available for free on the Internet. A real shamanic trance is a different thing, however.

Trance

These meditative states are portals to hidden healing energies. They may be induced by a practitioner, or, after practice, self-induced. **Past-life regressions** are a gentle form of trance. Certain gestures, sounds and rhythms can be used to create trances.

"Westerners assume that shamanic trance is a meditation or visualization, that the whole experience arises from the mind and is related to the 'imagination.' Shamanic trance journeys are an actual movement out of one body (the physical) and into another (the energy body). . . . Shamans are 'shape shifters' who learn to change their form at will . . . [so they can] slip through a crack between the worlds. . . ." Vicki Noble, *Shakti Woman*

Hypnosis

Both hypnosis and self-hypnosis influence our experience and behavior by directly changing what goes on in our brain. Psychologist David Oakley, using high-tech imaging, has shown that the brains of genuinely hypnotized people differ markedly from the brains of people faking hypnosis. Hypnotized brains have high levels of activity in the occipital lobes (visualization) and the left temporal lobe (verbal analysis). The "highly hypnotizable" have a rostrum area in their brain that is a third larger than usual.

Hypnosis is used scientifically to study amnesia. Is it a healing tool? Numerous anecdotal accounts claim hypnosis helps us to:
o   Lose excess weight
o   Increase the chances of quitting smoking
o   Counter addictions, including gambling
o   Improve our ability to focus and concentrate
o   Reduce anxiety and nourish calmness
o   Overcome or lessen many chronic problems including bulimia, migraine, and erectile dysfunction

"Healing from any illness is facilitated by identifying your power symbols and your symbolic and physical relationship to [them] and heeding any messages your body and intuitions are sending you about them."
Caroline Myss, *Anatomy of the Spirit*

Image Arts:
Color Therapy, Art Therapy, Mandalas, Archetypes

Color Therapy (chromotherapy, photobiology, photo-irradiation)

From ancient mages to modern scientists, it is obvious that looking at colors and being bathed in a color – whether from stained glass, gemstones, clothing, expressive art, the walls of a room, or imagining it – can change our mind and our mood in a myriad of ways. Exposure to colored light causes direct physical and emotional changes that nourish and support healing.

"Photobiology's roots in mysticism, which empower color with symbolism and magic, detract from its credibility."   Lindsey Gruson

Scientifically-validated uses for colored light:

o   Sitting under red light stimulates the sympathetic nervous system; in ten minutes blood pressure, respiratory movements, eye-blink frequency, and anxiety are measurably increased.

o   Blue light at 470 nanometers stimulates the parasympathetic nervous system, increasing relaxation and lowering hostility.

o   Photo-irradiation with blue light destroys 90.4 percent of antibiotic-resistant staph infections (MRSA). The longer the treatment, the better the results. [*Journal of Photomedicine and Laser Surgery*, April 2009]

o   In the twentieth century, babies with fatal neonatal jaundice got a blood transfusion. Now they get intense blue light. (But that irritates their nurses, who are soothed with gold light.)

o   Blue light on the backs of the knees eliminates both jet lag and sleep problems. [Institute for Chromotherapy, www.pantone.com]

o   After looking at red lights, athletes' physical strength increased 13.5 percent, and the electrical activity in their arm muscles increased 5.8 percent. [*American Health*, May 1988]

o   Prisoners put in a holding cell painted Baker-Miller pink had a reduction in muscle strength, and a significant reduction in violent and aggressive behavior – within 2.7 seconds. Sleep often occurred within ten minutes. [*Journal of Orthomolecular Psychiatry*, 1979]

"The light of Durga is red. The blue light is Krishna. . . ." Mother Meera

o Ultraviolet light is the standard treatment for psoriasis in the United States. In Russia, it is showered on coal miners to prevent black lung disease.

o Exposure to full-spectrum light (sunlight especially) influences brain chemistry, easing all types of depression.

"It seems clear that light is the most important environmental input, after food, in controlling bodily function." Richard J. Wurtman MD, MIT

Art Therapy

Color, form, pattern, line, and texture can be used to manifest our unspoken, unspeakable, desires and fears.

"Any drawing has a cathartic effect; that catharsis allows the symbol to move inner psychic energy and begin the healing process."
Gregg Furth, *The Secret World of Drawings*

Mind Medicine is symbolic. Our unconscious helps us create healing art, talismans, amulets, altars, mandalas: archetypes we can touch and smell and see. These symbolic pieces carry intention, and are magnified in their power by our imagination.

We enter the forest of the witch. We are swept into a shamanic trance. The storyteller is looking in our eyes. The air is perfumed. We become the hum of the singer, the rhyme of the poet, the passion of the flowers. We become the high priest/ess, the trees of the sacred grove, the altar itself. We hear the call that echoes in every cell: health/wholeness/holiness.

"Remember that creating an image in the conscious imagination is quite different from creating the energy itself. . . . Thinking light around you does not make light." Jack Schwartz, *Human Energy Systems*

Bernie Siegel has his patients draw their visions of various treatments to guide their choices. Elisabeth Kübler-Ross, in her five-day "Life, Death, and Transition" workshops, reviewed drawings made by each student as a prerequisite to their participation.

Change your drawing, change your life. In an art therapy session, feeling frustrated, I tore a hole in my drawing. "Better than tearing a hole in yourself," the therapist said. "Now something new can get in," she affirmed.

Mandalas

Creating or coloring mandalas – geometric images with a strong center – connects us to the collective unconscious, reveals our own psyche, and shows us the path to health/wholeness/holiness.

"[The] mandala . . . reacts upon its maker. Very ancient magical effects lie hidden in [it] . . . the magic of which has been preserved in countless folk customs."
                                    C. G. Jung, *Man and His Symbols*

Archetypes

These symbolic expressions of profound energies activate healthy beliefs and behaviors, according to Carl Jung. I agree.

Archetypal images from myths, fairytales, sagas, legends, religious texts include super-human beings, god/desses, elementals, shape-shifters, sacred plants, animals, numbers, and geometric forms.

My apprentices work with a personal archetype; me too. For decades, mine was Artemis, the wild, barefoot woman of the woods. As a crone, post-menopause, my new archetype is the Statue of Liberty. She wears a headband, as I do, and hers has energy spikes.

"Our psychological health and spiritual growth are largely dependent on recognizing [and] developing . . . the conflicting archetypes within us."
                                    Bill Whitcomb, *The Magician's Reflection*

Archetypes are **talismans** when pocket-sized. Archetypes appear in shamanic ritual, in the theater, and in **ceremony**. Ceremony creates a safe space where we can encounter and interact with intense energies and become archetypal (for a while). Intention and imagination, nourished by sound, color, and smell, weave together into a whole that is far greater than the sum of its parts.

Step 2 Time Limit

In every Step, we set a time frame, a time limit. When it is up, we may renegotiate a new time limit or add on another Step. Do not linger too long in Mind Medicine. It is easy to get lost in a dream and allow the best time for bold action to slip away.

Mind Medicine: Energy

Energy Medicine engages a vital force that is recognized world-wide, but doesn't exist as far as Science is concerned.

"Reiki, acupuncture, homeopathy, and similar methods may be 'feel-good interventions,' but they are an irrelevant and superfluous part. It is the kind attention of the practitioner that matters – and only that attention. . . . The ritual of reiki (or acupuncture, or whatever) is wasteful, distracting, and arguably unethical."   Steven Novella, neurologist, Yale

While it shares qualities with other Mind Medicines, Energy Medicine differs in two important ways. First, Energy Medicine goes from personal into relational. Someone else is involved, even if at a distance; we are in relationship. Second, that other person often uses light, non-manipulative touch. Serenity Medicine is alone medicine. Story Medicine is better with an audience, but works just fine on your own. Energy Medicine invites the other.

"The body is the meeting point of consciousness and reality, energy and matter, silence and mind."   Steven Harrison, *Stillness Speaks*

Experience Entrainment

1. Go to a beach (or rent a video). Watch the waves. Feel what happens to your breathing, what happens in your gut.
2. Listen to music with a very strong rhythm in the bass line. Or sit outside in a heavy rainstorm. Feel what happens to your heart; emotions may arise.
3. Sing or drum in concert with others. Feel what happens in your brain and nerves.

Experience Chi

1. Rub your hands briskly together until they are warm. Stop rubbing. Slowly separate the palms. The stretchy, tingly feeling is chi.
2. Play with the chi/qi. Move your palms together and apart. Can you make a ball of chi?
3. Place the ball of chi inside your own body, wherever you wish. Feel for entrainment before you let go.

Interaction with another person is essential to Energy Medicine. When energies resonate, sympathetic resonance entrains them so they move coherently and smoothly together. Entrainment is the engine of healing in vibrational medicine. Entrainment gathers disparate energies into wholeness.

Entrainment occurs in all wave forms, from those in the ocean to those of the heart, from the flights of birds to the electrical messages sent by our nerves. A skilled practitioner of Energy Medicine entrains with the complex, healthy energy of the Universe, and passes it on.

Entrainment cannot be forced or coerced, prayed to or pleaded with; it must be allowed, invited, opened to. When we feel safe enough to let go and flow, we can entrain with patterns of wholeness and vibrate with abundant health.

All matter is made up of atoms which are constantly vibrating. This vibration is known by many names including chi and qi.

Call It

ase
chi/qi
prana
life force
kundalini
essence
élan vital
divine spark
universal healing
energy
tachyon
orgone
veriditas
Wakan Tanka

Radiant, mutable, dancing, dynamic, spontaneous, creative, capricious, reliable, rising, efficient, unstoppable, mysteriously moving Energy

This energy, like a strong wind or a swiftly-flowing river, must be accommodated on its own terms. Engage it, embrace it, move with it, and it will carry you fast and far. Try to control it and you usually find yourself with more problems than you began with.

Engaging joins and connects. Engaging shares power. Engaging is an act of communion and an exchange. Engaging the energy allows the natural, healthy chaos of the universe to act through and in our beings, and to manifest as health/wholeness/holiness. Controlling the energy leads ultimately to balance, rigidity, stasis, and an idealized, non-real, un-whole, unhealthy self-image.

Energy Medicine practices may be hands-off, or there may be subtle, light, quiet physical touch without manipulation. The goal is to engage and entrain the energy of life in all its chaotic non-measurable splendor.

"Is it possible that chaos is health? And that . . . predictability and differentiability . . . is disease? When you reach an equilibrium in biology, you're dead. Health is not a static structure, but a dynamic system, capable of phase transitions."   Arnold Mandell, neuroscientist

Every form is filled with energy; energy acts through form. Energy is neither superior to, nor better than, form. Healthy energy; healthy form. Health is wholeness, not division into this and that, better and worse, higher and lower. Sickness, injury, disease, emotional storms, and trauma break us into pieces, and give us an opportunity to accept more of ourselves, to get more out of life, to be awed by the Great Mystery, to become more than we were.

When we are intent on getting rid of a problem, we position ourselves athwart the natural flow of energy. As the energy pushes against us, we feel weaker and weaker and less able to "control" it. When we join with and engage the energy, including the problem's energy, we absorb its power and grow stronger.

"The Human Energy Field [includes] electrostatic, magnetic, electromagnetic, sonic, thermal, and visual components." Barbara Ann Brennan

Energy vibrates in every remedy – homeopathic, herbal, or pharmaceutical – we take. The energy of the homeopathic remedy is magnified by dilution to act upon the most subtle parts of our organism. The energy of the pharmaceutical is reduced to a single vibration to limit and restrict actions. In contrast, single plant remedies, made with fresh plants and vodka, or dried plants and hot water, retain the *élan vital* of the original plant and provide a combination of constituents and chi that is an ideal way to initiate and support multidimensional healing in body, psyche, and mind.

"We are asked to exert mind over matter, to prove our strength by dominating our basic instincts, suppressing the raw energy of the core self. . . . But the victory of one part over another does not lead to wholeness, but further fragmentation."   Anodea Judith, *Eastern Body, Western Mind*

Energy Medicine eludes language, for it speaks from, and to, the deep nonverbal, nonlanguaged places of health/wholeness/holiness. We hear and sense and know these places, this energy, before we can talk, before we are born. If we could speak the language of this energy, perhaps its syllables are sound, color, odor, touch; its sentences are symbols; and its full story is ceremony.

Energy Medicine, like all Mind Medicines, is not limited to our mind. The results can be as physical as surgery or drugs. Energy Medicine engages us with the world outside our skin, shifting our perspective so we can manifest abundant health and wholeness.

Vitalism

This ancient healing belief (dating back at least to Aristotle) honors the "vital force" of both patient and remedy. Science, with its focus on devitalized drugs, views Vitalism as superstition. Vitalism lives on in the hearts and minds of many herbalists, alternative medicine practitioners, and even a few medical professionals.

Earth Energy

"We have never quite comprehended that we walk about in a sea of mild electromagnetism . . . [produced by the earth]."   Michael Persinger

Earth Energy is distinct from, but closely related to, life force energy/chi/prana. The earth itself generates electromagnetic energy which promotes abundant health. Aboriginal peoples use the channels (ley lines) and gathering points (nodes) of earth energy as special healing spots and often mark them with stones.

Earth energy is available everywhere, for free, to everyone, directly, through our feet, and indirectly, through the mineral kingdom. Wearing shoes reduces access to earth energy. Putting your bare feet on the earth, walking barefoot, and sleeping on the ground are easy ways to engage and absorb earth energy, as is forest bathing, an Earth Energy healing technique from Japan.

". . . rubber shoe soles reduce the drawing in of prana by fifty percent."
Choa Kok Sui, *Pranic Healing*

Forest Bathing/Shinrin Yoku

"Taking in the forest atmosphere" or forest bathing, is a well-studied example of Earth Energy Medicine.

Science confirms that engaging in *Shinrin Yoku*:

o Creates beneficial changes in the nervous system
o Increases intake of phytoncides that are directly antibacterial and antifungal; nourishes natural killer cells
o Counters/decreases anxiety, depression
o Reduces angry outbursts, hyperactivity
o Supports restful sleep
o Improves immunity
o Reduces blood pressure
o Accelerates recovery from surgery and illness
o Increases the ability to focus, esp. in children with ADHD
o Decreases levels of stress hormones (cortisol and adrenaline)

Shinrin Yoku, which can be as simple as visiting a forest and breathing, has become a cornerstone of preventive health care and healing in Japanese medicine and is covered by insurance.

Even one session of *Shinrin Yoku* increases the number of natural killer (NK) cells. Continued forest bathing increases levels of adiponectin – a hormone often low in those with metabolic syndrome, type-2 diabetes, and cardiovascular disease. Daily practice gives one deeper and clearer intuition, increased access to core energy, improved capacity to communicate with the land and the plants, stronger connection to chi and Eros, deepening of friendships, and an overall increase in joy and ease.

Forests, it is said, respond to human presence by increasing healthy electromagnetic fields that restore and nourish our nervous systems. And trees emit *phytoncides,* volatile oils which subtly affect the brain and nervous system (unlike essential oils, which are drug-like and a threat to health). In a forest, one feels both relaxed and filled with amazing energy. Lucid and creative. Pulsing with the joy of existence.

"Wilderness is a necessity." John Muir, mountaineer, environmentalist

Engaging the energy allows us to feel useful while acknowledging our helplessness.

Minerals

Ordinary rocks, semi-precious stones, gemstones, crystals, copper, silver, and gold vibrate with earth energy. The mineral kingdom, like the plant and animal kingdoms, is co-creative with all of life, including us. Mineral allies help us nourish abundant health.

Minerals absorb, store, amplify, convert, and transmit energy. Computers use quartz crystals in these exact ways. We can too.

While there are lots of ideas about which minerals affect which parts of the body or mind, any mineral form of earth energy can absorb problems, amplify creativity, and clarify intentions.

Minerals can be put on an altar, in a bowl of water, by your door, around your neck, wrist, or finger, in an amulet, in a charm, or used in any other way you desire. I have a friend who collects crystals bigger than he is, and he has let me see them and be with them. Each one is a stunning presence, each an entrainment into the beating heart of the earth, psychedelic as any light show.

Wisdom from Asia

Qi Gong and **Tai chi** are Lifestyle Medicines (pages 114-115) that help us engage with earth energy through our feet. Consistent practice "restores healthy flow of chi, and removes all problems." Practicing barefoot, or in cotton-soled shoes, increases abundant health. In Chinese hospitals, those who cannot stand and do the gentle movements receive benefit by watching others practice.

Feng Shui is a form of Chinese geomancy used to auspiciously align a city, site, building, or object with its surrounding earth energy fields. Feng Shui principles help us engage with and benefit from the earth energies we encounter in our homes, workspaces, and gardens. Beware. Charlatans outnumber true adepts since the severe repression against Feng Shui fostered by Mao.

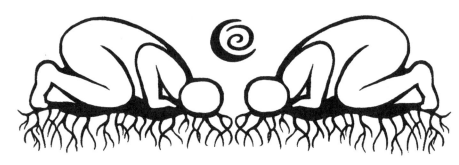

Touch
Healing with noninvasive contact

Touch is energy medicine. Touch heals. Mothers do it. Nurses do it. Lovers do it. Friends do it. Animals do it.

A large body of evidence finds touch essential to survival in infancy and an important component of optimum health at all ages. Touch can facilitate openness to pleasure and well-being. It increases our capacity to be fully alive and joyously embodied.

Deep touch, like Swedish massage or Rolfing, is not Step 2. Mind Medicine touch is nonmanipulative, nonjudgmental, noncorrective, and nonintrusive. And if that touch is infused with energy, so much the better.

Clinical trials have found that one-on-one touch support during chemotherapy, with or without any attempt at healing, consistently improves comfort and perception of well-being.

"When you approach the individual through the body, you enter directly into the archaic layers of the personality."
Thérèse Bertherat, *The Body Has Its Reasons*

Energy Medicine encourages us to connect with, trust, symbolize, enter into, and embrace the idea of a Universal healing energy that is abundant, free, and accessible.

The human hand is one of the most important tools for focusing, transmitting, and sharing Universal healing energy. With the lightest of touches, a practitioner entrains with the one asking for help and with life force energy. Here are a few ways to do that:

Alexander Technique
A hands-on technique that can help you identify and change physical and mental habits that cause pain, stress, and fatigue. Practitioners make subtle aligning adjustments which can be remembered and practiced by the recipient.

Performing artists and people living with chronic disease and pain benefit the most from Alexander work, but everyone enjoys the improved well-being and abundant health it fosters. Validated scientifically to relieve chronic back and neck pain.

Working with Alexander technique can:
- o   Improve posture, coordination, respiration, and balance in athletes and the elderly
- o   Reduce low back pain, general chronic pain, and stuttering
- o   Ease emotional challenges
- o   Improve respiratory muscle function
- o   Rehabilitate those with stress-related diseases, including rheumatism, high blood pressure, COPD, and sleep disorders
- o   Be as effective as beta-blocker medication in controlling the stress response during public performances

In a multiple-intervention study, after three months and after one year, those in chronic pain rated Alexander technique as the most helpful of all the interventions.

Aten Stunde   *aten*/breath, *stunde*/hour

The Breath Hour is done in total silence. Simple, light, touch directs energy, via the breath, into places that aren't breathing and vibrating. This superb manifestation of Mind Medicine is ideal for stressed adults, especially new parents.

Biodynamic Craniosacral Therapy

Practitioners "listen through the hands" with "subtle palpatory skills" to identify places where stress and trauma interfere with the rhythms of the *breath of life*. In a noninvasive way, they manipulate the skull to facilitate the body's own self-healing and self-regulating processes. It is hoped that the practitioner's clear quality of presence acts as a reflective mirror for the patient's "potential for change." Craniosacral therapy is most helpful for those with chronic sinus infections, headaches, jaw pain, neck pain, and shoulder pain. It is suitable for all ages, in acute or chronic cases.

Breath

Blowing and sucking are shamanic healing techniques that use the breath directly. The breath may be contained by the hands, blown through a hollow stem or a horn, or magnified by the inclusion of liquids blown on the body or short sharp sounds.

Feldenkrais

This form of touch therapy is unusual in that it can be self administered. Practitioners seek "not self-control through punishment, but self-exploration." There is no particular goal, no "perfect" body to create, no "ideal" person to become. I have been involved in this work for decades and feel it is as important as my weekly practice of yoga and Tai chi in creating abundant health.

"By becoming aware of our body we give ourselves access to our entire being – for body and spirit, mental and physical, and even strength and weakness, represent not our duality but our unity." Thérèse Bertherat

Hug for Health

The irrepressible Patch Adams MD says "All consensual hugs are therapeutic." If you are lonely, depressed, or anxious, give his Five Minute Hug a try. Hug standing up. Give and receive. No movement other than breathing. People who receive hugs regularly are 60 percent less likely to get a cold or the flu. And their tumors, if they have any, grow more slowly. [*Nature Comm.* July 2018]

Laying on of Hands

All cultures have "hand healers." Some specialize in healing burns or broken bones or trauma. Others claim miraculous cures of degenerative or chronic problems. Hand healing is an important part of Christian faith healing.

"Do not neglect the spiritual gift within you, bestowed on you through prophetic utterance with the laying on of hands. . . ." 1 Timothy 4:14

Mudras

Another way to initiate and enhance electromagnetic currents within the body is to put one's fingers in a certain pattern, known as a mudra. Mudras are usually done while sitting, with the hands resting easily on the thighs. They also may be practiced standing or lying down, anywhere, any time. Repetition brings rewards.

To begin: Release tension in your hands by shaking or rubbing them until the finger tips feel tingly/electrical and the palms are warm. Then move the fingers of both hands into a mudra. Hold the mudra for ten seconds at first, then for longer and longer times. Deepen and slow the breath. Relax the shoulders.

o   **Prana Mudra:** *Increase vitality; overcome disease.* Bring the thumb tips of both hands to rest on the tips of the little and ring fingers. Extend the remaining two fingers and connect with the flow of chi.

     o   **Vayu Mudra:** *Counter arthritis, trembling, and Parkinson's.* Curl the index finger toward the base of the thumb and meet it with the thumb tip; straighten the other fingers into the flow of chi.

     o   **Gyana Mudra:** *Sharpen memory; improve intellect; connect universal and individual consciousness.* Palms up, press index fingers and thumbs together; the other fingers touch and stretch into chi.

     o   **Anjali mudra:** *Express love, gratitude, honor, and respect for self and all creation.* Press the palms together in front of the heart/chest. Release the shoulders and experience the flow of chi.

     o **Prithvi Mudra:** *Increase strength and happiness.* Lightly press the tips of the thumb and ring finger together, keeping the other fingers straight.

     Traditional Chinese healers say: "In health the Qi flows smoothly; too much or too little Qi, that is disease."

     "Movement gives health and life. Stagnation brings disease and death."   Chinese proverb

Non-dual Therapies

Non-dual therapies – such as **mindfulness** and Judith Blackstone's **Realization Process** – engage our energy in subtle ways, foster a rich acceptance of our humanity, and offer deep healing from trauma, loss, and both physical and psychic pain.

Reiki

Pronounced ray-key, this Japanese therapeutic touch technique has been shown to help reduce stress, aid relaxation, and promote healing. Studies find that both real Reiki and sham Reiki groups feel improved well-being, indistinguishably. High-quality clinical trials of Reiki are lacking. A large trial of Reiki to relieve fibromyalgia found no benefit.

Rosen Method Bodywork

The "power of gentleness" helps clients "access the unconscious through touch." Reliably helpful for those with asthma, migraines, psychosomatic illnesses, and many chronic problems.

"What impressed me about the Rosen Method was the stillness, patience, and acceptance in the person who worked on me. His gentle but direct way of touching invited me to experience my physical presence from the inside and to live more consciously in it." Gordon Carrega, *Up Ahead*

Therapeutic Touch

This method of repairing a patient's "biofield" without actually touching them is popular among nurses, who introduced it into ICUs and pushed until it was accepted as part of the curriculum at institutions such as Yale. The most notable result is less anxiety and improved well-being in cancer patients. The Merck Manual reminds us that systematic reviews of existing studies have not found sufficient evidence to support therapeutic touch's effectiveness for treating any disorder. A 1998 study found practitioners unable to detect biofields.

"Polarity therapy seeks to cultivate sensitivity to and respect for the river of life energy within everything." Dr. Randolph Stone, *Polarity Therapy*

Chakras

Chakras are envisioned as turning wheels of colored energy found in the body. Every acupuncture point is a chakra. Energy workers visualize seven (sometimes 8) major chakras, located in a row from the tailbone to the crown. They also use the **aura** – the visible energy spectrum surrounding the body – as a diagnostic tool.

Psychic Surgery

Realistic but fake surgery activates the placebo effect at a primal level, the realm of wish-fulfillment. Our senses are so deeply engaged with dramatic extractions of "diseased tissues" (actually palmed eggs, blood clots, and other sleights of hand) that the psyche is enticed into believing the psychic surgeon has actually removed the disease. And, sometimes, what we believe becomes real.

Vibrational Medicine: Devices

Most Mind Medicine is done in the mind, or with light touch, but a variety of devices are believed to magnify, purify or intensify energy, including magnetic and electrical energies.

Dowsing

Those who divine or witch for water or lost objects say asking the right question is critical. Experienced dowsers say you always get the right answer, but the question may be wrong. Ask first: Can I? May I? Should I? Then: Is there need without greed? Then: Where is the water? How far down? Where is the lost item? Dowsers use T rods, L rods, bobbers, and pendulums of various sizes.

Electro-medicine

Electricity seems similiar to life force energy, giving it healing cachet. In the late 1800s, apparatuses of many sorts that applied various electrical energies were sold as a certain cure for all diseases. Electrical treatments today, especially those for mental health and pain, are invasive and thus Step 6.

Royal Raymond **Rife**, working in collaboration with doctors at the University of Southern California, claimed to cure 52 diseases, including cancer, typhoid, leprosy, streptococcus, typhus, and polio with his Beam Ray. In 1934, at the University of Southern California Medical School, Rife treated 16 terminal cancer patients with ultrasound for three minutes daily for three days, repeated at intervals for 3-4 months, achieving an amazing 100 percent remission rate.

Cancer viruses are "highly absorptive of ultrasound at their resonance frequencies." Ultrasound at the intensity used for physical therapy mortally wounds all cancers within a few seconds, but patients don't survive, since the liver and kidneys are usually overwhelmed by the immense amount of dead tissue created.

Today, digital Rife machines are widely available and used to help counter cancer, AIDS, Lyme disease, arthritis, muscle and joint pain, skin problems, and Morgellon's disease.

Whether or not Rife was as successful as he claimed, modern digital machines do not supply the same complex, multilevel layers of sound, ultra-sound, and electrical waves emitted by Rife's original analog machines. The Beam Ray, for instance, is an X-ray tube filled with helium, which emits high frequency, high intensity light pulses, plasma shock waves, and multi-pole oscillating electric fields into the patient's body. If you want to experiment with a Rife machine, pracitioners insist that it is worth the effort and expense to find and use an analog tube type, not a new machine.

Magnetic Therapy

Magnets and magnetic fields are used to ease pain from osteoarthritis, rheumatoid arthritis, chronic hip and knee pain, and fibromyalgia. But magnets are no more effective than placebos for relief of chronic low back and wrist (carpal tunnel) pain.

Twice-weekly magnetic stimulation of the pelvic floor eased incontinence in more than half of the women treated. There is evidence that magnetic therapy can deepen sleep and reduce nerve pain, especially diabetic foot pain.

The Earth produces a powerful magnetic energy that no doubt has effects on our health. But wearing or sleeping on magnets, using a magnetic-field-generating machine or drinking magnet-conditioned water is unlikely to have much effect.

Orgonomy

Freud's student Wilhelm Reich "discovered" a life force energy which he called *orgone*. Patients sit (naked) inside an Orgone Accumulator – a box made of alternating layers of organic materials (to attract orgone) and metallic materials (to radiate the orgone toward the center of the box). They hope to restore the flow of life force energy and "cure all mental and physical problems and reverse cancer." Reich believed that orgone was healing but could be deadly as well, and that man-made energy was disturbing it.

Radionics

Albert Abrams became a millionaire by leasing the radionic machines that he created in the early 1900s. Modern practitioners say Abrams' machines are useless, being nothing more than "obfuscated collections of wires and electronic parts," and that the practitioner's healing abilities are paramount.

Step 2: Mind Medicine
References & Resources

A list of all titles dealing with Mind Medicine would be a book unto itself.

Mind Medicine: Faith

Dossey, Larry. *Prayer is Good Medicine.* Harper Collins, 1996.
Lipton, Bruce. *The Biology of Belief.* Mountain of Love Press, 2007.
Oman, Maggie (ed). *Prayers for Healing.* Conari, 2000.
Teish, Luisah. *The Natural Woman's Book of Personal Charms and Practical Rituals.* HarperOne, 1988.
Yacoboni, Celeste. *How Do You Pray?* Monkfish, 2014.
* https://sciencebasedmedicine.org/the-power-of-faith-and-prayer/
* https://sciencebasedmedicine.org/reiki/
* www.nytimes.com/2006/03/31/health/31pray.html
* www.newsmax.com/Health/Headline/prayer-health-faith-medi-cine/2015/03/31/id/635623/
* www.nchi.nlm.nih.gov/pubmed/1659567
* http://onlinesurgicaltechniciancourses.com/2010/25-intriguing-scientific-studies-about-faith-prayer-and-healing/
* http://www.skeptic.com/
* http://quackwatch.org/
* https://news.yale.edu/2014/10/15/positive-subliminal-mes-sages-aging-improve-physical-functioning-elderly

"Data from 97,253 women participating in the National Institutes of Health's Women Health Initiative showed that those who scored high on optimism had significantly lower rates of heart disease, cancer, and mortality than women who scored high on pessimism." Hilary Tindle MD

Mind Medicine: Placebo

Benedetti, Fabrizio. *Placebo Effects: Understanding the mechanisms in health and disease* (2nd ed). Oxford University Press, 2014.
Cytowic, R. E., MD. "The Placebo Response: Not in Your Head but in Your Brain." *Psychology Today.* 9 Jan 2012.
Dispenza, Joe DC. *You Are the Placebo.* Hay House, 2015.
Harrington, Anne. *The Placebo Effect: An Interdisciplinary Exploration* (1st ed). Harvard College Press, 1997.

Moerman Daniel E. *Meaning, Medicine and the Placebo Effect.* (Studies in Medical Anthropology.) Cambridge University Press, 2002.

Sifferlin, Alexandra. "Placebo's New Power." *Time,* Sept 2018.

Zubieta, Jon-Kar, et al. "Placebo reins in pain in brain." *Journal of Neuroscience.* Aug 2005.

• http://programinplacebostudies.org/tag/harvard-placebo-studies/
• www.ncbi.nlm.nih.gov/pubmed/514753
• www.nejm.org/doi/full/10.1056/NEJMp1504023
• http://harvardmagazine.com/2013/01/the-placebo-phenomenon
• http://sitn.hms.harvard.edu/flash/2016/just-sugar-pill-placebo-effect-real/
• www.newyorker.com/magazine/2011/12/12/the-power-of-nothing
• www.rd.com/health/healthcare/placebos-can-work-people-know-not-real/

Homeopathy
Bach, Edward. *Heal Thyself.* CW Daniel Co, 1931.

Barnard, Julian & Martine. *The Healing Herbs of Edward Bach.* Ashgrove Press, 1995.

Dannheisser and Edwards. *Homeopathy, Illustrated.* Element, 1998.

Grossinger, Richard. *Homeopathy.* North Atlantic, 1998.

National Center for Homeopathy (NCH), 1500 Massachusetts NW #41, Washington, DC 20005.

Penselin, Gudrun. *Healing Spirituality with Bach Flowers.* 2016.

• www.homeopathic.com
• www.homeopathycenter.org (NCH, address above)
• www.quackwatch.org/01QuackeryRelatedTopics/homeo.html

Mind Medicine: Intention and Imagery

Word Art
Bennett, Robin Rose. *Healing Magic.* North Atlantic, 2014.

Cassileth, Barrie. *The Alternative Medicine Handbook.* WW Norton, 1998. (Detailed explorations of two dozen Step 2 techniques.)

Castaneda, Carlos. *The Art of Dreaming.* HarperCollins, 1993.

Cornell, Ann. *The Radical Acceptance of Everything.* Calluna, 2005.

Dossey, Larry MD. *Healing Beyond the Body.* Shambhala, 2003.

——. *One Mind.* Hay House, 2013.

Gawain, Shakti. *Creative Visualization.* Bantam, 1982.

Hay, Louise. *You Can Heal Your Life.* Hay House, 1984.

Ingerman, Sandra. *Soul Retrieval.* Harper, 1991.
Marchant, Jo. *Cure: The Science of Mind over Body.* Crown, 2016.
Moss, Robert. *Dreamways of the Iroquois.* Destiny, 2005.
Myss, Caroline. *Anatomy of the Spirit.* Random House, 1996.
Noble, Vicki. *Shakti Woman: Female Shamanism.* HarperSF, 1991.
Paladin, Lynda. *Ceremonies for Change: Creating Personal Ritual to Heal Life's Hurts.* Stillpoint, 1991.
Perkins, John. *Psychonavigation: Travel Beyond Time.* Destiny, 1990.
——. *The World Is As You Dream It.* Destiny, 1994.
Schulz, Mona Lisa. *Awakening Intuition: Using Your Body-Mind Network for Insight and Healing.* Harmony, 1998.
Shinn, Florence Scovel. *Writings.* DeVorss & Co, 1988.
Skully, Nicki. *The Golden Cauldron.* Bear & Co, 1991.
Tulku Thondup. *The Healing Power of the Mind.* Shambhala, 1999.
Walker, Barbara. *Women's Rituals, A Sourcebook.* Harper, 1990.
Whitcomb, Bill. *The Magician's Reflection: A Complete Guide to Creating Personal Magical Symbols.* Llewewllyn Publishing, 1999.
Pert, Candace. *Molecules of Emotion.* Scribner, 1997.
Weil, Andrew. *Health and Healing.* Houghton Mifflin, 1988.
Wier, Dennis. *Trance, from Magic to Technology.* TransMedia, 1996.
• www.law-of-attraction-haven.com (free books; free affirmations)

"Purpose is a combination of focusing toward, and flowing with, energies associated with a goal." — Ken Eagle Feather

Hypnosis
• www.scientificamerican.com/article/hypnosis-memory-brain/
• www.selfhypnosis.com/downloads/stop-gambling/

Image Art
Achterberg, Jeanne. *Imagery in Healing.* Shambhala, 2002.
Ardinger. Barbara. *Goddess Meditations.* Llewellyn Press, 1998.
Austen, Hallie Iglehart. *The Heart of the Goddess: Art, Myth, and Meditations of the World's Sacred Feminine.* Wingbow, 2018.
Beaucaire, Michal. *The Art of Mandala Meditation.* Orion, 2012.
Blair, Nancy. *Amulets of the Goddess Oracle.* Wingbow, 1993.
Campbell, Joseph. *The Mythic Image.* Princeton University Press. 1974. (Hundreds of multi-cultural archetype images.)
Cornell, Judith. *Mandala, Symbols for Healing.* Quest Books, 1994.
Elder, George R. *An Encyclopedia of Archetypes.* Shambhala, 1999.

Furth, Gregg. *The Secret World of Drawings; Healing Art.* Sigo, 1988.

Hillyer, Carolyn. *Weavers' Oracle.* www.seventhwavemusic.co.uk

Keyes, Margaret. *Inward Journey: Art as Therapy.* Open Court, 1987.

Koff-Chapin. *Drawing Out Your Soul.* Center for Touch Drawing, 1998

Marashinsky, Amy Sophia. *The Goddess Oracle:* Element, 1997.

McMurray, Madeline. *Iluminations, The Healing Image: Finding – and learning from – the inner artist for psychic growth.* Wingbow, 1988.

McNiff, Shaun. *Art As Medicine.* Shambhala, 1997.

Montano, Linda. *Art in Everyday Life.* Astro Artz, 1981.

Moon, Beverly. *Encyclopedia of Archetypal Symbolism.* Shambhala, 1999.

Noble, V. & J. Tenney. *Motherpeace Tarot.* Wingbow, 1986.

Pearson, Joel et al. "Mental Imagery: Functional Mechanisms and Clinical Applications." *Trends in Cognitive Science, Oct 2015.*

Color and Light

Gruson, Lindsey. "Color Has a Powerful Effect on Behavior." *New York Times.* Oct 1982.

Liberman, Jacob. *Light: Medicine of the Future.* Inner Traditions, 1990.

Ott, John. *Health and Light.* Pocket Books, 1973.

Phillips, Charles. *Transform Your Life with Color.* CICO, 2015.

St. Clair, Kassia. *The Secret Lives of Color.* Penguin Random House, 2017.

- www.ncbi.nlm.nih.gov/pmc/articles/PMC1297510/
  [Analysis of Chromotherapy; Its Scientific Evolution. Dec 2005.]
- www.mayoclinic.com/health/seasonal-affective-disorder/DS00195
- www.nmha.org/go/sad
- www.ehow.com/about_5366927_birren-color-theory.html

Mind Medicine: Energy/Vibration

Judith, Anodea and Goodman, L. *Creating on Purpose: Manifesting Through the Chakras.* Sounds True, 2012.

Brach, Tara. *Radical Acceptance.* Bantam Dell, 2003.

Brennan, Barbara Ann. *Hands of Light: Guide to Healing Through the Human Energy Field.* Bantam, 1987.

Bruyere, Rosalyn. *Wheels of Light: Chakra.* Bon Productions, 1989.

Chuen, Master Lam Kam. *The Way of Energy: Mastering the Chinese Art of Internal Strength with Chi Kung.* Gaia Books, 1991.

Coddington, Mary. *Seekers of the Healing Energy: Reich, Cayce, the Kahunas, and Other Masters of the Vital Force.* Healing Arts, 1978.

DeNicola, Alison. *Mudras.* US Games, 2017.

Eagle Feather, Ken. *Toltec Dreaming, Don Juan's Teachings on the Energy Body.* Bear & Co, 2007.

Ellyard, Lawrence. *Reiki Meditations for Beginners.* Lotus Press, 2008.

Gardner, Joy. *Color and Crystals: Chakras.* Crossing Press, 1988.

Gebhardt, Christa and Hansel, J. *Whole Again, The Homeopathic Way of Healing (13 Stories).* Narayana Verlag, 2006.

Gerber, Richard. *Vibrational Medicine.* Bear & Co., 1988.

Grey, Alex. *Sacred Mirrors.* Inner Traditions, 1990.

Gunther, Bernard. *Energy Ecstasy.* Newcastle, 1978.

Judith, Anodea. *Eastern Body, Western Mind.* Celestial Arts, 1996.

MacKinnon, Danielle. *Animal Lessons.* Llewellyn, 2017.

Motz, Julie. *Hands of Life.* Bantam, 1998.

Oschman, James. *Energy Medicine, the Scientific Basis.* Elsevier, 2015.

Paulson, Genevieve Lewis. *Kundalini and the Chakras; A Practical Manual for Evolution in this Lifetime.* Llewellyn, 1995.

Prendergast, John H. PhD. *In Touch: How to Tune In to the Inner Guidance of Your Body and Trust Yourself.* Sounds True, 2015.

Radha, Swami Sivananda. *Mantras.* Timeless Books, 2012.

Rankin, Lisa MD. *Mind Over Medicine.* Hay House, 2013.

Schwarz, Jack. *Human Energy Systems.* Dutton, 1980.

Smith, Fritz Frederick, MD. *Inner Bridges, A Guide to Energy Movement and Body Structure.* Humanics, 1986.

"The Resonating Universe," *Revision,* Vol 10, No. 1; Summer 1987.

Sui, Choa Kok. *Pranic Healing.* Weiser, 1990.

Usui, M. *The Original Reiki Handbook of Dr. Mikao Usui.* Lotus Press/Shambhala, 2000.

Villoldo, Alberto. *Shaman, Healer, Sage.* Hampton Books, 2000.

Wallace, Amy & B. Henkin. *Psychic Healing Book.* Wingbow, 1978.

Wood, Matthew. *The Magical Staff: The Vitalist Tradition in Western Medicine.* North Atlantic Books, 1992.

Wright, Susan. *The Chakras in Shamanic Practice.* Destiny, 2007.

• www.natureandforesttherapy.org/

Non-dual Therapies
Blackstone, Judith. *Being Here, A Guide for the Spiritually Sensitive Person.* Sounds True, 2012

Tull, Deborah Eden. *Relational Mindfulness.* Wisdom, 2018.

• www.mindful.org

Touch

Allison, Nancy (ed.). *Illustrated Encyclopedia of Body-Mind Disciplines.* Rosen Publishing, 1999.

Assefi, et al. "Reiki for the treatment of fibromyalgia: a randomized controlled trial." *J Alt Comp Med,* 2008.

Bertherat, Thérèse. *The Body Has Its Reasons.* Healing Arts, 1989.

Hammerschlag, et al. "A Systematic Review of . . . Nonphysical Contact Treatment." *J Alt Comp Med,* 2014.

Krieger, Dolores. *Accepting Your Power to Heal.* Bear & Co. 1993.

Monroe, Carolyn. "Effects of Therapeutic Touch on Pain." *Journal of Holistic Nursing,* 2009. (http://journals.sagepub.com)

Rosa, et al. "A close look at therapeutic touch." *JAMA,* 1998.

Rosen, Marion. *Rosen Methode Bodywork.* German ebook, 2010.

- www.rosenmethod.com
- www. acatnyc.org/the-alexander-technique
- www.amsatonline.org/research
- www.healthandyoga.com/html/meditation/mudras.aspx
- www.doyouyoga.com/7-common-yoga-mudras-explained-23667/
- www.bibletools.org/index.cfm/fuseaction/Library.sr/CT/BS/ k/235/Basic-Doctrines-Laying-On-of-Hands.htm
- www.craniosacraltherapy.org/Whatis.htm#

Devices/Electro-medicine

Brown, et al. "Efficacy of static magnetic field therapy in chronic pelvic pain." *Am. J. of Obstet. & Gynecol.* 2002 187(6):1581-7.

Chandi, Groenendijk, Venema. "Functional extracorporeal magnetic stimulation as a treatment for female urinary incontinence." *British Journal of Urology International.* 2004;93(4):539-42.

Colbert A. P., et al. "Magnetic mattress pad use in patients with fibromyalgia." *J. of Back/Musculoskeletal Rehabil.* 1999;13:19-31.

Sylver, Nenah PhD. *The Rife Handbook.* Barner Books, 2011.

- http://dowsers.org
- http://educate-yourself.org/gw/rifedeathofcancerindustry %20.shtml
- www.rifeenergymedicine.com/appbh.html
- http://lymebook.com/rifehandbook.htm

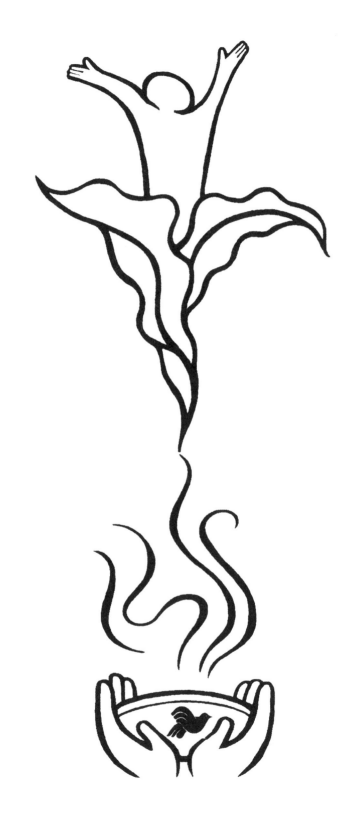

Step Three

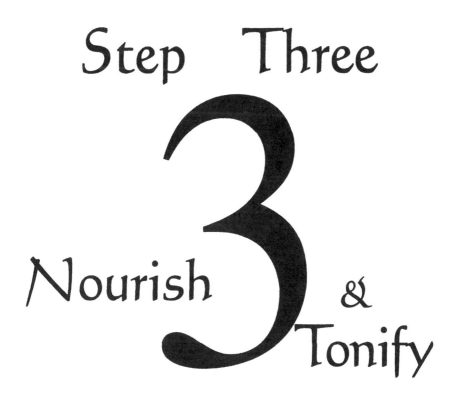

3

Nourish & Tonify

Lifestyle Medicine

"Harmony with the land and the universe is the goal of healing."
Paracelsus (1493-1541)

Nourish & Tonify

The heart of health is nourishment. Nourishment brings substance and energy, matter and vibration into our being. Through all our senses, by all our impressions, we are nourished.

The soul of health is tonification. Tonics create rhythmic pulses of movement, the pulsating patterns of life. Tonification strengthens us and keeps us flexible.

Nourishment adds to the substance (*blood*) of an organ or organism. Each intake nourishes. Ongoing and repeated intake maintains nourishment.

Tonification improves functioning (*chi*) of an organ or organism. Repetition tones; the more sustained the repetition, the greater the tone.

Nourishment has a form, a reality, a beingness of its own. It adds to our form, our reality, our beingness. Nourishment includes, but is not limited to, intake of: protein, minerals, sugars, water, light, images, sounds, touches, emotions, ideas, awareness.

Tonics act upon, and in concert with, that which is created by nourishment. Tonification builds the capacity to do, to work, to manifest. Tonification is regular rhythmical movement: breathing, dancing, walking, drumming, grieving, laughing, sawing, sweeping, singing, chanting, Tai chi, yoga.

Nourished: nurtured, sustained, cared for, cherished, fed, nursed, fostered, maintained, supported, provided for, aided, assisted.

Toned: flexible, elastic, resilient, fit, firm, sound, sturdy, healthy, sensitive, vigorous, vital, strong, energetic, tempered, vibrant.

Nourishment is substance, like earth; tonification is energy, like fire. Nourishment is the notes of the melody; tonification is the pulse of its rhythm. Nourishment builds "blood" (a concept, not a substance), provides the raw materials for life, and grounds us in a particular body. Tonification builds "chi" (life energy), sets our inner rhythms, fires our metabolism, and steadies our mood.

For healthy growth, nourish.   **For healthy energy, tonify.**

Benefits of Lifestyle Medicine

o   Lengthens healthy lifespan
o   Decreases cancer risks
o   Counters lifestyle diseases including type-2 diabetes
o   Improves balance, decreases falls
o   Strengthens bones
o   Improves memory
o   Promotes faster healing
o   Lessens likelihood of chronic problems
o   Puts a smile on your face
o   Increases satisfaction with life
o   Helps one through grief and tough times

Lifestyle Medicine is the heart and soul of abundant health.
It strengthens, sustains, enhances, and fortifies our health. The
first three Medicines are mental and emotional, thus, hard to study.
Lifestyle Medicine is measurable, quantifiable, thus, well studied.

Lifestyle Medicine is physical, fertile, creative, orgasmic. It
enters us. We drink it in. We open our mouths to it. We breathe it.
We open our skin to it. We soak it in. We absorb it. We become it.

Lifestyle Medicine demands our active participation. It requires
action and effort. In return, our range is increased, our horizons
broadened, our reach extended, our energy magnified, our mental
acuity expanded, and our stamina strengthened. An enhanced
ability to stretch and flex, physically and emotionally, is one of
the gifts of Step 3, and a marker of abundant health.

In Step 3 we in-corpo-rate (bring *in*-to our *corpus*-body) the elements of health, and increase our range of motion and emotion in
order to utilize what we have incorporated. Lifestyle Medicine
reminds us that abundant health is maintained and regained by
vigorously and rhythmically nourishing health/wholeness/holi-
ness in all aspects of ourselves.

Food and exercise are complex, emotionally laden subjects.
We are not designed to think about what we eat or how we move,
yet, for abundant health today, we must.

Grandmother Growth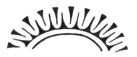

"I'm delighted you could join me today," laughs Grandmother Growth, grasping your hand and setting off at a brisk pace. You are quite certain she is two or three times your age; how can she be so vigorous, so vital, so filled with joy and energy?

You hear the bubbling sounds of a lively river, the happy sounds of children at play, and the contented *puka-puka-puk-puk* of a hen who's just laid an egg. Cooking smells waft on the breeze, making your mouth water. You grin in anticipation.

"Here. Change into this swimsuit. You can eat later." The wise woman holds out a big towel to shelter you. "Race you to the raft," she challenges, with amusement sparkling in her eyes.

Once there, the wise woman exclaims: "You think too much about what you eat. Don't change your diet; let your diet change you.

"Our ancestors lived long and healthy lives eating what the Earth gave them, with gratitude. For the most part, unless there was famine or they were injured, they were vigorous even in old age, without once measuring calories, worrying about carbs, fat, gluten or protein, or consulting a food-combining chart. Try it."

You watch the children on the shore flying their kites, your heart feeling both full and spacious as you wonder at her words.

Lifestyle Medicine Saves Lives

o **75 percent** of cardiovascular disease is preventable with three lifestyle modifications: eat well, exercise often, quit smoking.

o **90 percent** of type-2 diabetes in women is caused by excess weight, unhealthy diet, lack of exercise, smoking, and drinking alcohol. Excess body fat underlies 64 percent of cases of type-2 diabetes in men and 77 percent of cases in women.
Harvard School of Public Health

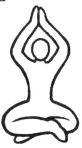

o ". . . **70 to 90 percent** of your lifetime cancer risk could be due to external factors [lifestyle]."
Yusuf Hannun MD

Nourish Wholeness

Nourishment is the basis of health and the fuel for healing.

Nourishment is more than what we eat and drink. Sights, sounds, smells, sensations, emotions, energies, stories, ceremony, safe space, affection, honesty, and beauty nourish us. Lifestyle Medicine nourishes our emotions and our spirit.

Abundant health is wholeness. To nourish wholeness, we nourish that which is bright, with joy and gratitude. To nourish wholeness, we nourish our shadow, with anger and grief. Opposites intermingle to create health/wholeness/holiness. We love all of ourselves. We nourish and strengthen all aspects of ourselves: good/bad, positive/negative, attractive/ugly, sane/crazy.

When we encounter "difficult" feelings – anxiety, abandonment, betrayal, deprivation, inadequacy, jealousy, desire, greed, rage, embarrassment, loss, fear, revenge – Step 3 advises us to "feed the demons." That is, nourish those emotions, listen to them closely rather than try to shut them down. *Respond to their needs.* If given a safe home in us, unsavory aspects paradoxically nourish abundant wellness.

Nourish the Problem

"After the birth of her third child in four years, my sister's postpartum depression was exceptionally severe," she confided. "How can you nourish that?"

"To build health, we nourish the person. To regain health, we nourish the problem," I replied. "Perhaps the nourishment she needs is alone time with her new baby. A 'lying in' period of 3-6 weeks, when mom is alone with the new baby and not responsible for the other children, is a custom in some cultures."

She gave me the strangest look: "That's what she did. She nourished her depression! She went away for three weeks so she could be alone with her baby. It cured her depression."

To some, this is absurd. They believe problems are caused by "bad" feelings, and that if you turn them into "good" feelings (by forgiving or accepting), you will get well. There is some truth to this, but changing your feelings doesn't guarantee a cure. Acceptance nourishes greater health and wholeness.

Muscles are toned by moving them. Emotions are toned by claiming them, by owning them. We prune away our desire to blame our emotional states on others, on outside events. Toned muscles support us; they are flexible and strong. Toned emotions alert us; they are intuition's messengers. Learn about emotional tonics on pages 118-122.

"I make a list of all the reasons that I know I will fail, and I sink into the feeling. I say it out loud, 'I don't want to do this. I can't do it.' I pout. I whimper. I hang my head and cry. An hour later, all the negativity is gone and I am ready to move on."   Thomas Stone, *To the Stars*

Do we have to overcome parts of ourselves to be spiritual or to be healthy? Putting ourselves down and thinking of any part of ourselves as bad or wrong nourishes fragmentation, not wholeness. To see everything within us, and everything around us, as sacred, may be the ultimate expression of Lifestyle Medicine.

Practice: *Bless yourself today, just as you are.*

Optimum nourishment is whole, storied, abundant, seasonal, accessible, local, varied, lovingly touched, wild, and sacred.

Eating Abundantly Well

- Enjoy your meals; make them sacred.
- Eat to connect: with your body, your family, your home, your friends, and Nature.
- Adjust your diet to the season.
- Eat at least one meal a day at the same time.
- Make your diet as wide as possible; eat all foods.
- Eat more fermented foods; eat more wild foods.
- Eat a variety of foods, at each meal, and over time.
- Honor your ancestors; what did they eat?

Nourishing the wholeness of the unique individual cannot be done in isolation. We are all woven together; we are all relations; all life is part of our impressions. Abundant wellness can't arise unless person and planet, family and community are deeply nourished and fully functional.

"[Let us mark the] distinction between whole grains and refined; between foods grown organically and those grown with pesticides and commercial fertilizers; between raw-milk dairy products from pasture-fed cows and pasteurized dairy products from confined animals fed processed feed; between fresh and rancid fats; between traditional fresh fruits and vegetables and those that have been irradiated . . . between range-fed meats and those from animals raised in crowded pens; in short, between foods that nourished our ancestors and the products that dominate the modern marketplace." Sally Fallon, nutrition researcher, author

Parasites for Health

Three weeks after six patients with inflammatory bowel diseases (including ulcerative colitis) drank a brew of worm eggs, five went into complete remission. "For all of our existence these parasites have been with us. We need them," says immuno-parasitologist Joel Weinstock (University of Iowa). The worms seem to suppress the part of the immune system that attacks healthy tissue, and their absence may trigger auto-immune reactions leading to rheumatoid arthritis and MS.

A Spoonful of Story

I arrived too late to eat before my talk, but was promised dinner afterwards. Hours later, my hostess offered me sprouts and carrot juice. I asked for cooked grain, cooked greens, a piece of cheese. She had none of these.

She did offer me a beer. And this story: A local man bought the old brewery and renovated it, got local farmers to grow barley and hops, hired others to drive the delivery trucks. I rarely drink beer, but I did that night. It was my dinner and I was deeply nourished.

A Story in Every Bite

When the food we eat is storied, it nourishes us more deeply. When images, words, rites, rhythms, legends and lore surround our food, we have more threads to weave into our own stories, more ways to reweave ourselves in wholeness.

These are the ways of our grandmothers, the wise women of old, the Ancient Ones. Each food has its own creation myth: A Hopi mother who is cut into pieces and buried rises to feed her family as corn. A young Seneca girl loses her pouch of "friendship beads" and brings us all the gift of sunflowers. The sacred belly of the mother is source, is life, is food and story. Food stories are mythical and magical; storied food feeds body and soul.

Eating food that lacks a story results in a subtle kind of starvation. Storied food gives us a rightful intimacy with that which nourishes us, a sense of our place in the spiral of the great give-away, and assurance that we can care for ourselves. Without it, our sense of self-worth suffers, our sense of purpose is unclear, unfocused.

When you harvest and eat wild foods, you get a story. Pick dandelion greens and put them on your hotdog. Make nettle soup from your backyard. Visit the sea shore and snack on seaweeds – they are all edible. Try protein-rich, tasty, crunchy wild insects.

"The Shona of Zimbabwe eat grasshoppers, flying termites, and caterpillars. In Botswana, whole green ants have a lemon-like flavor. About six species of snails are eaten. When eating grubs, hold the head, or they will bite your tongue."   Bill Mollison, *Permaculture*

  ## Golden Rules of Food Shopping
The goal of shopping is to purchase real food.

o *Real food has no ingredients.* (Butter is real food; margarine is not. Milk is real food; soy beverage is not.)
o *Or the ingredients are whole foods.* (Whole milk and culture are yogurt, not skim milk, milk powder, gums, thickeners.)
o *Real food changes.* It molds, sours, ferments, sprouts, and rots; it supports life. *Eat food that spoils, before it does. Avoid preservatives.*
o *Real food has little or no packaging.*
o *Real food is seasonal.* (And stored, frozen, fermented, preserved.)

The Spirit of the Food

Finding, gathering, cultivating, harvesting, preparing, cooking, and storing food has been women's work and women's genius since time out of mind. In earth-centered cultures, all of these tasks, plus those associated with hunting (men's genius) are interwound with sacred stories and teaching tales. This invisible, unmeasurable aspect of nutrition is not in any supplement, yet story is of utmost importance to abundant health.

> *"I want to touch now on another very important area in my life as a food gatherer. It is my job, my purpose, to insure that I gather certain food for my husband and my children. . . . If you put something right in it, your body feels it. Your spiritual self feels it. In order to make me complete, I need the right food from the land. I also need to prepare it myself. I have to harvest it myself."* Gwaganad, Haida Nation

Everyday foods are sacramental when they are baked from local grains, prepared with local greens and herbs, brewed with ancestral yeasts.

Everyday foods that are processed, pre-packaged, and mass-produced are insubstantial, unbodied, unspirited, and no longer capable of nourishing wholeness/health/holiness.

Characteristics of Healthy Traditional Diets

o Wild, or minimally cultivated, foods at most meals.
o Fermented foods, including yogurt, wine and beer, eaten daily.
o Salt used generously. Mineral and vitamin intake very high.
o Unheated animal protein – milk, fish, meat, eggs, insects – eaten frequently; few other foods eaten raw.
o Animal fats predominate; vegetable oils rarely used.
o Real foods (cod liver oil, molasses) counter deficiencies.

o *No* refined foods (white flour, white sugar, white rice).
o *No* protein powders (milk, soy, whey, egg, pea powders).
o *No* synthetic foods (coffee creamer, artificial sugar, margarine).

Varied and Various, Vivacious and Vital

The more vital we are, the more variety we can tolerate. Variety nourishes resilience and helps create flexibility. In his study of human nutrition, Dr. Weston Price observed that the native peoples who ate the most varied diets generally lived the longest, suffered the least degenerative disease, and had the healthiest teeth.

". . . despite their apparent disorderliness, indigenous gardens [are] polycultural masterpieces [with] up to seventy different plant species mixed chaotically, but never innocently."   Jeremy Narby, PhD, anthropologist

Humans are willing and able to eat almost anything. Coprolites (fossilized feces) reveal that our ancestors ate about 2000 different foods in their lives. Modern Americans sometimes eat as few as 100 foods. The more varied the diet, the greater the likelihood that all the macro- and micro-nutrients needed for optimum health will be present.

"Ancient nomadic cultures tended to leave organic wastes behind, restoring nutrients to the soil. . . . Modern, settled societies simply want to get rid of waste as quickly as possible. But the ability of . . . natural ecosystems to absorb modern synthetic wastes is [almost] nonexistent. . . . "
Michael Braungart, environmental chemist

A Healthy Diet

Our bodies have instincts which guide us to eat abundantly well, so long as there are no manufactured foods available. Any diet of whole, cooked foods that includes all the gifts of the earth – animal and vegetable – is a healthy diet. A diet that unnecessarily limits foods – like gluten-free (for non-celiacs), raw food, juice only, vegan, or Paleo – cannot create long-term abundant health.

If you want guidelines: DASH (Dietary Approaches to Stop Hypertension) is the best. If you want help losing weight, and keeping it off, Weight Watchers delivers consistently great results.

**You can't nourish the people apart from the land
or the land apart from the people.**

"It is totally unfounded to say that food enzymes [sold as supplements] are important nutrients or that their lack in any way influences health."
Manfred Kroger PhD, *Consumer Health: A Guide to Intelligent Decision Making*

Vitamins

Vitamins are groups of closely-related compounds that function together. To be functionally useful, vitamins require minerals, and sometimes other vitamins. They are often enzymatic.

Living things like plants and people make many vitamins, especially antioxidants. Humans make B vitamins in their intestines, vitamin D on their skin, and vitamin A in the liver. We can't make vitamin B_{12} (plants can't either, but cows can) or vitamin C; we must get them from food. And some vitamins require that we eat their precursors to make them: carotenes become vitamin A.

Processing and refining removes vitamins. White flour is white because the golden, vitamin E-rich wheat germ and the brown, B-vitamin-and-fiber-rich bran are gone. "Enriching" foods and taking supplements does not restore wholeness or nourish abundant health. **The only truly bioavailable vitamins are those in foods.**

Plants make vitamins in response to stress. Wild and organic plants are more stressed, thus richer in vitamins.

Plants continue to make vitamins after they are harvested. Storing, chopping, fermenting, and cooking trigger the production and liberation of vitamins in most vegetables, including tomatoes, corn, peas, beans, whole grains, leafy greens, and carrots.

Raw fruits/vegetables do not provide more vitamins. They supply little more than fiber (unless juiced) and vitamin C. Unwashed, fresh, raw greens in salads add healthy soil bacteria to the gut.

*"Antioxidants are more effective and better able to ward off cell damage when present in combination. They function as a team –
an antioxidant network – and having one or two star
players isn't enough."* Lester Packer, PhD.
world's foremost antioxidant researcher

Whole Foods, Whole People

Whole foods are unprocessed, unenriched, intact, and complete. When necessary, they are hulled, cut, peeled, seeded, skinned, frozen, ground, cooked, fermented, or dried. Whole foods vibrate with the rhythms of the places where they grow. They nourish with substance and energy, trace minerals and earthy stories.

Minerals

Well-mineralized tissues are the basis of abundant health.

Pure, elemental minerals are not usable by living things, though. We require our minerals in pairs. Pair the minerals sodium and chloride to get table salt. There are a host of possible pairs for every mineral. You can buy calcium lactate, calcium ascorbate, calcium carbonate, calcium gluconate, calcium citrate, calcium phosphate, calcium orotate, and calcium citrate malate.

Supplements supply just one pair, while plants contain dozens of different pairs, all of which nourish abundant, optimum health.

"The mineral composition of our body fluids depends entirely on our diet."
Paul Bergner, North American Institute of Medical Herbalism

**The longer food is cooked,
the more of its minerals are available.**

Wild Foods

Wild meat*	Wild eggs	Wild flowers
Wild mushrooms*	Wild grains	Wild shoots
Wild berries*	Wild seeds	Wild roots
Wild fish*	Wild leaves	Wild water
Wild shellfish*	Wild seaweeds*	Wild honey*

* Look for these at your local supermarket

Wild Foods Carry Beneficial Bacteria and Yeasts that

- Improve the mix of gut flora
- Ease inflammation
- Improve digestion
- Stabilize mood
- Protect memory
- Support the heart and cardiovascular system
- Favorably alter the chemistry of the blood
- Counter some of the adverse effects of drugs
- Help us survive, even thrive, in polluted environments

"The best thing about herbs is the fact that each contains thousands of biologically active compounds, hundreds in the ppm range. That gives your body a big menu from which to select what it needs. Cells will selectively grab minerals and vitamins that are needed."   Dr. James Duke, botanist

Wild Food

Wild food is our original food: food, as it were, from the Garden of Eden. Uncultivated, given from the earth's overflowing abundance. Wild food is a gift which we humbly receive. We partake of original innocence when we eat wild food. We recognize ourselves as children of the earth when we eat wild food.

Wild food is a holograph: complete, complex, resonant.

Wild plants manifest their right to choose where and when to grow, absorbing nutrition as they choose from the earth, the air, the sun and the rain. Eating wild food opens the senses and reveals the sacredness inherent in Nature.

Susun Says

✻ Optimum nourishment is inexpensive, delicious, easily grown or bought, and a delight to all the senses.

✻ Any improvement in diet improves health; and some people can be healthy eating anything.

✻ Traditional diets use hunted, gathered, herded, and cultivated foods. No traditional diets are vegan, raw, or vegetarian.

✻ Traditional diets create healthy, long-lived, spiritually-sound, emotionally-engaged people.

Child Eats Weeds

Four-year-old Sean wouldn't eat anything green, not even peas or bits of parsley on potatoes. Definitely not broccoli or salad. One afternoon, outside with mom, Sean copied her as she tasted garden plants and weeds. Sean wanted to taste them, too. Then Sean wanted to eat them. Still does, with mom and alone. At dinner, inside, it's still the same: no green will pass Sean's lips. But outside, plants are good green eats. Sean is on to something. How about you?

Wild food provides a remarkably varied, seasonal diet from local, abundant, and renewable resources.

Whatever our Paleolithic ancestors ate, it was all wild.

The biologically active macro- and micro-nutrients in wild foods are better antioxidants and better bone-builders than anything in a pill or capsule. Wild foods are much higher than cultivated foods in vitamins, minerals, essential fatty acids, protein and fiber, but much lower in sugar. Teosinte (wild corn) is 30 percent protein and 2 percent sugar, while cultivated sweet corn is 4 percent protein and 10-40 percent sugar.

Our cells know wild food, they know it from millennia ago, from tens of thousands of years before the first crops were planted, the first granary raised. Even a tiny amount of wild food – a mere mouthful or a single bite of some wild green, wild flower, or seaweed – will improve the bioavailability of nutrients from cultivated foods. Wild foods are the exact fit for our cellular receptors, those mysterious moving mandalas that gatekeep the integrity of each cell. Wild foods contain the original keys that open the locks to abundant nourishment, abundant health, and abundant fun.

Wild foods bring us closer to death, and that brings us more fully into life. Wild foods connect us intimately with the great give-away: I eat you and you eat me.

"There is no death that is not somebody's food and no life that is not somebody's death."   Gary Snyder, *The Practice of the Wild*

Great Give-Away
I eat you and you eat me.

All nourishment is a gift, a great give-away of life. Each breath is a gift, a great give-away. Food is a gift, a great give-away from the plants and animals. Today, I am gifted, I eat. Tomorrow, I will be the gift.

Lifestyle Medicine for Joy

• Relate with humans/animals.
• Keep physically fit.
• See to your financial security.
• Have a sense of purpose.
• Follow your bliss and enjoy your life.
• Connect often with caring, like-minded people.

Superstars of Nourishment

Adding any superstar of nourishment – including dark chocolate and green tea – to your diet will improve your health, but the easiest way to start is by adding nourishing herbal infusions. Their optimum nutrition will change your taste buds, making super healthy foods like yogurt, weeds, seaweeds, and mushrooms taste really good. Up to a quart a day is safe for anyone of any age.

☆ Nourishing Herbal Infusions ☆

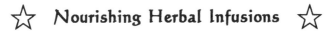

Benefits of drinking up to a quart of infusion daily include:

o   More energy; deeper sleep
o   Denser, more flexible bones
o   Less anxiety, better mood
o   Normalization of blood pressure
o   Healthier skin and hair
o   Improved eyesight, especially at night
o   Protection against chronic diseases
o   Less risk of diabetes; lessening of diabetic symptoms
o   Improved cardiovascular functioning
o   Increased joint flexibility
o   Better memory, sharper mental focus

Nourishing herbal infusions will change your life. To make one: Pour four cups (1 liter) boiling water over one ounce (30 grams) dry weight of the herb. Cover tightly. Steep at room temperature for 4-10 hours (or overnight). Strain, squeeze. Refrigerate. Drink cold or hot, with honey or anything else. I like miso in hot nettle.

Watch me make infusions on YouTube.

Stinging nettle, herb of energy, rebuilds kidneys, restores adrenals. **Oatstraw** makes nerves strong, helps sexy hormones. **Linden** is the world's best anti-inflammatory. **Comfrey leaf** is for flexible toughness in bones, ligaments, tendons, skin, and mucus surfaces of the digestive, respiratory and reproductive tracts. **Red clover** counters cancers. **Hibiscus** keeps us hearty. **Violet** leaf is ultra soothing. **Mullein** creates healthy lungs. **Astragalus** is the everyday adaptogen. **Hawthorn** keeps the heart youthful.

☆ Yogurt ☆

Benefits of eating a quart/liter of yogurt weekly include:
  o   Fewer bladder/vaginal infections
  o   Fewer sexually-transmitted infections
  o   Greater longevity
  o   Decreased cardiovascular event risk
  o   Significant decrease in risk of colon cancer
  o   18 percent lower risk of type-2 diabetes
  o   Enhanced immunity
  o   Less cancer overall
  o   Less asthma and allergies
  o   Cessation of diarrhea
  o   Less gut distress during chemotherapy treatments
  o   Reduction of arterial stiffness

Ingestion of yogurt is strongly linked to increases in the amounts and activity of immune cells like cytokines, antibodies, natural killer cells, phagocytes, and T-cells. Lactic acid bacteria in yogurt can suppress the growth of pathogenic bacteria.

Our first nourishment is mother's milk, pulsing with her heart-beat song. The cow is the avatar of the Great Goddess. Milk is her quintessential herbal medicine: cows (and goats and many other animals) eat herbs and turn them into milk.

Psychologist Stephanie Demetrakopoulos celebrates milk as spiritual love made visible, as the connective tissue that ties one generation to the next. I see milk-hating as woman-hating, and fear of milk is fear of the female principle. Full-fat milk and eggs are the most nourishing foods known. They are female products.

When milk is fermented into yogurt – thus removing the lactose – it is the perfect food for everyone. Raw milk cheese, and its byproduct, whey – fresh fluid, never powdered – are healing miracles for the gut. Pasteurized milk can be difficult to digest, but it doesn't cause mucus or colds.

Unpasteurized, raw milk is loaded with active enzymes, which benefit us. It sometimes harbors listeria, a bacterium dangerous to fetuses. The USDA and the FDA are currently trying to eradicate access to raw milk to protect those foolish folks who, like myself, prefer it. They do approve of organic, raw milk cheese though. You will find it at your supermarket. If not, ask for it.

☆ Coffee & Decaffeinated Coffee ☆

Benefits of drinking 3-5 cups of coffee daily include:
- o Longer lifespan; 17 percent lower risk all-cause mortality
- o Lower levels of inflammation (except after injury/surgery)
- o Less cardiovascular disease, heart attack, stroke
- o Clearer arteries; 41 percent less calcification
- o 40 percent less Parkinson's
- o 20-40 percent fewer gallstones
- o 4-8 percent less risk of type-2 diabetes
- o 50 percent less risk of dying of mouth and throat cancer
- o More mental alertness; protection against Alzheimer's
- o More physical endurance
- o 20 percent less likelihood of being depressed
- o 17 percent fewer basal cell carcinomas (skin cancer)
- o Fewer headaches, less pain altogether

The evidence for the health benefits of coffee is robust and consistent.

Coffee **doesn't**
- • Help you lose weight
- • Drive up blood pressure permanently
- • Dehydrate you, though it is mildly diuretic
- • Worsen incontinence
- • Make your heart palpitate

Caffeine, an alkaloid found in tea and coffee, but not in chocolate, is strongly psychoactive, and quite addictive.

The amount of caffeine in your cup of tea or coffee has a lot to do with how the plants were grown (shade-grown is highest in caffeine), when it was harvested (new leaves have more caffeine than older ones), how it was handled (chopping and grinding increase available caffeine), and how long it is brewed (the longer the brew, the more caffeine). (More on caffeine on page 163.)

Green tea has less caffeine than black tea, and both have much less than coffee.

"The psyche discovers itself by touching, diving into, being surrounded by the ground of being, matter-nature-mother." Stephanie Demetrakopoulos

☆ Black and Green Tea ☆
Camellia sinensis

Benefits of drinking three or more cups of tea daily include:

- Lower cholesterol
- Lower blood pressure
- Less diabetes
- Less heart disease
- Increased endurance
- Less skin cancer
- Stronger liver
- Mental clarity
- Less plaque buildup
- Higher HDL
- Lower LDL
- Lower triglycerides
- Improved circulation
- Stronger, healthier heart
- Fewer varicosities
- Less atherosclerosis
- Fewer heart attacks
- Less belly fat
- Better oral health
- Fewer sunburns
- Less dementia
- Fewer blood clots, strokes
- Denser, more flexible bones
- Alpha-wave-dominant mental state
- Increased flexibility of the arteries
- Better digestion and nutrient uptake
- Protection against a wide variety of cancers
- 31 percent less likelihood of having ovarian cancer
- Less likelihood of Parkinson's (normalizes dopamine)

Few foods excite scientists as much as green tea, with its phenomenal range of health benefits.

L-theanine, found in tea, but not coffee, is strongly associated with calmness, alertness, and focus.

Catechins, powerful anti-inflammatory antioxidants, account for as much as 30 percent of the dry weight of white or green tea. They act to ease pain and anxiety through the non-addicting endocannabinoid system. Catechins regulate food intake, making tea the ideal beverage for those wanting to maintain or lose weight.

Tea destroys or inactivates *herpes* virus within minutes (in vitro). As a bath/wash, it counters athlete's foot fungus and conjunctivitis.

Tea not only helps prevent cancer, it counters its progression, metastasis, and recurrence.

"It is better to be deprived of food for three days, than of tea for one."
Ancient Chinese proverb

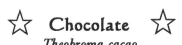

☆ Chocolate ☆
Theobroma cacao

Benefits of eating 1-3.5 ounces of dark chocolate daily include:
o   Less inflammation; less stress
o   Improved mood, memory, and immunity
o   Heightened sensory awareness
o   A sense of energetic calm
o   A healthier cardiovascular system
o   Reduced LDL cholesterol; increased HDL cholesterol
o   Lower blood pressure
o   Improved blood flow; fewer blood clots
o   Increased insulin sensitivity
o   Thinner blood; fewer strokes
o   Increased amounts of brain chemicals, including endorphins, dopamine, and serotonin

The brain on chocolate is the brain in love.

Unlike coffee and tea, chocolate does not contain caffeine. Instead, it has **penethylamine**, a pleasure-inducing stimulant, **theobromine**, a mild stimulant, and **anandamide**, a neurotransmitter that nourishes bliss and relaxes the nerves.

Ounce for ounce, chocolate has the most antioxidants of any edible plant. Throw away those supplements and eat a little 80 percent dark chocolate for abundant health. Or drink a cup of cocoa.

Chocolate is very good for your brain. Research done at Harvard Medical School in 2013 found older adults had improved blood flow to the specific brain regions devoted to memory when drinking two cups of hot cocoa daily.

Chocolate is usually sweetened, so it is calorie rich, but it doesn't seem to drive up body weight. In fact, those who eat chocolate at least twice a week have lower body mass index (BMI) than those who don't, even without eating less or exercising more.

Cacao is traditionally combined with psychoactive plants such as psilocybin, spices such as cinnamon, flavors like orange, and nuts or dried fruit. It is also turned into a molé sauce and poured over meat. Yum.

To date, no incidents of overdosing on cacao are known.

☆   **Weeds & Seaweeds**   ☆

Amaranth, Dandelion, Lamb's Quarter, Wild Mustard Greens
Alaria, Dulse, Fucus, Kombu, Nereocystis, Nori, Wakame

Benefits of eating any amount of weeds and seaweeds daily include:
- o   Increased life expectancy
- o   Healthier skin and hair
- o   Heavy metal removal, especially lead; safe for children
- o   Reduced estrogen load; lower risk of breast cancer
- o   Removal of radioactive isotopes
- o   Stronger immune activity
- o   Increased bone density
- o   Increased production of B-lymphocytes and macrophages
- o   Stimulation of T-cell production; better utilization of T-cells
- o   Improved thyroid functioning
- o   Lower serum cholesterol (inhibits bile acid absorption)
- o   Lower blood pressure (–10 after 2-3 months of 6-12 g/day)

Weeds – whether from the land or the sea – are abundant, accessible, free, mineral-rich, low-fat, beautiful, savory, and loaded with special antioxidants. Weeds are tuned to our needs; their nutrients are uniquely biologically available and active. They are optimum nourishment for abundant health.

Seaweed favorably alters estrogen and phytoestrogen metabolism. Eating 5 grams of *Alaria* seaweed a day increases urinary excretion of estrogen after 7 weeks. Regular use of *Fucus* seaweed lengthens the time between menstrual cycles.

Alginate and **chitin** – seaweed polysaccharides – heal wounds and soothe an esophagus harmed by reflux. These same polysaccharides block the interaction of cell walls with encapsulated viruses, like *herpes*, helping the immune system resist viral infection.

Those with metabolic syndrome usually use 4-6 grams dried seaweed daily for at least two months. Those with osteoarthritis pain reduced it with 2.5 grams of seaweed a day for twelve weeks.

Over-zealous ingestion of seaweed can increase serum thyroid hormone levels so much that the thyroid swells into a goiter.

Algin, an indigestible fiber found in some seaweeds, mobilizes and removes mercury, lead, cadmium, manganese, tin, zinc, and radioactive strontium-90 and barium through the feces. About 400,000 deaths a year are related to lead exposure.

☆ Mushrooms ☆

Maitake, Reishi, Shiitake, Turkey Tail,
Chaga, White Button, Enoki, Portabella, Oyster

Benefits of eating wild or cultivated mushrooms, fresh, cooked, or dried, or of taking mushroom/mycelium tincture include:

o Less inflammation
o Less heart disease
o Improved immunity
o Stronger macrophages
o Lower blood pressure
o Better brain function
o Reduced waist circumference
o More energy, especially in elders
o Increases in neutrophils, immunoglobin, NK cells, CD4
o Lower total cholesterol, LDL, and triglycerides
o Less gastric, esophageal, colon, lung, prostate cancers
o Significant reduction of breast cancer, esp. postmenopause
o Fewer infections, especially herpes, HIV*
o Protection against liver damage from hepatitis B
o Less asthma, fewer allergies
o Less anxiety and depression, esp. with terminal cancer
o Enhancement of standard cancer treatments**

o Less diabetes
o Less cancer
o Less joint pain
o Healthier hair/skin
o Higher HDL
o Healthier liver

* Extract/tincture of reishi has been shown to be more effective against bacterial infections – like *E. coli, M. luteus, S. aureus, Salmonella typhi, Proteus vulgaris,* and *B. cereus* – than most antibiotics.

** Improves patients' response to chemotherapy, elevates the body's self-defense, inhibits proliferation, adhesion, angiogenesis, migration, and invasion of cancer cells, repairs DNA fragmentation and chromosome damage, protects the liver and the gastric mucosa, and ensures a higher quality of life post-treatment. Reishi is proven to combat inflammatory breast cancer.

Mushrooms supply lots of potassium, beta-glucans, and some hard-to-get, but important nutrients: folic acid and selenium. Put fresh or dried mushrooms in the sun and they'll make vitamin D. (150-600 IU in thirty minutes. Chopped ones make more.)

"Microwave cooking inactivates much of the vitamin B_{12} in foods."
ScienceNews, 1998

☆ Tomato Sauce ☆

Benefits of eating one cup of tomato sauce or juice daily include:
- o Decreased risk of prostate and breast cancer
- o Less risk of cancer of the mouth, throat, lung, bladder, colon, stomach, pancreas, and cervix
- o Lower LDL cholesterol
- o Less heart disease
- o Better sight; prevention of cataracts & macular degeneration
- o Fewer sunburns and less skin cancer
- o Fewer colds, flus, infections
- o Less diabetes
- o Better bladder health
- o Less DNA damage

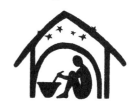

Lycopene is one of a powerful group of antioxidants found abundantly in tomatoes, sweet potatoes, mango, papaya, winter squash, red pepper, and watermelon. Heating, freezing, dehydrating, fermenting, and marinating in oil vastly increases the bioavailablity of all carotenes and carotenoids, including lycopene. Lycopene can stop the growth of cancer cell cultures in Petri dishes.

Well-cooked tomatoes strongly protect against all neuro-degenerative diseases. In general, despite raw food advocates' beliefs, vitamins are *increased* and minerals are *liberated* when plants are cooked. Study after study finds tomato sauce, soup, paste and cooked juice – but not raw tomatoes – full of health benefits.

It's really easy to make your own tomato sauce and freeze or can it for later use. To hasten the thickening of the sauce, I ladle out the tomato juice that rises to the top of the pot before I stir the sauce, and can that for a delightful winter beverage. To my mind, tomato juice is the only liquid worth drinking on board an airplane.

For a special treat, try Dried Tomato Paté; recipe on page 310.

"7.8 million deaths worldwide could potentially be prevented each year if people ate ten servings (800 grams) of fruits and vegetables each day."   *International Journal of Epidemiology*, 2017

Don't change your diet; let your diet change you.
Local wild foods, loving friends, and gratitude
nourish abundant health.

Tonify
Build Flexibility & Resilience

Good health is optimum functionality in the unique present moment. Tonifying builds free and flexible functioning. Tonification strengthens basic biological rhythms.

Pulse and unpulse. Tighten and relax. Healthy functioning is regular and rhythmical.

"In a healthy state, the body's structures are a multileveled series of interacting systems and subsystems that resonate harmoniously."
Gabriel Cousens MD, *Spiritual Nutrition*

Health is smooth, flowing, regular, and rhythmical. From our brain waves to our beating hearts, from our hormones to our muscles, we are rhythmical. We are spirals; we are waves.

Disease is erratic, flat, linear, and inflexible. Constant low-grade stress compresses, flattens, and destabilizes our rhythms.

Tonification resets our beat, expands our waves, and makes us more resilient. Tonfication resets our internal clocks, taps us into deep biological wholeness, plugs us into infinity.

"If you try to define life you will reach the inescapable conclusion that rhythms are among its most basic features. Every property used as an earmark of life – reproduction, respiration, irritability, and all the rest – is rhythmic. So why not include rhythmicity itself?" Jack Palmer, biologist

Lifestyle Medicine makes us fit enough and fed enough to surf the waves of fortune and dance to karma's tune. Abundant health is flexible enough to go with life's flow.

To create abundant health, we want to tonify all aspects of ourselves. **Physical tonics** – exercise, Qi Gong, Tai chi, yoga, and tonic and adaptogenic herbs – strengthen muscles and bones, heart and lungs, and even the internal organs. **Mental tonics** – reading, puzzles, games – enhance memory and concentration. **Emotional tonics** – drumming, chanting, singing, screaming, crying, laughing, and gratitude – tonify the psyche.

Stress

It is estimated that 98 percent of all disease is caused by stress. Tonification teaches us how to adapt to and utilize stress for health.

"Hardly a week goes by without new research tying stress to another major ailment."   Dr. Lee Berk, 2017

Stress keeps skyscrapers up. Tension holds up bridges. Tonification builds abundant health because it stresses us. Stress we move with keeps us healthy. Stress we don't deal with kills.

Many people respond to stress by sedating or stimulating themselves (Step 4). This erodes health. Lifestyle Medicine (Step 3) offers us a different response: to strengthen our health with tonics and herbal adaptogens.

Tonification is rhythmic stress. Tonification is effective use of tension. Tonification builds dynamic tension. It takes us to our edges and tests our boundaries so we may encompass more of life, with more energy, more joy, more enthusiasm, and more curiosity.

Sedation and stimulation give us a false sense of balance. Tonification and nourishment stretch us and unbalance us, reminding us that life is constantly changing. Balance evens out the extremes, countering healthy functioning. Imagine a balanced ocean: no waves or tides. Dead; lifeless. Imagine a balanced stream: no curves, no rapids. Boring.

Tonification teaches us to accept life and ourselves as we are. Lifestyle Medicine is not about becoming a perfect person, eating exactly the right thing and exercising to achieve a perfect body.

"We're living in an age of perfectionism, and perfection is the idea that kills. People are suffering and dying under the torture of the fantasy self they're failing to become."   Will Storr, *Selfie*

Tonification promotes restful sleep without the need for sedatives or soporifics. Tonification promotes alertness without the need for stimulants. Tonification helps prevent pain by keeping blood and chi flowing. It is the easiest way to prevent the chronic diseases of civilization: diabetes, obesity, joint failure, cardiovascular disease, fatty liver disease, cancer, and dementia.

Exercise

". . . the most effective, potent way that we can improve quality of life and duration of life is exercise." Mark Tarnopolsky, metabolic neurologist

Exercise is the classic tonic: garden, swim, dance, cycle, ski, lift weights, play ball, make love, paddle a canoe, cook a meal, ride a horse, make music, hike, sweep, take the stairs, sing, walk.

Benefits of exercising regularly include:
o Extension of life span (by at least five years)
o Reduction in overall mortality (by 12-39 percent)
o Reduction in risk of type 2-diabetes
o Lower blood pressure
o Reduction of cholesterol levels
o Improved circulation to the brain
o Improved memory and focus
o Reduction of stress
o Improved immune functioning
o Reduction in addictive behavior
o Faster wound healing
o Reduction in risk of edema
o Increased self-esteem
o Protection against many forms of cancer
o Reduction in risk of broken hip; improves bone mass
o Increased release of chemicals that dull pain
o Improved mood; counters depression, eases grief
o Reduction in risk of uterine cancer (by 30 percent)

". . . exercise is regenerative medicine – restoring and repairing and basically fixing things that are broken." Marcas Bamman, exercise physiologist

---

✳ Don't Sit There. Get Up! ✳

Sitting for more than six hours a day increases the risk of diabetes, cancer, heart disease, and high blood pressure, no matter how much, how hard, or how long you exercise.

Researcher Richard Rosenkranz says: "All you need to do to reduce the risk of prolonged inactivity is stand up and walk slowly. You don't need exercise, just some increased activity."

Walk *You already do it.*

The easiest, most enjoyable, and best way to derive the benefits of exercise is to walk! More is always better, but surprisingly few steps make big differences in overall health and longevity if you make it a habit. When can you walk instead of sit? I walk while I read to my grandchild when she is far away. I walk during my weekly blog talk show. *Hint:* Get a walking partner. *Hint:* Avoid hand or ankle weights; they slow you down.

Any walk is a tonic. For abundant health, **walk barefoot** and **walk outside**. Bare feet absorb the healing properties of the herbs they tread on. Bare feet channel *chi* from the earth into all the meridians. Healing reflex points in the feet are activated as bare feet stretch and adapt to changing terrain. *Hint:* Walk on a lawn. *Hint*: NuFoot shoes are like walking in socks.

Increase tonification and prevent muscle stiffness by taking 25 drops of St. Joan's wort (*Hypericum perforatum*) tincture in a glass of water before and after exercise.

Trager Approach/Mentastics

Non-intrusive movements jiggle, rock, and swing you in gentle rhythmic ways to release physical and mental patterns, ease pain, facilitate relaxation, and increase mobility. *Mentastics* is a Lifestyle Medicine that leads us to explore how to move with the least tension and effort possible, freely and easily. Trager tablework is Step 4, Alternative Medicine. Trager practitioners are trained to bring curiosity, playfulness, and effortlessness to their work, to avoid causing pain, and to increase ease through a full range of sensations.

"A shift in the body is a shift in consciousness." Joseph Heller
student of Ida Rolf and Brugh Joy, author of *Body Wise*

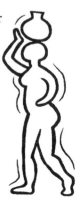

No Time to Exercise?

If you are willing to push hard – and rest deeply – you can get an hour's worth of fitness in 10 minutes. Here's how. Go as hard as you can, as fast as you can, get breathless, for 1 minute. Reduce speed to moderate for 1 minute. Repeat 4 more times. Rest.

Yoga

Yoga is the "yoke" joining body, mind, and spirit. Physical postures (asanas) and breath (pranayama) build strength, balance, flexibility, focus, and resilience. Yoga works for every body – when you find a style that works for you. *Hint:* Do yoga in the afternoon. *Hint:* Do yoga at normal temperatures. *Hint:* A vigorous class once a week for ten years is ten times better than a daily class for a year.

Cumulative benefits of a consistent yoga practice include:
o   Increased muscle strength and flexibility
o   Improved balance; fewer falls
o   Less joint pain; more mobility; less arthritis
o   Deeper respiration; fewer allergies
o   More energy and vitality
o   Weight reduction; healthy metabolism
o   Improved heart and circulatory health
o   Protection from injury; better coping skills
o   Less inflammation; less back pain
o   Better, deeper sleep; slower aging
o   A more positive outlook on life; less anxiety, depression
o   Mental clarity and calmness, better memory and focus
o   Increased body awareness
o   Relief from chronic stress patterns
o   Reduction of cortisol levels; less damage from stress
o   Lower blood pressure, heart rate, fasting blood glucose
o   Relief from Post Traumatic Stress Disorder (PTSD)
o   Lower total cholesterol and LDL cholesterol

Time Limit for Lifestyle Medicine

We create 20-40 million new cells every minute. The cells that work the hardest – liver, blood, gut – die and are replaced the fastest. Tonification and nourishment improve these cells quickly and then all of your other cells improve too. Changes are often noticeable within a week, significant changes within 3-6 weeks. If not, go on to the next Step.

In acute conditions, Lifestyle Medicine moderates the side effects of Pharmaceutical and Deep Medicines. Lifestyle Medicine prevents/minimizes chronic conditions and disease progression.

Breema

Union of body and mind through natural flowing movements, without exertion or contortion, to release pain and improve energy.

"You want to get rid of your garbage . . . but where are you going to throw it? There's only one existence."   Breema homepage

High-Intensity Interval Training

An effective way for older people to build muscle, regulate insulin, cut fat, and increase heart health in one minute a day.

Functional Fitness Training

Long used in rehabilitation after stroke, surgery, or a heart attack, the whole-body movements improve tone more than strength training does, while increasing balance and flexibility.

Tai Chi   *Meditation - make that: medi-cation - in motion*

These flowing series of poses, practiced regularly, provide as much tone as resistance training or brisk walking, with less effort. *Hints:* Wear loose clothing and flexible shoes. Join a group.

Cumulative benefits of a consistent Tai chi practice include:

o   More strength, flexibility, stability, poise
o   Better sleep, stronger immune system, healthier heart
o   Fewer falls; less injury from falls; improved bone health
o   Improvement in overall feeling of well-being
o   Reduction of knee osteoarthritis, chronic pain, Parkinson's
o   Enhancement of reasoning and memory
o   Lessening of fibromyalgia pain, fatigue, depression

"A growing body of research is building a compelling case for tai chi as an adjunct to standard medical treatment for . . . many conditions commonly associated with age."   Peter M. Wayne, director Mind-Body
Research Program at Harvard Medical School

✳ Tonify: Set Life Rhythms ✳

• Eat at least one meal at the same time every day.
• Exercise or meditate at a regular time, at least once a week.
• Expose uncovered, closed eyes to the sun 10-15 minutes a day.
• Sleep in the dark; turn off nightlights, monitor lights, clocks.

Qi Gong   *Jogging without running*

The "Mother of all exercise" gives powerful benefits that other exercises do not, as it awakens one's "true nature," and helps develop your human potential. It may be practiced standing, sitting, lying down, or in your imagination (once you know how to do it). The deep rhythmic breathing, calm meditative state, and slow flowing movements are unsurpassed at:

o Reducing depressive symptoms
o Improving quality of life during radiation treatments
o Boosting circulation
o Generating healing electromagnetic fields
o Harmonizing life force energy (chi)

Orgasm

For abundant health, tonify the blood-rich pelvic organs. Regular orgasms – alone, partnered, with a vibrator – directly increase the tone of the bladder, the prostate, the uterus, and important core muscles that keep us upright. Seven orgasms a week is my goal; one a day or all at once, whatever works.

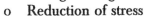

Benefits of regular orgasms include:

o Reduction of stress
o Improvement in immune functioning
o Improvement in cardiovascular health
o Increased lung function
o Fewer inner and outer signs of aging
o More happiness; less moodiness
o Relief from menstrual pain
o Greater compassion

Hellerwork/Structural Integration

This combination of interactive dialog, soft tissue work, and movement awareness replaces habitual ways of moving with more elegant, grounded ways, while nourishing and tonifying the whole person, no matter what age or level of ability.

"Hellerwork assumes that we are responsible for our bodies; that we have a choice; that life can be better from now on. Anyone can experience him/herself as a full manifestation of spirit in the simple acts of daily life."
Joseph Heller, creator of Hellerwork

Music, the Great Tonic

"Life is identical with sound." Sophie Drinker, *Music and Women*

"Sound spins a bridge between matter and spirit; our voices, riding on the breath, connect us into the current at the source of life." Molly Scott

Music, preferably live, preferably involving you, preferably rhythmic, nourishes abundant health and is an amazing tool for healing. Music is frequency, pitch, vibration, rhythm, emotion, sound, timbre, tune, inflection, phrasing, accent, and spirit.

"When the right vibrations are matched with the right intent, there is no limit to the healing power of sound." Jonathan Goldman, *Healing Sound*

You don't have to sing or play an instrument to benefit from music. Just hum. In many traditions, the original sound of creation is a hum. **How to Hum:** Say "uh-huh" and let the "huh" become "hum" by closing your lips. Put your hand lightly on the top of your head and hum there. Breathe and repeat. To go deeper, investigate humming different tones. Ha. Ho. Huh. Hee. Notice where each tone vibrates. When tones become words, you are chanting. Chants are musical affirmations.

Want company? There are a host of humming and chanting downloads, CDs, and YouTubes to sing along with. (See page 135.)

"One of the paradoxes of rhythm is that it has both the capacity to move your awareness out of your body into realms beyond time and space and to ground you firmly in the present moment." Michael Drake, *Shamanic Drum*

Listen to Music, Chant, Sing
Contemporary research shows music:
o   Lowers blood pressure and heart rate
o   Reduces the sensations of pain
o   Increases melatonin levels
o   Slows production of stress-related hormones, like cortisol
o   Increases endorphin levels
o   Oxygenates the cells
o   Increases lymphatic circulation
o   Boosts production of immune factors: immunoglobulin A, interleukin-1, and natural killer (NK) cells

Drum

"Drumming is the healthiest, most accessible and fastest way to reconnect with ourselves. "   Dr. Barry Bernstein, *Healthy Sounds*

One of the most enjoyable forms of tonic exercise is drumming. It is physical; it is mental; it connects us to the universal language of emotion. The drumbeat is the sacred heartbeat, the heartbeat of the mother.

Scientific studies find drumming:

o   Reduces stress
o   Induces deep relaxation
o   Encourages deeper sleep
o   Eases trauma, PTSD
o   Promotes self-esteem
o   Improves concentration
o   Lowers blood pressure
o   Accelerates physical healing
o   Eases chronic pain (increases endogenous opiates)
o   Releases emotional trauma
o   Helps reintegration of self after trauma
o   Induces synchronous brain activity
o   Can help retrain the brain after a stroke
o   Generates dynamic neuronal connections throughout the brain even after significant damage
o   Boosts the immune system
o   Increases well-being; even 15 minutes of drumming doubles alpha brain waves, creating euphoria and contentment
o   Is a valuable treatment for adrenal stress, fatigue, anxiety, asthma, arthritis, migraines, cancer, paralysis
o   Is especially helpful, calming, focusing, and healing for anyone dealing with Parkinson's, physical disabilities, autism, attention-deficient disorder, Alzheimer's, multiple sclerosis, Down syndrome, developmental disablities, emotional disturbances, mental illness, addiction, trauma, prison, and homelessness

"Group drumming tunes our biology, orchestrates our immunity, and enables healing to begin." Barry Bittman MD, Music & Wellness Institute

"Drumming integrates nonverbal information from the lower brain into the frontal cortex, producing feelings of insight, understanding, integration, certainty, conviction, and truth, which surpass ordinary understandings and tend to persist long after the experience, often providing foundational insights. . . ."   Michael Drake, shamanic drummer

In the drum circle, everyone gets to speak, everyone is heard, and everyone is an essential part of the whole – all at once.

Drumming and chanting are simple, effective ways to change your mind: from depressed to expansive, from confused to clear, from grieving to accepting, from estranged to connected.

"Our embodiment of stress becomes so habitual that we are no longer aware of it or, worse, perceive it as normal."   Mary Bond, *Body Mandala*

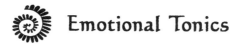 ## Emotional Tonics

Music is a tonic for the emotions. So are direct emotional expressions like laughing, crying, raging, feeling gratitude, and being with animals.

Laugh

Laughter is as important as diet and exercise in creating abundant health.

"Laughter appears to cause all the reciprocal, or opposite, effects of stress."   Dr. Lee Berk, medical researcher

Laugh out loud and notice your belly muscles, and you'll see why Norman Cousins calls laughing "internal jogging." We breathe more deeply when, and after, we laugh. People have cured themselves of horrible disorders, and helped themselves heal from terrible trauma, by watching funny videos and chortling, guffawing, and giggling for hours and hours, day after day.

"Laughter is the tonic, the relief, the surcease for pain." Charlie Chaplin

We begin to laugh as early as three months, and by our first birthday, we are laughing 300 times a day. We're 30 times more likely to laugh in the presence of other people than when alone.

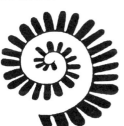

Laughing, the jest medicine, has been shown to:
o   Create closeness and strong, positive bonds
o   Lessen inflammation
o   Increase HDL cholesterol
o   Increase feel-good endorphins
o   Lower blood pressure
o   Lower cholesterol
o   Relieve depression
o   Aid digestion
o   Break the pain-spasm cycle
o   Increase vascular blood flow and oxygenation of the blood
o   Diminish physical and emotional pain
o   Improve tone of the muscles of the diaphragm, abdomen, lungs, face, legs, and back
o   Reduce stress hormones: cortisol, epinephrine and adrenaline
o   Increase the number, activity, and rate of response of gamma-interferon, natural killer (NK) cells, and T-cells
o   Increase immunoglobulin in saliva
o   Trigger production of dopamine and endorphins
o   Improve alertness, creativity, memory, concentration
o   Improve the quality of life for terminal patients
o   Offer relief to those undergoing painful treatments
o   Improve self-esteem and satisfaction with life

Laughter is the yin *to stress's* yang.

Patch Adams MD, of Gesundheit Institute, prescribes clowning around, being foolish, looking silly, playing at life, laughing, hugging, and enjoying yourself.

". . . work with these people [the Seneca nation of the Iroquois] . . . seemed more like a game where the thrill of it all kept the thought of fatigue away. Everyone laughed or sang and picked as fast as their two hands could touch the berries."   A. C. Parker (1834-1910)

Humor therapy is as effective as antipsychotic drugs in managing agitation in patients with dementia, with no adverse side effects.
Hearing laughter triggers brain areas that cause involuntary movement of facial muscles, making us smile.
Fifteen minutes of laughter burns about 40 calories.

"Laughter is the fireworks of the soul." Josh Billings, American humorist

Humor works fast. Less than a half-second after exposure to something funny, gamma brain waves – associated with deep states of meditation – move through the cerebral cortex.

"Laughter is intellectually creative in its very nature. Inherent in humor is the element of discovery. Humor teaches and reveals new understanding. Its creativity opens new realizations and opposes the dead-ending constricting and defeating results of violence and warfare. Mirth opens our minds. . . . Humor gives us a choice." William Fry MD, humor guru

Cry, Rage

Grief and anger are also emotional tonics, if not used indulgently. We may think of ourselves as weak if we cry, keen, wail, mourn, and weep, but it softens us where we are too hard. We may be frightened to express our rage, but it liberates us.

"All noises – even those which seem ugly – are valuable. . . . You will never eradicate the shadow in your voice, and thank heavens, for the shadow lies in the seat of the soul."   Paul Newham, *The Singing Cure*

ABCs of Anger
with thanks to Gordon Cook

A anger: At the moment, for a moment. "Infantile" rage.
The healthiest anger; gets things moving; very effective.

B anger: Before, something upset me. I brooded on it until it exploded. I have been collecting grievances; here they are.
Not so nice but not terrible either; clears the air.

C anger: As a child I swore no one would treat me like this and now you are going to get my childhood wrath.
Often unrelated to the present; confusing and scary.

D anger: Danger. Deflected and destructive. Since the object of my anger has too much power over me, I will be angry at you.
Unrelated to actual events; violent; a risk to health and life.

E anger: Existential anger. Fury at life as it is: chaotic, unfair.
Fairly useless, quickly becomes D anger at others and self.

Grieve and rage and your energy flows, pulsing with health. You are present in the moment, alive. Cope with it, stuff it, deflect it, put it off, and you automatically create stress and block the free flow of energy necessary for abundant health. You are living in the future; you are caught up in the past.

Emotional tonics, like all tonics, challenge us, helping us stay connected and emotionally flexible as we age. Laughing, crying, and raging – in fact, any strong emotion, including awe – is vigorous exercise for the brain, whether in real life or in imagination, as when reading or watching a movie. Not everyone has to rage out loud, but we all need to rage.

"The easiest way to discharge old pain by yourself is to find a movie that makes you cry. Don't fight it. Sink into it. Get a VCR, rent the movie, lock yourself in a room away from interruptions, and watch the part that makes you cry over and over."   Thomas Stone, *Cure by Crying*

My time with Elisabeth Kübler-Ross was deep learning in the power of rage. Person after person came forward to rage, scream and cry. Instead of denying their anger about the losses and injustices of life, Elisabeth encouraged them to work it out, to beat a phone book with a rubber radiator hose. Instead of turning their rage inward, where it would hurt them, they used their feelings, their voices, and their muscles to make space for abundant health.

"The inability that many of us have to grieve and weep properly for the dead is deeply linked with the inability to give praise for living." Martín Prechtel

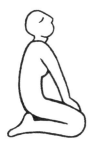

Be Grateful

"Gratitude is very powerful. If there were a drug that did [what it does], whoever patented it would be rich." Susan Peirce Thompson, cognitive scientist

Give me "An attitude of gratitude," said my Seneca Nation Wolf Clan Grandmother, Twylah Nitsch, She-Whose-Voice-Rides-the-Wind. When I was resentful, self-pitying, or ungrateful, I was sent to have a long talk with a big tree. "Gratitude is generated from within. It is not about what is happening outside," said the tree. "Being alive is awesome."

Benefits of gratitude practices – such as gratitude journaling, gratitude lists, thank-you notes, thoughts of gratitude before sleep, and inner bows for small services – include:

o   Lower lifetime risk of depression, anxiety, substance abuse
o   Higher HDL, lower LDL, lower C-reactive protein
o   Lower blood pressure; less plaque buildup in the arteries
o   Stabilization of heart rhythm
o   Less hemoglobin A1C, a key marker of glucose control
o   Better sleep for those in chronic pain
o   Deeper and more restorative sleep for all
o   More energy; better immune response, less inflammation
o   23 percent decrease in cortisol levels
o   41 percent less depression in at-risk patients after 6 months
o   Stronger impulse control, less addiction
o   Stronger interest in self-care

"Joy . . . [is] basic to flourishing. . . . [And] gratitude is the foundation for joy, since gratitude is the relationship-strengthening emotion, and joy is fundamentally and foundationally about connection."
Robert Emmons, PhD, gratitude scientist, *Thanks*

Pet Therapy

Animal relationships help us deal with grief, depression, anxiety, loneliness. Animals accept our feelings. Many a time I have leaned my head against the side of one of my goats and wept, feeling uncensored, loved, and accepted in a deep and simple way.

As little as fifteen minutes a day of animal therapy:
o   Relieves depression, anxiety, PTSD (by 87% in 6 weeks)
o   Focuses attention; improves learning, helps autistic people
o   Increases levels of oxytocin, the love hormone
o   Increases levels of serotonin; reduces cortisol levels
o   Lowers blood pressure; reduces risk of heart disease
o   Significantly lowers stress and anxiety of cancer patients undergoing radiation/chemotherapy treatments

The effects are strongest and longest with daily contact. Dog owners are more likely to survive major health challenges than others. If owning a pet is too much responsibility, consider volunteering at a local animal shelter. Or contact Pet Partners.

Light Tonic & Dark Tonic

"Light, the belt of heaven, holds together the circle of the universe." Plato

Exposure to light and periods of dark are important tonics. Too much or too little light or dark disturbs health in many ways. More or less light or dark can restore health. John Ott, pioneer light researcher, believed exposing the closed eyes to sunlight for five minutes a day was vital to abundant health.

Light is sometimes waves, other times, vibrating particles. We can see visible light, which has a spectral hue, or color temperature and a wavelength. We have evolved with, and are adapted to natural light wavelengths, which are warm and relaxing. Electric lights, electronic devices, and computer screens emit cool, blue or white hues that promote tension, alertness, and wakefulness.

More medical uses of colored light are on page 64.

o   Six weeks of 7000 lux bright light between noon-2:30 p.m. relieved symptoms of bipolar depression in 68 percent of individuals; no side effects. [*American Journal of Psychiatry*, Oct 2017]

o   Early morning bright light had no effect on bipolar depression, but did relieve seasonal affective disorder (SAD).

o   Israeli women in neighborhoods with outside artificial lights bright enough to read by at night had a 73 percent higher risk of developing breast cancer. [*Chronobiology International*, Jan 2008]

Visible Light Visualization

Imagine sunlight striking a prism over your head and seven waves of color streaming out. The shortest, fastest wave – violet – is absorbed into your crown. Your forehead absorbs indigo; your throat takes in blue; your heart receives green; your solar plexus drinks in yellow; the belly is drenched with orange. The longest, slowest wave – red – fills the root chakra.

Unabsorbed colors tinge the aura, coloring how we see and act in the world. Clear sight, clear speech, clear thought, and clear action are the result of absorbing the entire spectrum of colors.

Natural light alternating with natural dark sets our circadian rhythms for health. Getting natural light is not difficult: Go outside, sit or lie down, and let the sun fall on your closed eyes. Indoors, use full-spectrum or Blues Buster bulbs.

Getting natural dark is more difficult.

"... we are all exposed to electric light at night, whereas before electricity ... people got twelve hours of dark whether they were asleep or not."
Susan Golden, Center for Research on Biological Clocks

Melatonin production requires complete darkness.

Exposure to light at night (light pollution) is a problem in both the city and the country. It suppresses production of melatonin, leading to chronic health and sleep problems.

Melatonin is a brain chemical best known for inducing sleep. It also strengthens immune function, suppresses tumor growth, lowers cholesterol, acts as a powerful antioxidant, and nourishes hormonal wellness by its beneficial impact on the functioning of the thyroid, pancreas, ovaries, testes and adrenals. As always, your own melatonin is far superior to any pill.

Effects of light pollution include increased risk of:
o Depression   o Breast cancer
o Sleep disorders   o Obesity
o Insomnia   o Diabetes
o Cardiac problems
o Cancers of the endometrium, ovaries, prostate, colon, skin, and non-Hodgkins lymphoma

"Researchers estimate that up to 30% of breast cancers are secondary to light at night suppressing circadian rhythm – placing it on the same level of severity as the effects of tobacco smoke on lung cancer."   Mario Motta MD

An investment in a sleep mask and black-out curtains is an investment in abundant health. And, please, change night lights for motion sensor lights, which go on only when needed.

There is black light and clear light, but there is no white light.

Herbal Tonics, Adaptogens

"Herbal tonics are to the cells what physical fitness is to the body."
Neva Jensen, *Herbal Health Guide*

An herbal tonic is an herb or mixture of herbs taken daily for long periods of time to gently improve the functioning of a specific organ, a bodily system or tissue, or the brain. Herbal tonics that normalize functioning and help us resist the effects of stress are called *alteratives* and *adaptogens*.

Tonic herbs tonify; they do not cleanse. The claim that tonic herbs detoxify the liver, the kidneys, or the blood, is inaccurate.

Herbal tonics nourish and strengthen. They don't "stop working" after a while. And they are not stimulants.

✳ Herbal Tonics Build

- Strong circulation of all fluids (blood, lymph, mucus)
- A relaxed, powerful liver
- An alert, effective immune system
- Clear, connected thought processes
- Sensitivity to all stimuli
- Emotional depth
- Digestive ease
- Endurance and hope
- Sexual responsiveness

Tonic herbs contain constituents that astringe cellular membranes, causing them to tighten, then relax, tighten, then relax, just as exercise tightens and relaxes the muscles. This increases blood flow to the cells, just as exercise increases blood flow to the muscles. When more nutrients are available to the cells and muscles, overall health improves.

Both stimulants and tonics increase functioning, but their effects are different. Better functioning from tonification is maintained without the tonic, while increased functioning from stimulation disappears when the stimulant is withdrawn.

Regular rhythmic dosing of about 100 doses a year increases tonifying effects. Daily for two months on and two off is traditional. But daily every other week works just as well.

It is the overall length of time – hopefully years or decades – that one uses an herbal tonic that counts, as the effects are cumulative. Small to moderate doses, taken consistently, are best.

Types of Tonic Herbs

Tonic herbs act slowly. They are used as teas, infusions, or tinctures. Most tonic herbs are safe to take with drugs.

Food tonics such as blueberries, garlic, nettle, shiitake, seaweed, and oats supply high-quality nutrients to build strong immunity, moderate blood sugar swings, and charge every cell with antioxidants. Eat them often and in quantity.

Soothing tonics like marshmallow, fenugreek, linden, and astragalus soothe irritated tissues, calm agitated nerves, and bring ease to digestion and respiration. Use them daily, as desired.

Astringent tonics like barberry, oak bark, Oregon grape, and witch hazel are used externally, or in small amounts internally, to tighten varicose veins, hemorrhoids, prolapses, bladder problems, edema, and sinuses. Use as needed, not daily.

Bitter tonics are the daily drink of most people on this planet: coffee, black and green tea, maté, and chocolate. They aid digestion, tone up the liver and gall bladder, and influence healthy hormones. Best taken before or after meals, daily or as desired.

Adaptogens

Adaptogens are herbs that don't have specific actions on specific organs or problems. They are generalists. Adaptogens have a normalizing, stress-proofing influence on our whole being.

Primary Adaptogens

- o American ginseng root
- o Amla berries
- o Ashwagandha root
- o Astragalus root
- o Codonopsis/dang shen root
- o Cordyceps
- o Goji berry
- o Eleuthero/Siberian ginseng
- o Fo ti/He shou wu
- o Jiaogulan
- o Panax ginseng root
- o Reishi
- o Rhodiola root
- o Schisandra berry
- o Shiitake
- o Stinging nettle
- o Tulsi/Holy basil

Adaptogens aid longevity and help ameliorate the effects of aging. They increase our resilience and help us resist disease.

Adaptogens improve our ability to adapt to new stresses and different stressors. Adaptogens are frequently anti-inflammatory and antioxidant.

Studies find consistent use of adaptogens:

o   Increases physical and mental stamina/performance
o   Enhances healthy longevity
o   Diminishes inflammatory responses
o   Nourishes immune functioning
o   Reduces likelihood of all infections, colds, flu
o   Decreases incidence of cancer
o   Decreases risk of chemically-induced cancer
o   Reduces harm from medical and environmental radiation
o   Reduces side effects, increases effectiveness of chemotherapy
o   Alleviates adverse effects of long-term stress
o   Improves adrenal functioning; lowers cortisol levels
o   Increases general sense of well-being
o   Decreases anxiety and depression
o   Improves digestion and deepens sleep
o   Improves endocrine and neuroendocrine functioning

If you are under fifty and eat whole, well-cooked foods, drink nourishing herbal infusions daily, are physically and socially active, and get enough sleep, you will only need adaptogenic herbs in times of extreme stress, trauma, and transition.

If you are older than fifty, or don't eat well, don't drink nourishing herbal infusions at least four times a week, and spend too much time sitting in front of screens, then you'll probably benefit from daily use of adaptogenic herbs.

Moxibustion

The burning of moxa (*Artemisia chinensis*) is an ancient tonifying technique from China. Moxibustion is called the mother of acupuncture. In direct moxibustion, moxa is burned directly on the point to be activated. Indirect moxibustion, which is off the body, is my preference: Light a moxa stick and hold it near the point/ tsubo to be treated. Move the stick in spirals until strong heat is felt, then stop. Can be repeated daily to tonify inner organs.

Lifestyle Green Allies

for	to Nourish	to Tonify	to Soothe
Adrenals	nettle	codonopsis	relaxation
Bladder	**yogurt**	**cranberry**	**cornsilk**
Bones	comfrey leaf	exercise	boneset
Brain	**coffee, tea**	**sage, ginkgo**	**chocolate**
Circulation	nettle	hawthorn	hot bath
Digestion	**slippery elm**	**dandelion**	**mint**
Eyes	lycopene	amla	Bates*
Fertility	**red clover**	**raspberry**	**wld carrot seed**
Gall bladder	dandelion	yellow dock	gentian
Gums	**seaweed**	**yarrow**	**myrrh**
Hair	seaweed	nettle	burdock oil
Hearing	**oatstraw**	**yarrow**	**skullcap**
Heart	motherwort	hawthorn	passionflower
Immune system	**mushrooms**	**echinacea**	**usnea**
Intestines /colon	slippery elm	comfrey leaf	yogurt
Joints	**comfrey lf**	**exercise**	**CBD salve**
Kidneys	nettle	corn silk	asparagus
Liver	**dandelion**	**seaweed**	**burdock**
Lungs	mullein leaf	ground ivy	wild cherry
Lymphatics	**chickweed**	**cleavers**	**poke (stim)**
Mucus surfaces	comfrey leaf	linden flowr	marshmallow
Nerves	**oatstraw**	**St. J's wort**	**valerian rt**
Ovaries/testes	red clover	oatstraw	vitex berry
Pancreas	**dandelion**	**elecampane**	---
Pineal	violet	---	angelica
Pituitary	**vitex**	**ginkgo**	**cronewort**
Prostate	oatstraw	saw palmetto	seaweed
Skin	**seaweed**	**burdock rt**	**heat**
Stomach	yogurt	dandelion	potato
Teeth	**horsetail**	**yarrow**	**birch**
Thyroid	seaweed	chickweed	iodine
Uterus	**red clover**	**raspberry lf**	**life root**
Veins	nettle	witch hazel	horsechestnut

© 2020 Susun S. Weed

* Bates Method of Eyesight Improvement

Step 3: Lifestyle Medicine References and Resources

Nourish

Agriculture Handbook Book #456: Nutritional Value of Foods in Common Units. Dover reprint, 1986. Original by USDA, 1975.

Bergner, Paul. *The Healing Power of Minerals.* Prima Pub, 1997.

Bonvie, Linda. *Badditives: Harmful Food Additives.* Skyhorse, 2017.

Caldecott, Todd. *Food As Medicine.* Self-published, 2012.

Dunne, Lavon. *Nutrition Almanac, 3rd Edition.* McGraw Hill, 1990.

Fallon, Sally. *Nourishing Traditions Cookbook.* New Trends, 2001.

———. *Nourishing Broth.* Grand Central, 2014.

Gittleman, Ann Louise. *Beyond Pritikin.* Bantam, 1988.

Johnson, Cait. *Cooking Like A Goddess.* Healing Arts Press, 1997.

Keith, Lierre. *The Vegetarian Myth.* Flashpoint, 2009.

Margen, S. MD. *Wellness Encyclopedia of Food/Nutrition.* Rebus, 1992.

Katz, Sandor. *Wild Fermentation.* Chelsea Green, 2003.

Morris, Risa. *Herbal Feast.* Keats, 1998.

Ornish, Dean MD. *Love and Survival.* HarperCollins, 1999.

Papas, Andreas. *The Vitamin E Factor.* Harper Perennial, 1998.

Pedersen, Mark. *Nutritional Herbology.* Pedersen Press, 1996.

Pollan, Michael. *The Omnivore's Dilemma.* Penguin Press, 2006.

———. *Food Rules: An Eater's Manual.* Penguin Press, 2009.

———. *Cooked: A Natural History of Transformation.* Penguin Press. 2013

Price, Weston. *Nutrition and Physical Degeneration.* Keats Pub, 1945.

Salatin, Joel. *Holy Cows and Hog Heaven: The Food Buyer's Guide to Farm Friendly Food.* Polyface, 2004.

Scott, Anne. *Serving Fire: Rhythms of the Hearth.* Celestial Arts, 1994.

Shanahan, Catherine MD. *Deep Nutrition.* Flatiron, 2016.

Sokolov, Raymond. *Why We Eat What We Eat.* Summit, 1991.

Watson, Karol MD. "Multivitamins to Reduce Cardiovascular Mortality: Still No Evidence." *NEJM.* July 2018.

Weatherford, Jack. *Indian Givers.* Fawcett Columbine, 1988.

Yeager, Selene. *New Foods for Healing.* Prevention, 1998.

Youmell and Morrill. *Weaving Healing Wisdom.* Lexingford, 2017.

Ziegler, Ekhard & L. J. Filer. *Present Knowledge in Nutrition, 7th Edition.* International Life Science Press, 1996.

"Ultra-Processed Foods Linked to Cancer." *The BMJ*. Feb 2018.
* https://dashdiet.org
* www.nutritionletter.tufts.edu/
* www.westonprice.org
* https://cspinet.org/nutrition-action-healthletter
* www.environmentalnutrition.com/

Wild Food

Bullman, S. et al. "Bacteria Might Be a Cause of Colon Cancer." *Science.* 15 Dec 2017.

Cocannouer, Joseph. *Weeds, Guardians of the Soil.* The Devin-Adair Company. 1980. (Original publication 1950.)

Gittelman, Ann Louise. *"Beyond Probiotics: The missing link in your immune system* [soil bacteria]." Keats, 1998.

Falconi, Dina. *Foraging and Feasting.* Botanical Arts Press, 2013.

Phillips, Roger. *Wild Foods.* Little Brown & Co., 1986.

Robinson, Jo. *Eating on the Wild Side.* Little Brown & Co. 2013.

* www.nytimes.com/2016/12/29/well/eat/a-gut-makeover-for-the-new-year.html
* www.nature.com/articles/s41575-018-0061-2
* http://response.jwatch.org/*Probiotic therapy with* Bifidobacterium *species prevented or ameliorated autoimmune colitis in mouse model.*

Yogurt

"Yogurt for Heart Health." *Bottom Line Health.* July 2018.

"Yogurt May Reduce Type 2 Diabetes." *Harvard Gazette.* Dec 2014.

Don't Buy It: Soy Products

Soy products, with the exception of miso and tamari, contain phytates and tripsin inhibitors which prevent utilization of key minerals, such as calcium and zinc, and of vitamins, especially vitamin B_{12} – which is already notably low in many diets. Other components disturb thyroid functioning. Soy powders and isoflavones added to food are manufactured by DuPont Chemical.

I use miso and tamari every day, tofu and tempeh rarely, and soy beverages, soy cheese, soy burgers, and soy dogs, never.

- www.aboutyogurt.com/index.asp?bid=21
- http://ajcn.nutrition.org/content/71/4/861.full
- https://translational-medicine.biomedcentral.com/articles/10.1186/s12967-018-1410-1

Coffee & Tea
- www.medicalnewstoday.com/articles/270202.php
- www.ncbi.nlm.nih.gov/pubmed/23465359
- www.healthline.com/nutrition/top-13-evidence-based-health-benefits-of-coffee
- www.ncbi.nlm.nih.gov/pubmed/16507475
- www.ncbi.nlm.nih.gov/pmc/articles/PMC4055352/

Blue-Green Algae
Alternative Medicine, 2nd ed. Institiute for Natural Resources, 1998.
Blue Green Algae Alert. *American Health*. October1996.
"Super Blue Green Not So Super." *Nutrition Action.* July/Aug1998.
"Why Florida's Cormorants Looked Drunk." *ScienceNews.* Nov 1998.
Ruscigno, Matt. "Is chlorella beneficial?" *Environ. Nutr.* Feb 2014.
Stainbrook Karen. "My Poor Little Lake." *NYS Conservationist.* April 2014.

"I went from never thinking about where my food came from to thinking about it all the time." Michael Pollan

Don't Buy It: Blue-Green Algae

Analysis of blue-green algae (spirulina/chlorella) finds trivial amounts of vitamins, minerals, amino acids. The highest dose has fewer vitamins than half a cup of broccoli. Its vitamin B_{12} cannot be absorbed by humans. A 2013 study found blue-green algae to have minimal effect on the elimination of stored chemicals/toxins.

The euphoria some people experience after ingestion is due to algal nerve poisons, chemically related to, but more dangerous than, cocaine. In some algae it is stronger than cyanide. Blue-green algae is renowned for killing pets and wildlife. Exposure causes negative health effects including allergic reactions. Spirulina grows most abundantly in water contaminated with sewage and chemicals. Pricey pond scum. Drink nourishing herbal infusions instead.

Chocolate
Experimental Biology, annual meeting, April 2018.
- www.ncbi.nlm.nih.gov/pubmed/?term=26026398
- www.medicalnewstoday.com/articles/270272.php

Seaweed
American Journal of Nutrition. 139: 1–6
Cerier, Leslie. *Sea Vegetable Celebration.* Book Pub. Co., 2001.
Lewallen, Eleanor & John. *Sea Vegetable Gourmet Cookbook.* Mendocino Sea Veg Co, 1996.
- www.ncbi.nlm.nih.gov/pubmed/24697280
- www.drugs.com/npp/seaweed.html
- www.berkeley.edu/news/media/releases/2005/02/02_kelp.shtml

Mushrooms
- www.cancer.gov/about-cancer/treatment/cam/hp/mushrooms-pdq
- http://foodforbreastcancer.com/foods/mushrooms
- www.realmushrooms.com
- www.hostdefense.com

Mushrooms inhibit aromatase, needed for estrogen production. Their lectins recognize cancer cells and prevent them from dividing.

Tomato
- www.townsendletter.com/Jan2006/tomato0106.htm
- www.eurekalert.org/pub_releases/2001-08/acs-spn081401.php
- https://academic.oup.com/jnci/article/94/5/391/2520089

Alcohol
Schwarzinger, Michael MD. "Dementia and Alcohol." *Bottom Line Health.* May 2018.
Lancet 2018. doi:10.1016/SO140-6736(18)31310-2

"Alcohol is a colossal global health issue." The Lancet, 2018

One-third of depressed people in the SMILES study who ate more whole grains and less refined grains, more vegetables and less fried food, more nuts and fish and less processed meat, more olive oil and fewer sugary drinks, and less alcohol for 12 weeks "achieved depression remission."
[*BMC Medicine,* Jan 2017]

Don't Buy It: Sugar

"There is growing evidence that sugar leads to cravings and withdrawal [and elevates dopamine], which are the hallmarks of addictive disorders. You can see it on an MRI." Aura Schmidt, UCSF

o Sugar may be addictive.
o Sugar is worse for your heart than saturated fat or salt.
o And as bad for your liver as alcohol.
o It raises blood pressure and cholesterol, even in children.
o A soft drink a day, especially if artificially sweetened, triples the 10-year risk of a stroke.
o A soft drink a day shortens lifespan as much as a pack a day.
o In adults, especially women, sugar decreases protective HDL.
o Sugar interferes with sound sleep.
o Consumption is strongly linked to Alzheimer's.
o It increases the risk of depression and auto-immune diseases.
o It vastly increases the risk of being obese.
o It causes cavities, inflames the gums, increases tooth loss.
o Cancer cells love it, especially squamous cell carcinomas.
o 75 percent of packaged foods contain added sugars.
o Fruit juice is extremely high in sugar, even if it's natural.
o The average American eats 65 pounds of sugar a year.
o Sugar is sucrose, fructose, corn syrup, maltose, dextrose, amazake, cane juice, fruit juice concentrate.
o Sucralose, saccharin, and aspartame are worse for health.
o Honey, maple syrup, sorghum, agave syrup are natural, but they are still sugars.

Sugar

Walvin, James. *Sugar. The World Corrupted: From Slavery to Obesity.* Pegasus, 2018
"25 Ways Sugar is Making You Sick." *Reader's Digest.* April 2018.
"The Scoop: Sugar and Cancer." *Environmental Nutrition.* June 2018.
"Artificially Sweetened Beverages. . . ." *Stroke.* 20 April 2017.

The aim is to set free the divine light which is mysteriously present and shining in each one of us.

Exercise/Move It!
"Activity Increases Longevity." *J of Am Geriatrics Society*. Nov 2017.
Bourman, Sherry. *Walk Yourself Well*. Hyperion, 1999.
Bond, Mary. *The New Rules of Posture*. Healing Arts Press, 2007.
Buchanan, Patricia PhD. "Feldenkrais Method."*Bottom Line*, 2018.
Chia, Mantak. *Multi-Orgasmic Woman*. Rodale, 2006.
———. *Healing Love: Cultivating Female Sexual Energy*. Destiny, 2005.
Furchgott, Roy. "One Workout You Must Do." *AARP*. Nov 2018.
Graves, Ginny. "Working Out Saved My Life." *Health*. Nov 2017.
Heller, Joseph. *BodyWise*. Tarcher, 1991.
Knaster, Mirka. *Discovering the Body's Wisdom*. Bantam, 1996.
"Lifestyle Interventions Cut Need for Antihypertensives Within 4 Months." www.abstractsonline.com. Sept 2018.
"Qi Gong Stimulates Healing Energy." *Healthy Years*. April 2018.
"Tai chi helps Parkinson's patients." *Harvard Health*. April 2012.
Valdez, Natasha Janina. *Vitamin O (Orgasms)*. Skyhorse, 2015.
Wang, Chenchen MD. "Tai chi for fibromyalgia." *Tufts*, June 2018.
Wayne, Peter PhD. *The Harvard Medical School Guide to Tai Chi*. Harvard Health/Shambhala, 2013.
"Yoga Reduces Stress." *Psychoneuroendocrinology*. Dec 2017.
- www.thewalkingsite.com
- www.nufoot.com
- www.trager.com
- www.ncbi.nlm.nih.gov/pmc/articles/PMC3023168/
- www.verywell.com/can-yoga-help-my-eating-disorder-4113359
- www.verywell.com/top-health-benefits-of-yoga-3566733
- www.breema.com
- www.taichihealth.com
- www.treeoflifetaichi.com
- https://nccih.nih.gov/health/taichi/introduction.htm#use
- https://qigong.com/home
- www.ncbi.nlm.nih.gov/pmc/articles/PMC3085832/
- www.hellerwork.com
- http://stretchcoach.com/articles/pnf-stretching/
- www.functionalmovement.com
- https://jamanetwork.com/journals/jamainternalmedicine/fullarticle/225987
- www.apa.org/monitor/2011/04/orgasm.aspx
- www.liveabout.com/benefits-of-masturbation-2982830

"The effects of music on exercise are so profound that it becomes a type of legal performance-enhancing drug." Costas Karageorghis PhD

Music

Campbell, Don. *Healing Yourself with Your Own Voice.* Sounds True Audio, 2005.

Crouch, Michelle. "13 Incredible Ways Music Benefits You." *Reader's Digest.* June 2018.

Drinker, Sophie. *Music and Women.* Zenger, 1948, 1977.

Gardner, Kay. *Sounding the Inner Landscape: Music as Medicine.* Element Books, 1997 (1990)

Gass, Robert. *Chanting: Spirit in Sound.* Broadway Books, 1999.

Goldman, J. *Vocal Toning the Chakras,* Sounds True Audio, 2005.

———. *The Humming Effect.* Healing Arts Press, 2018.

Hoffman, Janalea. *Rhythmic Medicine: Music with a Purpose.* 1999.

Oliveros, Pauline. *Sonic Meditations.* Smith Publications, 1970.

Patel, Aniruddh. *Music and the Brain.* Great Courses, 2015.

Sacks, Oliver MD. *Musicophilia: Tales of Music and the Brain.* Vintage, 2008.

Shenandoah, Joanne. *Matriarch: Iroquois Women's Songs.* Silver Waves Records, 1997.

Thiel, Lisa. *Journey to the Goddess,* 1994; *Mother of Compassion,* 2002.

- www.healingsounds.com/the-healing-power-of-cosmic-hum/
- www.healthysound.com/
- www.imnf.org [Institute for Music and Neurological Function]
- www.MollyScott.com *Creative Resonance Institute*
- www.rhythmicmedicine.com
- www.scientificamerican.com/article/psychology-workout-music/
- www.soundstrue.com [sound healing collection]

"I have seen deeply demented patients weep or shiver as they listen to music they have never heard before, and I think . . . there is still a self to be called upon even if music, and only music, can do the calling."
Oliver Sacks

Drumming

- https://project-resiliency.org/resiliency/the-benefits-of-drumming/
- www.healingdrummer.com/
- www.thoughtco.com/drum-therapy-1729574
- www.rootstorhythm.com/health.html

Emotional Tonics
Briar, Jeffery. *Laughter Exercises for Health.* Creative Arts Press, 2011.
Chemaly, Soraya. *Rage Becomes Her.* Atria, 2019.
Childre, Doc and Deborah Rozman. *Overcoming Emotional Chaos.* Jodere, 2002.
Cooper, Brittney. *Eloquent Rage.* St. Martin's, 2019.
Kataria, Madan. *Laughter Yoga.* Penguin Press, 2012.
Levine, Stephen and Ondrea. *Embracing the Beloved: Relationship as a Path of Awakening.* Doubleday, 1995.
Lyle, Lesley. *Laugh Your Way to Happiness.* Watkins, 2014.
Plant, Judith (ed). *Healing the Wounds.* New Society, 1989.
Prechtel, Martín. *The Smell of Rain on Dust: Grief and Praise.* North Atlantic Books, 2015.
Provine, Dr. Robert. *Curious Behavior: Yawning, Laughing, Hiccupping, and Beyond.* Belknap, 2012.
Stone, Thomas. *Cure by Crying.* Cure by Crying, Inc., 1995.
Cornell, Ann. *The Power of Focusing.* New Harbinger Press, 1996.
- www.care2.com/greenliving/8-health-benefits-of-laughter.html
- www.everydayhealth.com/womens-health/health-benefits-of-laughter.aspx
- http://humor.ch/inernsthaft/fry2.htm
- www.humorproject.com/
- https://laughteryoga.org
- www.patchadams.org
- https://time.com/5026174/health-benefits-of-gratitude/

"It may be that to laugh in the face of death is courageous, but to laugh in the face of life is absolutely heroic."   Rabbi Moshe Waldoks

Animals
"The Healing Power of Animals." *UCLA Healthy Years.* June 2015.
Oaklander, Mandy. "The science of pet therapy." *Time.* 17 April 2017.
Wolt, Hannah. "The Pet Prescription." *Prevention.* Feb 2013.

Light & Dark
Chepesiuk, Ron. "Missing the Dark: Health Effects of Light Pollution." *Environmental Health Perspectives,* Jan 2009.
Ott, John. *Health and Light.* Pocket Books, 1973.

Don't Buy It: Alcohol

Alcohol has long been believed to be health-promoting. Christened *aqua vita*, the water of life, alcohol is the basis of herbal tinctures, and a social lubricant in many cultures. But is it healthy?

o   Chronic heavy drinking (more than 3 drinks a day for women; more than 4 a day for men) is responsible for 57 percent of early-onset dementia, even if the heavy drinking ceases.

o   Drinking 1-2 drinks four or more times weekly increases the risk of premature death by 20 percent.

o   Moderate alcohol consumption does reduce risk of heart-related problems, but the increases in cancer and mortality risk outweigh that benefit.

o   The amount of alcohol in a dose of **herbal tincture** is less than a tenth of an ounce. At this level it does not interact with opioid medicine. Alcoholics and Muslims can safely use tinctures.

Wurtman, R. J. "Effects of Light on the Human Body." *Scientific American*, July 1975.
• www.ncbi.nlm.nih.gov/pmc/articles/PMC2627884/

Adaptogens
Winston, David. *Adaptogens*. Healing Arts Press, 2007.
Yance, Donny. *Adaptogens in Medical Herbalism*. Healing Arts, 2013.

The wise woman does not steal inevitable and useful pain. The wise woman sees problems as allies of wholeness. The wise woman nourishes the flow, the fluidity, the clarity. The wise woman adds pieces back to the puzzle, enhancing wholeness.

"Difficult, despised areas of life, like addiction and depression, are not just problems to be resolved. They actually point to treasure. They are signposts, indicators that something valuable and positive is hidden away, waiting to return to one's wholeness."
Ann Weiser Cornell, *The Power of Focusing*

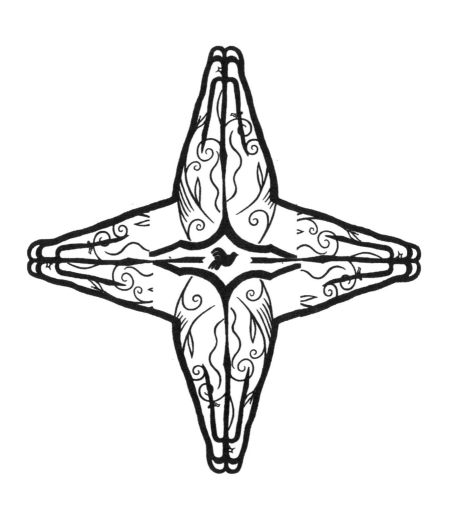

The Great Divide 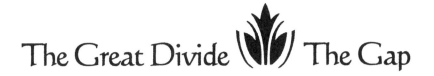 The Gap

Welcome to the Gap. We stop. We reflect on the Medicines that build health: Serenity, Story, Energy, and Lifestyle Medicines. We look ahead, wondering about the Medicines that save lives: Alternative, Pharmaceutical, and Deep Medicines.

A gap is a space. The Gap is the space between the first four Medicines, the ones that keep us abundantly well, and the last three Medicines, the ones that protect us from death. We pause.

A gap divides things. The Great Divide separates the Seven Medicines into a safe half and a dangerous half. It separates the Medicines that build health from those that erode health.

The first four Medicines improve health with little or no harm. They are true preventative medicines. The last three Medicines injure health, sometimes to the point of disability or death, while aiming to preserve or lengthen life.

The Gap alerts us and warns us. It reminds us that mortal danger lies on the far side where diagnostic scans and screening tests – posing as preventative medicine – can ruin your health. In pursuit of staying alive, we resort to drugs, knives, radiation, chemicals. Trying to stave off death, we are severed, disconnected, dislocated, scattered.

The first four medicines become complementary, integrated medicine on the far side. On their own they build health. With dangerous medicines, they are our salve, from *salvus* – Latin for "safe and healthy" – our wholeness, *sarva* – Sanskrit for "entire."

The last three Medicines can resolve distress, fight disease, restore and normalize function, ease pain, counter cancer, and sometimes enable miracles; nonetheless, they damage our health. Adding serenity, story, energy, substance, and resiliency – the gifts of the first four Medicines – to Alternative, Pharmaceutical, and Deep Medicines promotes abundant health and wholeness.

The Gap is a natural barrier. It slows us down, gives us time to question what we are doing. The Great Divide gives us an overview, a place to look back as well as forward. Here we can rest, review what we have done, and prepare for what lies ahead.

Do I have a Serenity Medicine practice? Is fear dictating my choices? *Before crossing the Great Divide, I check to see that I am rooted and centered and in touch with All that I am.*

Do the stories I tell myself – and the stories I hear from others – promote wholeness and expansion? Am I limiting myself and shutting down? *I have free will to choose. I can change my mind. I don't have to believe everything I think or what others believe.*

Am I agreeing to and relying solely on high-tech diagnosis? Have I investigated other ways of knowing? *What are my dreams telling me? What emotions am I afraid to talk about? What do I sense?*

Am I empowering myself and getting the care I want? Am I doing what I am told unquestioningly? *I can be my own expert. Patience is a virtue only when nothing else can be done.*

Am I using Mind Medicine against myself by imagining the worst? Or am I creating abundant health with every thought, and engaging the energy of health/wholeness/holiness with every breath? *I am a beloved child of the universe. I am a unique manifestation of ancient atoms and timeless energies.*

How can Lifestyle Medicine enrich me? What small change will bring more abundant health? More family time? More walking? More beans? More cooked greens? More nourishing herbal infusions? *Even the best diet can get a little better. Get more from your exercise by doing less – more often. Stretch . . . your muscles, your mind, your imagination, your boundaries, your heart.*

Do I need to cross the Gap? How can I get the most benefit from the last three Medicines? How can I protect myself from the inherent harms of these Medicines? *Set time limits. Set a return date. Do not linger on the far side of the Gap. Be proactive. Take a friend.*

High on the Great Divide, the winds swirl and whirl. Dust devils and tornados of pain, anxiety, stress, depression, poverty, loneliness, and low self-esteem can sweep us over the Gap. Spiraling vortexes of mindfulness, gratitude, relationships, non-dual thinking, and self-worth keep us abundantly well and help us integrate healthy behavior/thoughts if we must make a perilous journey to the far side.

As a means of maintaining health, and as preventative care, medicines on the far side generally do more harm than good. Though it is difficult to believe, every remedy on the far side of the gap injures us in some way – less if use is infrequent, more with larger doses and repeated or habitual use.

Ordinary health care for most Americans is strictly on the far side of the gap: Pharmaceutical and Deep Medicine, with a little Complementary/Alternative Medicine thrown in, is all there is.

With a few exceptions, practitioners of Alternative, Pharmaceutical, and Deep Medicines are not focused on your health. They are solving a problem, keeping you alive, and, often, making sure they are not sued.

When brought to the far side of the gap, the first four Medicines become complementary, integrated medicines.

The two sides of the divide work well together. Not only do the first four Medicines create a healthy being who is less likely to suffer side effects from drugs, dyes, radiation, anesthesia, surgery, and infections, they are superb at moderating and countering the damage from far side Medicines.

A cartoon in the *New Yorker* shows a glowing, smiling, calm patient. "Are you messing around with Alternative Medicine?" the doctor asks.

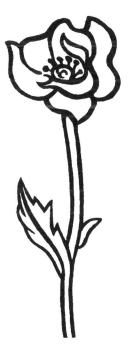

Yes. Yes, we are. Medical studies attest to the effectiveness of the first four Medicines for maintaining abundant health. Serenity Medicine, Story Medicine, Energy Medicine and Lifestyle Medicine are especially effective in restoring and maintaining healthy blood pressure, cardiovascular tone, mood, blood sugar, muscular and mental strength, flexibility, and concentration.

The complementary, integrated medicine revolution has helped a growing number of health professionals lay aside their beliefs that Mind Medicine and Alternative Medicine are nothing more than false hope and misguided good intentions. When healers, doctors, and patients come together with integrated medicine, we are all much nearer to being abundantly well.

Standardized Herbs?

For centuries herbalists, alchemists, and scientists have searched for active ingredients in plants. Active ingredients – such as alkaloids, glycosides, volatile oils, and lectins – can be concentrated into drugs that are lethal at a high enough dose.

The remedies of the near side have few or no active ingredients. They feed wholeness, foster flexibility, and restore energetic connections. They are safe; they may work slowly; they make deep change. The amount used is variable and non-critical as there are few side effects even with repeated use and large doses.

The remedies of the far side have active ingredients. Active ingredients stimulate, sedate, poison, and kill. They create strong, immediate, measurable physical reactions. They combat diseases and problems, promptly and vigorously. They *always* have detrimental side effects.

Metabolizing and excreting active ingredients can damage the kidneys, liver, heart, and the environment. Some active constituents in plants and drugs can cause genetic mutations that lead to cancer.

Due to the great likelihood of harm, remedies from the far side of the Gap need to be precisely measurable and replicable. Doses must be specific and overdoses are feared.

Since the amount of active ingredient in any given plant varies – sometimes by a lot, due to soil fertility, weather, harvesting conditions, and method of preparation – those used to drugs believe that herbal safety requires standardization, so each dose is the same.

But standardizing herbs is like standardizing wine. The sanitized, standardized product lacks personality, individuality, wholeness. Ideally each remedy *is* slightly different, allowing the normal variations in plant compounds work synergistically with our bodies to promote individual, not standardized, health.

"Clinical guidelines are meant to standardize medical care in ways that improve quality and reduce risks. But the idea of standardized medicine is problematic. . . . Guidelines can have a profound leveling effect. . . . What's more, guidelines largely represent the beliefs and opinions of their expert authors, who have to compromise to reach a consensus. . . . They are intended to help you and your health care provider make decisions, not to dictate them."   John Swartzberg MD, UC Berkeley

Health/wholeness/holiness – in herbs, bodies, and spirits – is complex, unique, and exquisitely variable. Standardization can make an herbal remedy *more* druglike, more dangerous, and more likely to have side effects and interactions with other remedies.

Variation is a hallmark of health.

Grandmother Growth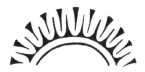

"Now isn't this view worth that climb?" beams the wise woman. She hums a melody you can't quite recall. She is hardly out of breath, while you find it hard to catch yours: from the climb, from the elevation, and from the views.

"We are on the highest ridge of these mountains," she continues, with a glowing smile as you plop down on the rocky ledge.

The wind picks up. It lifts her hair and blows it back from her high forehead. The leaves in the trees rustle as though they were agreeing with her. In the distance water gurgles and splashes.

"Close your eyes and feel the earth energy pathways, the ley lines, that meet here. Let the manna, the nourishment, of this special spot seep into you and touch you."

After a timeless time, she arises, takes your hand, and together you walk out onto a precipitous point. Hawks soar beneath you. In every direction, wave on wave of mountain and hill, valley and chasm, river, stone, and tree spread around you.

She turns you toward the east.

"Soften your focus. Magnify your awareness. Feel the energies. The wind carries memories of the Medicines we have visited. Imagine Serenity Medicines bubbling up and flowing down the mountain to the great Sea-of-Well-Being. Envision Story Medicines dancing and tumbling through the hills. Sense Mind Medicines and faith rippling and murmuring along the way. Enjoy the laughter and sighs and thrills of Lifestyle Medicine as it chuckles and slides along, investigating, sensing, and experiencing.

"Taste the verdant lushness. Touch laughter, grief, emotion, children playing freely. Submit to ordered, elegant, cozy, chaos, where time is told not by watches, but by light and shadow, warmth and frost. Everything you see and sense is inhabited by spirits and quickened by the ancestors. Everything around you, including you, is a conduit of energy and a container of memory."

Sunset is in full bloom when she turns you toward the west.

"Open your eyes wide, wide, wide. Open your ears. Open your senses. Be alert. Be aware. Be deeply grounded. You have seen where we came from, now observe where we are going. The way up was hard, the way down is easy, or so it seems.

"There is Alternative Medicine with its hot springs and glacial lakes. And Pharmaceutical Medicine, known for its hidden rapids and dangerous sandbars; it ends at the Loch of Endless Longing. The most turbulent of all, Deep Medicine, crashes over a steep cliff into the Ocean of Forgetfulness."

Even in the gloom of full dusk, you can make out slick, sharp stony ledges, dry ridges, steely cliffs, scarps, and scree slopes that carve the gray, somber land below you into a maze. From far below come the sounds of a carnival, a circus. Eerie, half-seen rainbows flicker. A metallic sheen comes off the water below.

As if reading your mind, the wise woman whispers: "Not all waters on the far side of

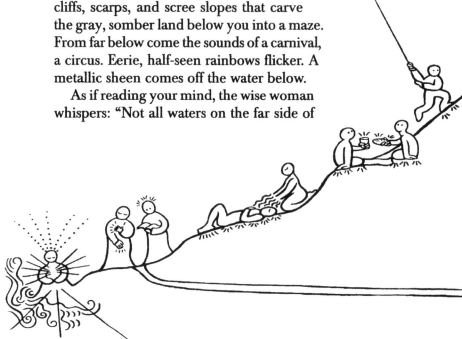

the Gap are safe to drink. Some are harsh and bitter, some cloyingly sweet, some too hot."

The wind is suddenly chill. You realize how very tired and hungry you are. The wise woman turns you to the north.

"There's our cabin. We need to be well-rested and well-nourished to deal with the hazards and challenges we're going to encounter as we visit the last three Medicines."

A gust of wind throws sleet in your face as you follow the wise woman toward the warm cabin, simple food, and refreshing sleep.

In the morning, you are eager to set out, but the wise woman will have her mug of herbal brew first. You sit down beside her at the table on the porch.

"Beware!" she croaks in a mock scary voice.

"Be aware that we will meet false faces on the other side of the Gap. Are you ready? Instead of self-acceptance, you will find drugs to change your mood, and surgery to make you feel better about yourself. Are you ready? Instead of real energy, there will be stimulants. Instead of relaxation and self-knowledge, sedatives and antidepressants. Are you ready? Instead of real herbs, plant medicines are made as drug-like as possible. Can you refuse? You could be poisoned in the name of health, injured in the quest for healing, judged by machines. Are you ready?

"We could be injured. We could be lost. There is no guarantee that we will return. Shall we go?"

You shiver at her words and arise.

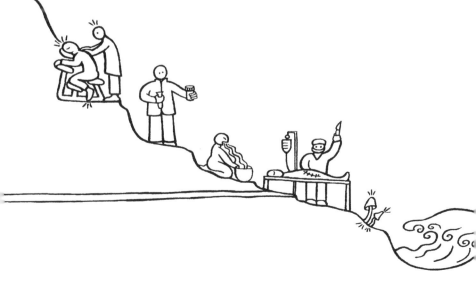

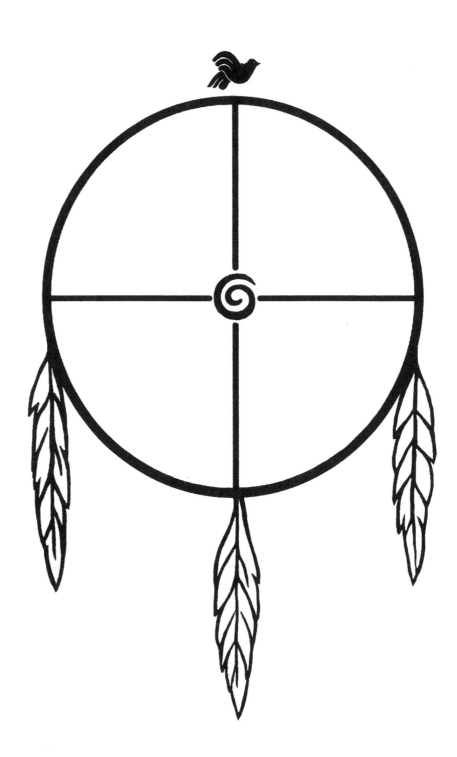

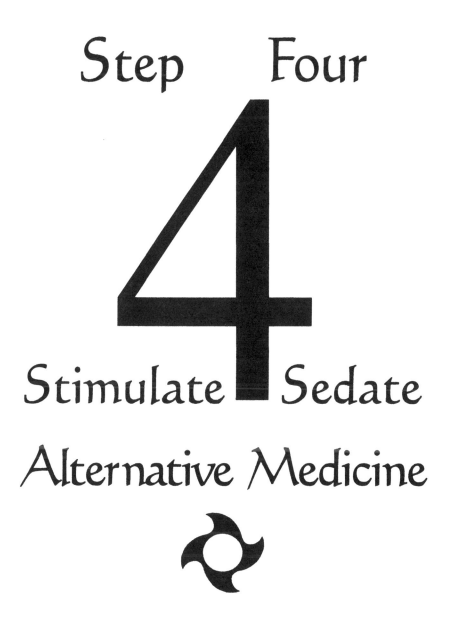

Step Four

4

Stimulate | Sedate

Alternative Medicine

"*Stimulants are the perfect drugs for capitalism. They . . . squeeze time out of the body.*" Dale Pendell, *Pharmako/Dynamis*

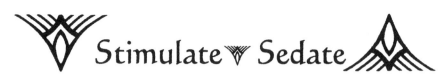

Stimulate ⩔ Sedate

day & night   hot & cold   up & down   yang & yin   go & stop

Stimulants and sedatives disturb normal functioning of organs and organisms: stimulants produce unnaturally strong action, sedatives produce unnaturally deep relaxation.

Stimulants directly influence the activity of a living organism or one of its parts by exciting a sensory organ or by evoking muscular contraction, nerve firing, or glandular secretion.

Sedatives directly influence the activity of a living organism or one of its parts by calming or tranquilizing a sensory organ, muscular contraction, nerve firing, or glandular secretion.

Stimulants and sedatives may be required to maintain life in extreme situations, if organs and organisms can't self regulate.

Stimulants energize, excite, invigorate, quicken, increase, animate, arouse, revive, agitate, provoke, stir up, inflame, force.

Sedatives calm, ease, alleviate, tranquilize, quiet, relax, soothe, palliate, numb, depress, suppress, knock out, oppress, deaden.

Stimulants and sedatives are especially useful in chronic situations when entrenched patterns of distress predominate.

Stimulants: aphrodisiacs, bitters, cathartics, caustics, cholagogues, diuretics, euphoriants, emetics, emmenagogues, galactagogues, irritants, laxatives, purgatives, rubifacients.

Sedatives: analgesics, anesthesias, anodynes, antispasmodics, astringents, demulcents, emollients, hemostatics, hypnotics, nervines, narcotics, relaxants, soporifics, tranquilizers.

Stimulants and sedatives alter mood, relieve pain, and increase pleasure. Most organisms seek them, sometimes to the point of addiction. Natural stimulants and sedatives generally taste bad or are available in limited quantity, which limits their use. When these

outer & inner   far & near   light & heavy   sharp & dull   full & empty

active ingredients are synthesized, addiction is encouraged due to lack of taste and ease of access.

Modern life puts stimulants (like energy drinks and coffee) and sedatives (like over-the-counter pain-killers and alcohol) within easy reach of everyone. They push out real nourishment. Reliance on Step 4 undermines health. The goal is to use stimulants and sedatives in the smallest dose for the shortest time needed.

Stimulants: sugar, pepper, coffee, tea, soft drinks, chocolate, ginger, guarana, some anger, loud music, fast dancing, some sexual acts, processed foods.

Sedatives: pain-killers, alcohol, valerian, poppy heads, warm bath, warm milk, quiet music, rain, TV, reading fiction, over-eating, orgasm.

The ill effects of consistent use of stimulants and sedatives are cumulative: the higher the dose and more frequent the use, the greater the harm.

Minimal use of Step 4 for a minimal time yields the greatest benefit.

Stimulated: blown up, boosted, compulsive, delirious, energized, freaked out, frenzied, hysterical, hyped up, intoxicated, jazzed, manic, over the top, speedy, wired, wound up.

Sedated: downed, depressed, impassive, tranquilized, calmed, quieted, controlled, detached, laid back, stagnant, catatonic, hypnotized, palliated, groggy, deflated, stultified, zoned.

Practices That Stimulate & Sedate • chiropractic • Swedish massage • hydrotherapy • extreme heat/cold (sauna and cold plunge) • shiatsu • acupuncture • pranayama • reflexology •

Herbs That Stimulate & Sedate: • black cohosh • blue cohosh • cannabis • catnip • chamomile • cinchona • cramp bark • hops • lobelia • pennyroyal • peppermint • sage • skullcap • thyme

According to the *Physician's Desk Reference for Herbal Medicines*, **cannabis** *sedates* nausea, convulsions, pain, perception of time, body temperature, blood pressure, intra-occular pressure, bacterial growth, and tumor growth. It *stimulates* appetite, heart rate, sensory impressions, bronchial dilation, anxiety and panic.

Grandmother Growth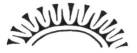

You feel the hair on the back of your neck stir, rise. You know she is near, the wise woman. She fascinates you. She scares you. You want to see more of her. You want her to leave you alone.

You hear a muted roar in your ears, like a distant, constant thunder. You feel a mist on your face. Your nerves are jittery; you feel all on edge and out of sorts. You wish you had a smoke, a drink, anything, anything to make you forget your nervousness. You feel impatient, pressed for time, eager to do whatever has to be done, and then get on to the next thing, whatever that is.

"Don't you remember a thing, empty head?" comes the growl you were anticipating. "Breathe. Breathe out. Good. Now sigh. Use your voice and sigh. And open your eyes wide. Look at me and listen carefully.

"You have crossed the Great Divide and you now stand in another world. A world that is dangerous, deadly. You must stay attentive, consider well, and act with care. You will be forgiven for your mistakes, but you will pay for them.

"Some of the danger is obvious. Like the waterfall just around the next bend. To avoid being swept away by it, we will climb down beside it, then cross behind it. There we enter a maze of paths crossing into alternative realities. Many are dead ends that take you nowhere, leaving you stranded and confused, with empty pockets and little hope.

"Some, however, are yellow-brick-roads where adventures await and all your desires are fulfilled. Find the road that rises up to meet you. Feel the blessings under your feet. Get a grip on yourself, dear child. Stop hyperventilating and scaring yourself silly. Plenty of chills, thrills, and high-speed adventures await us. Keep your eyes open wide. Keep your ears alert. Keep your heart expanded. Keep breathing. Remember your power. Follow me."

airy & heavy   dead & alive   front & back   wide & narrow   true & false

Benefits of Alternative Medicine

o Greater sense of personal control over one's health
o Fewer, less severe side effects compared with drugs
o Connects one to Nature and natural processes, rooted
o Often effective when the standard of care is not
o Creates excitement, feels pioneering
o Holistic techniques involve the whole person

Alternative Medicine includes a wide range of beliefs and practices. Some herbalists, acupuncturists, and massage therapists practice in the Wise Woman tradition. Osteopaths, and some herbalists and massage therapists practice in the Scientific tradition; Dr. Weiss (German) adds purified alkaloids to his herbs. Naturopaths, Ayurvedic and anthroposophic doctors, most herbalists and massage therapists, homeopaths, and chiropractors practice in the Heroic Tradition. But whatever the philosophy, stimulating and sedating – chi, blood flow, nerve impulses, etc. – is the task at hand.

Strange as it seems, Alternative Medicine does not build health. We are on the far side of the gap; our health can be compromised, especially when supplements, drugs, essential oils (Step 5), cleanses, colonics, or vitamin drips (Step 6) are part of the treatment.

Step 4 remedies are often dramatic and usually fast acting. They appeal to the part of us that wants a quick fix. They may provide a wild agitation or a strange calm.

Step 4 remedies let us push past our limits: increase our energy, stay up to study, drive all night, conquer weakness. And Step 4 remedies let us push past the demands of our emotions: turn ourselves off, swallow our distress, drown the pain.

The stimulants/sedatives of Step 4 harm with constant use or overuse. There is a hierarchy of harm within this Step, just as the Steps themselves are ordered by likelihood of harm. So I divide Step 4 into ten increments: 4.0 (tonic) to 4.9 (drug-like).

The wise woman uses 4.0 to 4.4 remedies, with nourishing and tonifying constituents. Heroic healers like the dramatic effects of remedies in the 4.4 to 4.8 range. Scientifically-inclined practitioners use remedies of 4.8 and up.

Addiction

Our lives are saved. Hooray! Our mood is altered. Whoopee! We are addicted. Uh-oh.

It is hard to believe that something that appears so serene in one place, can, a little further along, sweep you away. Hard to know how dangerous it is, and where the dangers are hidden. That bywater is a safe place to swim; this one swirls into a whirlpool that few escape. That ant will share your lunch with you, no problem; that one will put you to bed for a day if it stings you.

Step 4 remedies push us and our organs past normal functional limits, unlike tonics and adaptogens, which nourish the foundations of health. Step 4 remedies increase and decrease flows of both blood and energy throughout the body, but do not nourish abundant health.

When we and our organs become accustomed to a stimulant/sedative, which can happen quickly, the amount needed to achieve the same effect increases, which decreases sensitivity, endlessly.

We crave the stimulant/sedative. The dose gets higher, the dosing more frequent. The rebound is more depressed, more manic. When the stimulant wears off, we are more tired than before. When the sedative loses effect, we are more frantic than before. The worse we feel, the stronger the need to take the "remedy" again. We are drawn into addiction dose by dose, day by day.

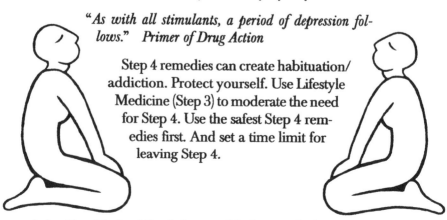

"As with all stimulants, a period of depression follows." Primer of Drug Action

Step 4 remedies can create habituation/addiction. Protect yourself. Use Lifestyle Medicine (Step 3) to moderate the need for Step 4. Use the safest Step 4 remedies first. And set a time limit for leaving Step 4.

shakey & stable   hard & soft   intense & boring   rough & smooth   funny & sad

Alternative Medicines

According to the Mayo Clinic National Center for Complementary/Alternative Medicine, the most commonly used alternative medicines are naturopathy, aromatherapy, massage, herbs, meditation, Ayurveda, homeopathy, Chinese medicine, acupuncture, reflexology, chiropractic, and Reiki.

Not all alternative medicines are Step 4. Some – like homeopathy, acupuncture, and Reiki – are Mind Medicine, Step 2. Many alternative practitioners rely on supplements and herbs in capsules, and that's Step 5. Chelation therapies, extreme detoxification regimes, colonics, and IV drips of vitamins are Step 6.

My favorite examples of Alternative Medicine – acupuncture, herbs, massage, naturopathy, osteopathy, reflexology, spinal manipulation, hydrotherapy, and cognitive behavioral therapy – are here, along with my warnings about aromatherapy.

Step 4 remedies may be mild or powerful, best used often or best used rarely. These differences are an advantage, and a source of confusion. They allow a wide range of effective treatments for a wide range of people.

Relieve Menstrual Cramps
Explanation of Steps in text at right

Step 3.9	Warm bath, nettle infusion
Step 4.0	Hot water bottle, rocking
4.1	Motherwort tincture, acupressure
4.2	Crampbark tincture, massage
4.3	Ginger tea, Calif. poppy tincture
4.4	Black cohosh tincture, shiatsu
4.5	Catnip smoked, valerian capsules
4.6	Wild yam tincture, acupuncture
4.7	Pennyroyal tincture
4.8	Belladonna tincture (caution!)
4.9	Ergot fungus *(do not use)*
5.0	Opium, hashish *(illegal)*

• Remedies at 4.0 – 4.2 are safest and can be used often.

• Remedies at 4.3 – 4.5 are used for short periods to relieve acute distresses.

• Remedies at 4.6 – 4.7 are best used only as needed.

• Remedies at 4.8 – 4.9 are used only when all other options have failed.

Acupuncture (needles, auricular, shiatsu, acupressure, cupping)

Chinese, Japanese, and Korean herbalists and healers have many ways of stimulating and sedating the flow of chi (vital energy) in the body through specific tsubos (energy points) along meridians (paths).

Moxibustion, one of the oldest of these techniques, tonifies chi. Cupping, and the related gua sha, have also been in use for thousands of years to stimulate and sedate, as has shiatsu (acupressure). Acupuncture is the newest technique, since it depends on a modern skill, the ability to make a thin steel needle.

Current research has found acupuncture helpful:

o   Against migraines, tension headaches
o   Against pain after dental surgery
o   To calm chronic pain, menstrual pain, fibromyalgia
o   To lower blood pressure, reduce angina pain
o   To counter dependence on opioid drugs
o   As a restorative after chemo/radiation therapy
o   Against Parkinson's [Chinese studies show benefit]
o   Blue Cross/Shield covers acupuncture for pain management

Stimulating the point P6 (directions at MSK website, link on page 167) with pressure, needles, or electro-acupuncture, but not with wristwatch-like electrical devices, is especially effective against nausea and vomiting:

* After surgery
* During and after chemotherapy
* When dealing with motion sickness

Is it safe? Mostly. Do choose someone with experience, the more the better. And consider the use of moxibustion or cupping instead of or in addition to needles.

"Qi, the organizational force of the body, moves according to simple laws, yet like water, it carries with it different properties depending on its location. . . . Lakes are still, clouds rise, oceans roll, rivers flow. Acupuncture relies on this uniformity of Qi whilst celebrating its different manifestations."   Daniel Keown MD, *The Spark in the Machine*

"The World Health Organization has recognized acupuncture as effective in treating mild to moderate depression."   Andrew Weil MD

Aromatherapy

Aromatherapy is portrayed as a safe way to enjoy and benefit from herbs. It is not. Essential oils, whether diffused into the air, used in personal care products, or added to herbal remedies, act like drugs and hormones, disrupting the health of every cell in the body.

Essential oils destroy bacterial cells, true. But every healthy cell in the body is also injured. Essential oils kill energy-producing mitochondria in the cells. Aromatherapy can interfere with the immune system, increase insulin-resistance, and raise cholesterol.

Essential oils are made by extracting, concentrating, and purifying the volatile oils found in plants. Aspirin is made by extracting, concentrating, and purifying a plant compound (salicin) found in willow. The processes are the same; the result is the same: the creation of a drug. *Essential oils are drugs, not herbal medicines.*

Essential oils are antifungal (kill yeasts), antibacterial (kill bacteria), and anti-microbial (kill microbes). Our gut flora/microbiome is made up of yeasts, bacteria, and microbes. Essential oils injure them, whether applied to our bodies or diffused into the air.

Essential oils disrupt hormone signals, especially in the young. Essential oils strip varnish off finished furniture and melt some kinds of plastic on contact. **I avoid essential oils completely.**

Is it safe? No. One ounce of most essential oils is a lethal dose. It is unsafe even to have essential oils in the household with children. Babies have been poisoned by mouthing closed bottles.

In addition to problems true for all essential oils, there are problems with specific oils; e.g., tea tree oil can destroy the nail bed.

Instead: Try **Natural Scent Therapy**. Add the aromatherapy herb you want – lavender or orange, cinnamon or clove, or any other dried **herb** – to a pan of boiling water and boil for five minutes. Turn off heat. Inhale. Ah. Put a real lavender plant – or rosemary, or rose geranium, or lemon balm, or any other aromatherapy plant you like – in the massage room; your touch releases the aroma as needed. Infuse aromatic herbs in coconut oil instead of buying scented lotions. *Brush your teeth* and rinse your mouth with yarrow tincture, instead of commercial toothpaste or mouthwash, all of which, no matter how "natural," contain essential oils.

Herbal Medicine

Plants feed us and shelter us, clothe us and delight us, and they are our allies in health and healing. All animals know the healing herbs; all primates use them. Written human records on how to prepare and apply herbs go back at least six thousand years.

To me, herbal medicine is the ideal Alternative Medicine, the crown jewel of self-care. Free and accessible, herbal medicine is people's medicine. It's the health care that's right outside your door – even if you live in a city.

My primary use of herbs is as nourishing herbal infusions (Step 3). And I use herbs exclusively – refusing drugs and hi-tech tests – for most chronic and acute conditions.

I have used herbs successfully for the past fifty years for

o   Oral health: countering gum disease, cavities
o   Cardiac health: lower blood pressure and cholesterol
o   Hormonal health: more fun for more years
o   Relieving chronic and acute pain
o   Soothing injuries: bee stings, broken bones, lacerations, incisions, burns, bruises
o   Countering infections of all sorts, from strep to MRSA
o   Preventing and easing coughs, colds, and the flu
o   Dealing with digestive upsets
o   Countering tick-borne diseases
o   Sending lethargy packing
o   Ending anxiety
o   Coping with fertility
o   Conquering cancer

Is herbal medicine safe? Most herbs are safer than most drugs. For safety's sake, follow these three simple rules: Don't take herbs in capsules or pills. Take one herb at a time. Only use herbs you are familiar with.

Green blessings are all around you. Visit my YouTube channel and get started today. It's easy and fun.

"They call me doctor, nurse, teacher, I don't have a piece of paper that validates my education. It's my own people that validate my life's work."
Doña Enriqueta Contreras, Zapoeteca shaman

Tonic? Stimulant? Sedative?
Up & Down in Herbal Medicine

Herbalists often use the terms "tonic" and "stimulant" interchangeably. For instance, Dr. Christopher's classic text, *School of Natural Healing*, highlights twelve tonic herbs, most of which are stimulating. Eight of them (75 percent) are purgative, emetic, laxative, and/or cathartic. Surely vomiting and diarrhea are not tonifying, and the herbs that cause that are stimulants, not tonics.

Dr. Christopher's liver tonic formula includes four potentially poisonous herbs (goldenseal, bitter root, cayenne, Culver's root), an astringent (quaking aspen bark), a mild stimulant (ginger), and a dangerous plant, even in reasonable doses (quinine/ *Cinchona*). Herbs that actually tonify the liver include thistle seed, and dandelion, yellow dock, or burdock roots; each as either tea or tincture.

The difference is important. Tonifying herbs (Step 3) are generally safe taken in any dose and used as often and as long as desired. Stimulant/sedative herbs (Step 4) must be used more cautiously.

Herbs and other Step 4 remedies stimulate *and* sedate. Drugs (Step 5) are stimulants *or* sedatives. Drugs generally have a direction of action, while Step 4 remedies can go both up and down.

Some Step 4 remedies are one way sometimes and the other at other times: One can take a cold shower to calm down, or to invigorate. Reading can put you to sleep, or cause your pulse to pound.

Some Step 4 remedies do both in sequence, first one and then the other: Alcohol agitates and irritates, then sedates and depresses. A hot bath stimulates circulation, and that relaxes the bather.

Some stimulate at one dose and sedate at another: Tiny doses of *Lobelia inflata* (puke weed) excite the nerves and increase vasodilation, while very large doses are said to cause a death-like paralysis.Short deep massage strokes stimulate, while long surface strokes are relaxing.

Some have one effect on some and the opposite effect on others: Twenty percent of people find valerian irritating; the rest fall asleep. Cannabis makes some mellow and others paranoid. Kava kava root can put you out or help you dance all night, your choice.

Some herbs stimulate and sedate all at once. Coca leaves are a local anesthetic and a cerebral stimulant. Aromatic mints stimu-

Stimulants, Irritants, Energetics
from safest to more dangerous

Step 3.9	Nettle infusion, ephedra tea
4.0	Peppermint, tulsi, rosemary, oregano, thyme tea
4.1	Ginseng tincture, ginkgo tincture
4.2	Horseradish, chocolate, garlic, yarrow
4.3	Ginger, eucalyptus, mustard, galangal
4.4	Maté, buchu, licorice
4.5	Tea (black or green), lobelia tincture (small dose)
4.6	Coffee, coca leaves, poke root, guarana
4.7	Cinnamon, cardamom, cloves, myrrh
4.8	Nutmeg, black pepper, cayenne
4.9	Goldenseal, kola nut, ephedra capsules
Step 5.0	Vitamin supplements, energy drinks
5.5	Vitamin B_{12} injections, amphetamines

Eighty percent of American adults drink 3-5 cups of coffee every day.

Sedatives, Soporifics, Hypnotics
from safest to more dangerous

Step 3.5	Warm milk, warm bath, oatstraw infusion
3.7	Linden infusion, dill seed tea, gentle rocking
3.9	Chamomile tea, motherwort tincture, lullaby
4.0	Lavender, catnip, or lemon balm tea
4.3	California poppy tea, oats tincture, passionflower
4.4	Skullcap tincture, poppy pod tea, CBD tincture
4.5	Cannabis smoked, valerian root tincture
4.6	Hops tincture, kava kava root infusion, feverfew tea
4.7	Lobelia tincture (large dose)
4.8	Wild lettuce sap, poppy pod tincture
4.9	Saffron tea, opium
Step 5.0	L-tryptophan pills, opiates
5.2	Essential oils
5.5	Sleeping pills, opioids

Sedatives make you sleep; *soporifics* aid sleep; *hypnotics* make you sleepy.

late digestion and relax the nerves. Kava kava enhances mental activity while gently relaxing the muscles.

And the effect of the herb can be switched from one effect to the other by preparing it differently: Hot teas are more stimulating, cold teas are more sedating. Herbal vinegars are more exciting, herbal honeys are more soothing.

"What goes up must come down," is certainly true in Step 4. The greater the dose and the longer the use, the more true it is.

Because stimulating/sedating herbs have such different effects, they are often considered inferior to drugs, and their use with drugs is feared. I believe the variances of plants are more life-like and healthier than the standardization of drugs, and they can be used together safely. When using Steps 4 and 5 at the same time I:

- o Use herbs in water, vinegar, and alcohol, not in capsules.
- o Use herbs that also nourish and/or tonify.
- o Use one herb at a time. (See page 304.)

"Valerian, particularly simple valerian tincture, has an adequate [calmimg] effect only if given in sufficiently large amounts. [Use] A whole teaspoon . . . if necessary, several times a day. Indeed, sometimes 2 teaspoons at one time [are used]."   Rudolf Fritz Weiss, MD, herbalist

Make An Herb More Dangerous
from safest to least safe

Step
3.0	Eat a little of the fresh herb.
3.3	Make tea with fresh herb; preserve herb in honey.
3.5	Infuse fresh herb in oil; make tea of the dried herb.
3.7	Make a vinegar from the fresh herb.
3.8	Make a dried herb infusion, steeped overnight.
3.9	Make a decoction by boiling the dried herb.
4.0	Tincture the fresh herb in 100-proof vodka.
4.2	Tincture the dried herb in 198-proof alcohol.
4.9	Take the dried herb in a capsule.
5.0	Take a standardized tincture of the herb.
5.2	Inhale, apply, bathe in, or ingest the essential oil.
5.5	Synthesize a drug based on the herb.

Massage Therapies

Massage comes in hundreds of forms. The most common are:

Swedish massage – Long strokes, kneading, deep circular movements, vibration and tapping relieve muscle tension.

Deep tissue massage – Slow, forceful, penetrating strokes help muscle and connective tissue unbind and heal.

Comfort Touch – Gentle, sensitive strokes are ideal for the very old, the very injured, and the very traumatized.

Maya abdominal massage – Deep, rocking moves for pelvic health.

Pressure point massage – Deep, long-held pressure breaks up tight muscle fibers that form after trauma. Includes: shiatsu, reflexology, and Trigger Point Myotherapy, created by Bonnie Prudden.

"Simple enough to be taught to a child. Arm, shoulder, and neck pain all surrender [to trigger point therapy]."   Bonnie Prudden

Massage is increasingly considered medically valuable for relieving a wide range of acute and chronic conditions:

o Stress	o Headaches
o Myofascial pain syndrome	o Pain
o Anxiety	o Hypertension
o Digestive disorders	o Fibromyalgia
o Injuries	o Soft tissue strains
o Insomnia related to stress	
o Temporomandibular joint pain (TMJ)	

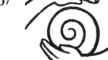

Massage has been shown to:
o Increase oxygenation of muscles
o Increase joint and muscle flexibility
o Increase overall strength
o Speed rehabilitation after trauma, surgery, cancer care
o Improve breathing
o Counter chronic pain
o Significantly lower heart rate, cortisol and insulin levels
o Promote feelings of caring, comfort and connection

Is massage safe? Yes. A license guarantees the therapist has been trained; but training varies widely. Massage shouldn't be painful. Speak up if something hurts you. *Hint*: Massage can be emotional. Look for a safe and comfortable ambiance.

Naturopathy

Naturopathic Medicine is one of the most accepted and most popular Alternative Medicines in North America. The best naturopaths use an eclectic mix of Steps 0 through 5 to create an individualized treatment for each person and situation.

There is a tendency to use the Steps globally (all at once) rather than sequentially (one at a time), and a strong reliance on the soft drugs of Step 5, with numerous supplements "prescribed" – and often sold at the office.

"Naturopathic medicine is not a single modality of healing, but a comprehensive array of healing practices, including diet and clinical nutrition, homeopathy, acupuncture, herbal medicine, hydrotherapy, therapeutic exercise, spinal and soft-tissue manipulation, physical therapies involving electric currents, ultrasound, and light therapy, therapeutic counseling, and pharmacology."   Burton Goldberg, the Voice of Alternative Medicine

Naturopathic practitioners are taught:

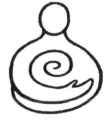

o   Nature is the best healer
o   Treat the cause, not the effect
o   Do no harm
o   Treat the whole person
o   Teach self-care for health
o   Emphasize prevention

Most naturopaths are taught to view themselves as "MDs with green coats," and herbs as supplements or "green drugs." This is Step 4 leaning toward Step 5.

Heroic Tradition naturopaths focus on balance, cleansing and the elimination of toxins. Toxins lurk in food (gluten, lactose), in the environment (pollutants, chemicals, radioactivity, hormones, heavy metals, pollen), and within our bodies (stagnant blood, estrogen-dominance, energy blockages, constipation, parasites). These ideas can be very dangerous to your health.

Is naturopathy safe? Yes. But. NDs are neither trained nor prepared to give you adequate warnings about the dangers of the supplements they prescribe and sell, while MDs (and pharmacists) are required by law to know, and alert you to, the side effects, interactions, and dangers of the drugs they prescribe and sell.

Osteopathy

Osteo is bone. Osteopathy supports self-healing by removing tension or restriction from the musculo-skeletal system and by strengthening the musculo-skeletal framework.. Osteopaths combine joint manipulation, postural re-education, and physical therapies such as myofascial releases, cranial manipulation, and functional releases to restore structural balance and good energy flow.

Osteopathic treatments have been shown to ease:

o Chronic pain	o Traumatic pain
o Menstrual pain	o Postural defects
o Digestive disorders	o Chronic stress
o Joint pain, arthritis	o General weakness
o Back pain	

Is osteopathy safe? Yes. In the US, osteopaths may include Step 5 remedies as part of the treatment plan; you can refuse.

Have Regular Bowel Movements
from safe aperients to more dangerous purgatives

Step
3.5 Eat whole grains (with their bran); eat prunes.
3.7 Exercise; have a regular time for your bowel movement.
3.8 Eat plantain seeds/husks (psyllium, Metamucil) as needed.
3.9 Bite your lower lip with your upper teeth for 30 seconds.
4.0 Drink more coffee; take burdock or dandelion tincture.
4.3 Use a dropperful of yellow dock root tincture daily.
4.4 Sip peppermint infusion as needed.
4.5 Supplement with oat bran or methyl cellulose (Citrucel).
4.6 Both cascara sagrada and aloes are laxatives. Careful.
4.7 So is senna (Fletcher's Castoria, Senokot).
4.8 Black walnut hull tincture can be cathartic.
4.9 Turkey rhubarb root tincture in large doses purges.
5.0 Mineral oil, castor oil, milk of magnesia, or Epsom salts purge.
5.9 Mercury is the ultimate purgative.

"Metallic mercury may be taken in considerable amount, acting merely as a purgative."   Kings Dispensary, 1898

Reflexology

This special type of foot massage stimulates 7200 nerve endings in the foot. You can receive a reflexology treatment or easily treat yourself by walking barefoot on sand, moss, or smooth rocks.

National Cancer Institute and National Institutes of Health studies find weekly thirty-minute reflexology treatments can:

o   Reduce pain
o   Relieve and counter headaches, migraines
o   Decrease overall stress response
o   Normalize and improve immune response
o   Reduce systolic blood pressure
o   Enhance relaxation and deepen sleep
o   Decrease anxiety and depression, improve mood
o   Counter PMS (premenstrual syndrome)
o   Complement standard cancer care and palliative care

Is reflexology safe? Yes. Reflexology points are often very tender. It is fine to complain when the pain is too intense.

Coffee vs Caffeine

Caffeine is an addictive, stimulating, water-soluble alkaloid, found in plants such as coffee, tea, and maté, in commercial products, and in drugs. It enters the blood 30-45 minutes after consumption, is in the brain within an hour, and throughout the body within 2 hours. The amount in breast milk matches or exceeds blood plasma levels. Most caffeine is metabolized by the liver; only 10 percent is excreted through the kidneys. Ten grams is a lethal dose, but as little as 1.5 grams can cause agitation, anxiety, tremors, rapid breathing, and insomnia. Withdrawal aggravates these symptoms.

But coffee – and tea – contain hundreds of other active constituents, including beneficial ones like antioxidant polyphenols. They are true herbal tonics, not drugs, so we tend to drink them daily.

Caffeine

in 5 oz of
cola soda = 15-25mg
black/green tea = 25-90mg
coffee = 50-150mg

per dose
Over-the-counter stimulants; No Doz = 100mg+
OTC diuretics = 100mg

Spinal Manipulation(Chiropractic)

Spinal manipulation – forceful pressure on the spine – and spinal adjustment – soft, stretching pressure on the spine – has been practiced for at least 5000 years:

o   To relieve pressure on joints
o   To reduce inflammation
o   To improve nerve function
o   To ease neck and shoulder pain
o   To resolve headaches
o   Against chronic back pain
o   To facilitate movement
o   To increase circulation
o   To relax muscles
o   To improve muscle function

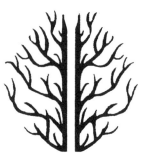

In order for the body to function well, there must be a flexible cohesiveness among the muscles, joints, bones, and neuromuscular system.

o   Spinal manipulation eases low-back pain as much as most pain medications, and as well as heat.

o   An Agency for Healthcare Research and Quality analysis found spinal manipulation more effective than placebo and as effective as medication in reducing the intensity of low-back pain.

o   Six weeks of gentle, stretching adjustments relieved neck pain in about three-quarters of participants.

It is estimated that there are more than 100 different types of spinal manipulations and adjustments used worldwide. Chiropractors, osteopathic physicians, physical /occupational therapists, and "bonesetters" are trained in spinal manipulation. Most practitioners also use other Step 4 techniques including ice and heat, electric stimulation, traction, activators, and ultrasound. Many practitioners also sell various supplements (Step 5).

Of special interest: **Network Chiropractic** gives the gentlest spinal adjustment. **Proprioceptive Neuromuscular Facilitation** is spinal flexibility training you learn to do with a partner.

Is a spinal adjustment safe? Mostly. Choose someone trained and licensed. Rare serious complications include stroke caused by neck manipulation, herniated disks, or compressed nerves.

Hydrotherapy

Any treatment using water – from an herbal bath to a high colonic/enema – can be called hydrotherapy. Most hydrotherapy immerses all or part of the body in hot water, often agitated with jets. Whirlpools, hot tubs, and Jacuzzis provide hydrotherapy.

Hydrotherapy can:
o   Decrease muscle spasms and increase range of motion
o   Relieve arthritis, tendinitis/bursitis, fibromyalgia
o   Strengthen weak muscles; increase circulation
o   Promote wound healing
o   Alleviate lupus, type-2 diabetes, and osteoporosis
o   Relieve stress at a cellular level
o   Lower blood pressure; increase endorphins
o   Relieve chronic pain: headache, back pain, joint pain
o   Soothe emotional pain, swelling, trauma, injury, stiffness

Is hydrotherapy safe? Only with extremely strict hygienic upkeep. A study of private and public hydrotherapy tubs found fecal bacteria in 95 percent, fungi in 81 percent, and staphylococcus in 34 percent, leading to urinary tract infections, skin infections/rashes, eye and ear infections, fungal infections, and pneumonia.

"The hydrotherapist seeks to normalize the quantity of blood circulating through a given area during a given period of time. In some cases this will mean an increase in circulation and in other cases a reduction."
                                                  Wade Boyle ND, *Nature Doctors*

Hot & Cold

"Heat is generally available, relatively inexpensive and safe, and, when effective, gives almost immediate and obvious [pain] relief."   Sidney Licht

Step 4 remedies are safer than drugs for relieving pain, and one of the safest techniques is the applicatin of heat and cold.

Heat, especially hot water and poultices of heated herbs, has a long history of use to sedate pain. Numerous studies find mud baths and mineral baths highly effective against pain and stiffness from osteoarthritis. Heat also stimulates circulation to injured tissues and prompts healing.

Neither heat nor sweating can remove toxins from the body.

Apply/increase heat with:

- Steam room
- Mineral bath
- Hot water bottle
- Hot rocks
- Moxibustion

- Sauna
- Cupping
- Heating pad
- Hot oil
- Poultices: hot onion, apple, herbs

- Sitz bath
- Hot sand
- Yoni steam
- Hot wax

Middle-aged men who take 4-7 saunas a week, compared to once a week, cut their risk of developing hypertension by 46 percent. Frequent saunas correlate strongly with reduction in the risk of sudden cardiac death and all-cause mortality.

Apply heat, or *cold if there is swelling, redness, or inflammation,* with:

- Fomentations
- Mud baths

- Soaks
- Foot baths

- Compresses
- Facials

Water Healing

Step 0:   Float in water, alone, with no sound, in the dark.
Step 1:   Relax in a tub of water; return to the womb.
Step 2:   Bathe with a holy number of herbs in blessed water.
Step 3:   Swim; take a bath in mineral water; visit a sacred spring.
Step 4:   Experience a steam bath, a sauna, or a Watsu session where water temperature and pressure can be varied.
Step 5.   Bathe with essential oils.
Step 6:   Be bombarded with needle-sharp sprays of water to cure hysteria/insanity. Be waterboarded (torture).

Cognitive and Dialectial Behavioral Therapies

Behavioral therapies (CBT and DBT) such as mindfulness training, can create fast, lasting, results by identifying destructive self-talk and by restructuring beliefs and behaviors. A therapist is recommended, but not absolutely required. Online help (see Resources) is available for those with anxiety, phobias, obsessive compulsive disorder, insomnia, depression, awful thoughts.

"Innovation medicine seeks to dismantle the hierarchical approach by emphasizing disruption and creativity – elements that are not restricted to any particular geographic area or clinician." Adam Kadlec MD, 2017

Step 4: Alternative Medicine References and Resources

Goldberg, Burton. *Alternative Medicine, the Definitive Guide*. Celestial Arts, 2002.

Acupuncture
Blum, Jeanne. *Woman Heal Thyself: Forbidden Pressure Points*. Charles Tuttle, 1995.

Ohashi, Wataru. *Do-It-Yourself Shiatsu*. Penguin Putnam, 2001.

Sachs, Judith and Judith Berger. *A-Z Guide to Healing with Pressure Points: Reflexology*. Dell, 1997.

Zhao L et al. "Acupuncture reduces angina." *JAMA Internal Med.* 29 July 2019.

- https://www.mskcc.org/cancer-care/patient-education/acupressure-nausea-and-vomiting [how to find N6]
- https://nccih.nih.gov/health/acupuncture
- https://www.pacificcollege.edu/news/blog/2014/09/20/many-benefits-chinese-cupping

Aromatherapy
- https://www.ncbi.nlm.nih.gov/pmc/articles/PMC3873673/
- https://kuumbamade.com
- https://www.nejm.org/doi/full/10.1056/NEJMoa064725 [Prepubertal gynecomastia linked to lavender and teatree oils]
- https://irp.nih.gov/catalyst/v21i6/the-human-microbiome-project
- https://www.ncbi.nlm.nih.gov/pubmed/22367888
- www.sciencedaily.com/releases/2016/06/160606200431.htm
- https://www.nature.com [search essential oils; 20,000 articles]
- https://skeptoid.com/blog/2014/04/05/essential-oil-claims-the-dangers-keep-on-coming/

Herbal Medicine
Alfs, Matthew. *300 Herbs, Indications and Contraindications*. Old Theology, 2003.

Bellebuono, Holly. *Women Healers of the World. The Traditions, History, and Geography of Herbal Medicine*. Helios, 2014.

Buhner, Stephen Harrod. *Plant Intelligence and the Imaginal Realm.* Inner Tradition, 2014.

Buhner, Stephen. *Sacred Herbal Healing Beers.* Sirius Press, 1998.

——. *The Lost Language of Plants.* Chelsea Green, 2002.

Christopher, John. *School of Natural Healing.* Atlantic, 1991 (1976).

Duke, James. *Green Pharmacy.* Rodale, 1997.

Elliot, Douglas. *Roots.* Chatham Press, 1976.

Foster, Steven, Rebecca Johnson, T. Low Dog MD, D. Kiefer MD. *Guide to Medicinal Herbs.* National Geographic, 2010.

Foster and Johnson. *Desk Reference to Nature's Medicines.* National Geographic, 2006.

Grieves, Maude. *A Modern Herbal.* Dover, 1971 (1931).

Hoffmann, David. *Medical Herbalism.* Healing Arts Press, 2003.

Hutchins, Alma. *Indian Herbalogy of North America.* Shambhala, 1991.

Levy, Juliette de Bairacli. *Common Herbs for Natural Health.* Ash Tree, 1997 (1974).

Lewis, Walter and Memory. *Medical Botany.* Wiley & Sons, 1977.

Lust, John. *The Herb Book.* Dover, 2011 (1974).

PDR for Herbal Medicines. Medical Economics, 2000.

Pendell, Dale. *Pharmako/Dynamis.* Mercury House, 2002.

Silverman, Maida. *A City Herbal.* Ash Tree, 1997 (1977).

Weed, Susun. *Healing Wise.* Ash Tree, 1989.

Weis, Rudolf Fritz, MD. *Herbal Medicine.* AB Arcanum, 1988.

Wichtl, Max/Bisset (trans). *Herbal Drugs and Phytopharmaceuticals: A handbook for practice on a scientific basis.* CRC Press, 1994.

Willard, Terry. *Textbook of Advanced Herbology.* Wild Rose, 1992.

Wood, Matthew. *Seven Herbs, Plants as Healers.* North Atlantic, 1997.

Massage

Knaster, Mirka. *Discovering the Body's Wisdom.* Bantam, 1996.

Prudden, Bonnie. *Pain Erasure.* M. Evans, 1980, 2006.

• https://www.mayoclinic.org/healthy-lifestyle/stress-management/in-depth/massage/art-20045743

Naturopathy

Lindlahr, Henry. *Nature Cure.* Nature Cure Pub. Co, 1922.

Vasquez, Alex DC, ND. *Chiropractic and Naturopathic Mastery of Common Clinical Disorders.* 2009.

Osteopathy
Chaitow, Leon. *Osteopathic Self-Treatment.* Thorson, 1990.

Reflexology
- www.ncbi.nlm.nih.gov/pubmedhealth/PMH0026897/
- www.mayoclinic.org/healthy-lifestyle/consumer-health/expert-answers/what-is-reflexology/faq-20058139

Spinal Adjustments
- https://www.ostpt.com/spinal-manipulation-adjustment/
- www.healthline.com/health/back-pain/spinal-manipulation
- https://nccih.nih.gov/health/pain/spinemanipulation.htm

Hydrotherapy, Hot & Cold
American Journal of Hypertension, re: saunas, SatEvePost 1/2, 2018.

Boyle, Wade ND, André Saine ND. *Lectures in Naturopathic Hydrotherapy.* Buckeye Naturopathic Press, 1988.

Lehman, Justus, MD (ed). *Therapeutic Heat and Cold, 3rd ed.* Williams & Wilkins, 1982.
- https://www.sciencedaily.com/releases/2017/09/170929093346.htm

Cognitive Behavioral Therapies *Online help for:*
- Anxiety, Phobias, OCD: MayoClinicAnxietyCoach
- Insomnia: (Free) CBT-iCoach/Stanford University
- Improving Mood: (Free) DepressionCBTSelf-HelpGuide; Moodkit ($5)
- Awful Thoughts: Cognitive Diary CBT SelfHelp (Free for Android); ThoughtDiaryPro ($5)

". . . new insights of neuroscience are exciting beyond measure, but there is always a certain danger that the simple art of observation may be lost, that clinical description may become perfunctory, and the richness of the human context ignored."   Oliver Sacks

"... *sedative-hypnotic agents ... produce a dose-related behavioral depression, progessively producing anxiolysis [calming], release from inhibitions, sedation, sleep, unconsciousness, general anesthesia, coma, and, ultimately, death. ...*" Robert Julien MD, psychopharmacologist

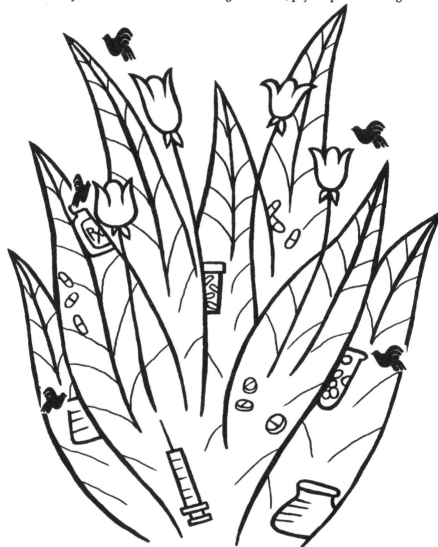

"*[Alkaloids are a] large and diverse group of chemicals including analgesics, narcotics, [and] central nervous system stimulants. ...*"
Dr. Terry Willard, herbalist, author

Step Five

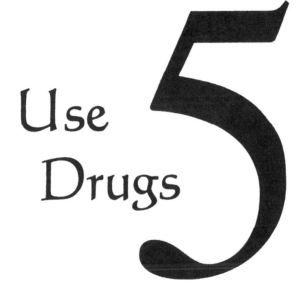

Use
Drugs

Pharmaceutical
Medicine

"When you get right down to it, there is no such thing as a safe drug."
HealthNews

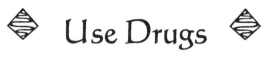

Use Drugs

Extract, Concentrate, Purify

Step 5 offers us pure, clean, white, standardized drugs. The Food and Drug Administration defines drugs as "articles intended for use in the diagnosis, cure, mitigation, treatment, or prevention of disease in man or other animals; and articles (other than food) intended to affect the structure or any function of the body of man or any other animal." By this definition, a hug is a drug.

I define a drug as a substance that is not a plant, nor made from a plant. Drugs are synthesized from hydrocarbons or created from constituents identified in plants. There are:

o Prescribed drugs
o Over the counter drugs
o Hormones, steroids
o Herbicides, pesticides
o Essential oils
o Vitamin supplements
o Cosmetic ingredients
o Industrial chemicals
o Psychoactive drugs

o Black-market drugs
o Food drugs
o Anesthesias, narcotics
o Opiates, opioids
o Antibiotics
o Solvents
o Flavors
o Dyes
o Emulsifiers

Plants become drugs when these three steps are taken:

1. **Extract** the constituent you desire. A tincture is an extract, but it is not a drug.

2. **Concentrate** the constituent you have extracted; remove the water or alcohol you used to extract it. Decoctions are concentrated by evaporation of water but are not drugs.

3. **Purify** the concentrated extract; remove specific constituents and standardize.

Side Effects Are Called

• Adverse drug reaction (ADR)
• Unforeseen drug interaction
• Medication misadventure
• Drug-induced suffering

Drug Benefits

o   Fast-acting
o   Very specific
o   Saves plants
o   Easy to take
o   Easy to prescribe
o   Incredibly profitable

Pharmaceutical Medicine is part of our lives. Drugs are everywhere. In 2017 there were 695 million prescriptions written for the five most popular drugs; 4.45 billion prescriptions total. Some drugs we want and ask for. Some we take because we are curious. And some because we are told, and we believe, we must.

Beware. Step 5 is dangerous. Go back to Step 4 if/when you can. Drugs injure as they help. Even properly-prescribed drugs can kill. Even correctly-used drugs can cause permanent physical and psychological problems. Drugs disturb mood, mental status, and sleep patterns. Drugs can cause severe, sometimes fatal, short-term reactions. Drugs taken for one problem can cause another.

"Far more people die each year from adverse reactions to prescription and over-the-counter medications than succumb to all illegal drug use."
Stephen Fried, *Bitter Pills*

". . . a well-educated empowered patient is critical for ensuring safe, appropriate use of prescription medications. . . . " Michael Carome MD

More than 4 million adverse drug reactions are reported yearly in the United States. More than 100,000 are fatal.

"The risk of an adverse drug effect is 50 to 60 percent if four drugs are taken chronically [daily], and almost 100 percent with eight or nine drugs."
Douglas Zipes MD, Distinguished Professor of Toxicology, Indiana U.

"More [Americans] die each year from reactions to the drugs they get in the hospital than are killed in automobile accidents. (And ten percent of all auto accidents involve drivers impaired by medications.)" NIH, 2017

Grandmother Growth

"Hold out your arms," the wise woman urges. "Put on this coat."
You comply. You've seen so many things with this old woman.
You trust her completely. And you're eager for another adventure.

"Put on these gloves, this hat, the mask and the goggles," she
says in her fiercely caring way. "We must protect ourselves."

She picks up a small glass Petri dish and a large glass bottle. As
she holds the Petri dish above her head, an indigo ray pulses from
it, rippling across the nearby wall's gleaming surface, revealing a
door. From deep within the flask in her other hand, a slender silver beam flows out, seeking and finding the keyhole.

The door opens. "Follow me; don't wander," grandmother
warns. "We are safe only if we follow the guidelines precisely,"
she admonishes. She looks down and your eyes follow hers to the
highly polished floor with glowing golden lines. You feel elated,
energized, outside yourself, outside of time.

When you look up, you are alone. Where *did* the wise woman
go? And why? You feel your heart beating faster and your mind
starting to whir. Almost without volition you find yourself walking. Ahead of you is another door.

On the door is a sign:

> BETTER THAN NATURE,
> BETTER THAN LIFE,
> TRUST US.

The room is white, glowing, attractive, safe, sterile, unpolluted.
"Here I am," you hear her say. "Refined!"

*In 1903, seeking to make unprescribed drugs illegal, the American
Medical Association and the American Pharmaceutical Association de-
clared: "Who kills the body of a man is an angel, compared to he who destroys
the soul by administering a drug without prescription." The law was
passed and two years later addictive soul-destroying opium and morphine
became the most-prescribed drugs in the United States.*

Pharmaceuticals Kill

In 2000, the Institute of Medicine reported that there are more than two million adverse drug reactions (ADRs) every year in the US. Drug reactions kill more than 100,000 hospitalized Americans and at least 350,000 patients in nursing homes each year. Scary drug reactions bring millions to emergency rooms yearly, where 8-10 percent of cases are ADRs. A 1999 study in *The Lancet* found adverse drug reactions the fourth leading cause of death in the US and this remains true twenty years later.

The actual damage to health and life caused by drugs is probably much greater. Doctors are supposed to make a "spontaneous report" if they observe an adverse reaction to a drug, but British physicians – who knew they were being observed – reported only 6 percent of the adverse drug reactions they encountered. It is estimated that 90 percent of all adverse reactions, and as much as 99 percent of serious adverse reactions, are **never** reported.

"While adverse reaction reporting is terrible in the United States, it is even worse in most of Europe, Asia, and South America."
Dave Flockhart MD, pharmacologist; Ana Szarfman, FDA

Women are significantly more likely to have adverse reactions than men. And doctors are less likely to report women's adverse reactions to drugs, believing it's "all in her head."

Step 5 Time Limit

Use drugs as little as possible for as short a time as possible. If that is not possible – and it is easier than modern medicine thinks to get off most drugs – at least prevent or moderate side effects by using complementary integrated medicines. I find it safe and effective to use non-encapsulated herbs with drugs, gradually lessening the amount of drug, as Alternative Medicine, Lifestyle Medicine, Mind Medicine, Story Medicine, and Serenity Medicine create abundant health.

Take Drugs

There are thousands of drugs in current use including: acetaminophen, acyclovir, allopurinol, alprazolam, amlodipine besylate, amoxicillin, ampicillin, amphetamines, apomorphine, aripiprazole, ascorbic acid, aspartame, aspirin, astemizole, atenolol, atorvastatin, azithromysin, benadryl, birth control pills, BPA, buprenorphine, bupropion, caffeine, calcium carbonate, calcium channel blockers, carvedilol, cephradine, cephalexin, ceftazidime, chloramphenicol, chloroquine, chlorpheniramine, cialis, cimetidine, ciprofloxacin, citalopram, clopidogrel, clonidine, cobicistat, cocaine, codeine, cortisone, cyanocobalamin, cyclobenzaprine, dl-alpha tocopherol, diazepam, dilantin, diphenhydramine, dimenhydrinate, doxycycline, duloxetine, efazolin, elavil, epinephrine, erythromycin, escitalopram, essential oils, ethambutol, fenofibrate, fentanyl, fexofenadine HCl, flagyl, fluoroquinolone, fluticasone, fluoxetine, folic acid, furamide, furosemide, gabapentin, glyphosate, heroin, hydrocodone, hydrochlorothiazide, hydromorphone, ibuprofen, isoniazid, kanamycin, lafaxine, lisinopril, loratadine, losartan, LSD-25, medendazole, melatonin, meloxicam, meperidine, metformin, methadone, methylphenidate hydrochloride, metrifonate, metronidazole, metoprolol, montelukast, morphine, neuraminidase inhibitors, niclosamide, nitrous oxide, nystatin, omeprazole, organophosphate, oxycodone, oxytocin, phenobarbital, penicillin, prednisone, potassium chloride, pravastatin, probenecid, procaine, pyrazinamide, quinolones, ranitidine, retinol, ribavirin, rifampin, ritalin, saccharine, selenium sulfide, sildenafil, streptomycin, sulfadimidine, scopolamine, simvastatin, sofosbuvir, spectinomycin, spironolactone, synthroid, tamoxifen, tamsulosin, tenofovir alafenamide, tetracycline, thalidomide, thiabendazole, thiamphenicol, thiabendazole, tramadol, trazodone, trimethoprim, ulipristal acetate, varenicline, venlafaxine, ventolin, warfarin, zolmitriptan, zolpidem.

"The surgeon who uses the wrong side of the scalpel cuts his own fingers and not the patient. If [only] the same applied to drugs. . . ."
Dr. Rudolf Buchheim (father of pharmacology), 1847

Are Herbs Drugs?

My Merriam-Webster dictionary says a drug is, among other things, "a substance other than food intended to affect the structure or function of the body." If herbs are foods, then they aren't drugs by this definition. What makes an herb a drug? Processing.

Many drugs are based on molecules first seen in plants. Some drugs are still made directly from plants. The herb itself is not the drug, even if it can be made into a drug.

"In order for a plant to be functionally poisonous, it must not only contain a toxic compound, but also possess effective means of presenting that compound to an animal in sufficient concentrations; the compound must be capable of overcoming whatever physiological or biochemical defenses the animal may possess against it. The presence of a known poison principle, even in toxicologically significant amounts, in a plant does not automatically mean that either man or a given species of animal will ever be effectively poisoned by the plant."   JM Kingsbury, *Deadly Harvest*

Drugs are synthesized or extracted from natural materials, concentrated, and purified. Common foods and herbs that are safe to eat can be poisonous when specific constituents are extracted, concentrated, and purified. Mint is safe, but its extracted essential oil contains more than two dozen poisons.

Drug vs. Herb

A drug has a direction of action. An herb has a sphere of action.

A drug is linear and specific. An herb is spiralic and inclusive.

A drug fixes the process. An herb joins the process.

Drugs are "substances that produce significant changes in the body, mind, or both, especially at small doses." Drugs, even in tiny doses, can cause unexpected violent physical reactions. Drugs – even legal, prescribed drugs – can kill.

Most plants, even those that contain poisons, are safe. All drugs, even those that are necessary, have detrimental, sometimes lethal, side effects.

Drug Safety

- *Do I really need this drug?* Will it make me healthy? Is it only to allay the side effects of another drug? Have I already used Serenity, Story, Mind, Lifestyle, and Alternative Medicines?

- *Fill out a drug worksheet* (www.worstpills.org/public/drug sheet.pdf). Review your need for each drug 2-3 times a year. Include eye drops, suppositories, hormones, patches, food supplements, herbal capsules, over the counter (OTC) drugs.

- *What do I know about this drug?* Read the package insert. Consult a Physician's Desk Reference. Talk to others who are taking it.

- *Talk to your pharmacist.* Pharmacists are very knowledgeable about drugs, their interactions, and their adverse effects.

- *Is there a similar, older drug that is safer?* Drug salesmen and TV ads encourage use of the newest, less well-tested drugs.

- *Avoid new drugs.* Most have been taken only for a few months by fewer than 5,000 people. Adverse effects may take years to develop and may occur in only one out of 10,000 people.

- *Ask about withdrawal or rebound effects.* Some drugs make your condition worse when you withdraw from them.

- *Use the lowest effective dose.*

- *Understand all instructions, including what to do if you miss a dose.*

- *Be sure the prescription and the label on your bottle match exactly* – especially when getting refills.

- *Don't be shy about reporting side effects.* Assume any change in your physical or mental state is caused by a new drug. If a drug makes you feel worse, stop taking it and call your doctor.

- *Buy from a known source.* Ten percent of all drugs sold in the global market contain too much, too little, or no actual active ingredient. Some are contaminated with heavy metals.

- *Avoid:* Compounding pharmacies, on-line pharmacies, "Canadian" pharmacies, small pharmacies with very low prices, and "unregulated, ineffective, and harmful bio-identical hormones."

"A whole range of widely-used drugs across all fields of medicine have been represented as safer and more effective than they are, endangering people's lives and wasting public money."   Fiona Godlee, *BMJ*, 2012

Hierarchy of Harm

"First, do no harm," is the basis of the Six Steps of Healing. Each Step is potentially more harmful than the one before it. As we saw in Step 4, once we cross the Gap/the Great Divide, there is also a hierarchy of harm *within* each step. That is, not all drugs are equally harmful. We can choose safer Step 5 remedies to get the same results with fewer side effects.

When we extract, concentrate, and purify/isolate just one ingredient from a plant, we lose the natural buffering constituents and make it more drug-like and more likely to cause harm.

Extractions are made from fresh or dried plants, with alcohol, glycerin, vinegar, or honey. Juicing fresh plants extracts little or nothing. Buffering constituents are usually retained in extractions.

Extracts are generally safe (with caution). Cod liver oil (overdoses of vitamins A, D). Flaxseed oil (often rancid). Golden seal tincture (harsh on the gut). Hashish (habit-forming). Opium (addictive).

Concentration involves boiling for extended times (fresh or dried), distilling (fresh or dried), or solvent-washing (fresh or dried) plant material. Buffering constituents are often degraded, destroyed, or

Spend Less on Drugs

Instead of supplements, drink nourishing herbal infusions.
Instead of essential oils, use natural scent therapy.
Instead of drugs, use Lifestyle Medicine and herbs.

If you choose to use a drug:
Ask for a generic
Avoid combinations
Tell your doctor lower price matters to you
A double dose pill costs less; cuts your cost if you cut it in half
Ask about Medicare MTM programs

Publix, Harris Teeter, and Meijer offer free generic versions of prescription medications – including metformin, antihypertensives, antibiotics, and anti-allergy meds – regardless of your financial resources. Price Chopper offers free diabetes meds.

discarded. Potentially posionous constituents are greatly magnified. Concentrates are more drug-like than extracts and more likely to interact badly with drugs or cause direct harm.

Use concentrates only in extreme need. Eat cooked greens instead of bottled chlorophyll or wheat grass juice; make fresh plant tinctures instead of buying standardized, more drug-like, extracts.

Purification/Isolation of the active ingredient from an extract or concentrate needs a chemistry lab, solvents, and the ability to do thin-line chromatography. In the lab, a complex group of constituents which buffer, help, and interact with each other in ways we do and don't understand, is reduced to one pure and isolated thing. The most active, most potentially poisonous part is isolated and we have a crude drug – and side effects.

The farther from the earth the food or remedy is, and the nearer to the chemical lab and processing plant, the more dangerous it is to our health, as in this progression: Cod liver oil, a natural source of vitamin A, is considered safe. Supplements of natural beta carotene (one of the factors of vitamin A) create health problems. Vitamin A supplements increase hip fracture rates. Synthetic vitamin A, retinol, can be deadly.

Purified/isolated foods and remedies are best used at the smallest possible dose for the shortest possible time, like any other drug.

Synthetic drugs are inherently more dangerous than other drugs because synthesis creates harmful substances called isomers.

Plants & Drugs

Eat a little foxglove; you'll be nauseated, but alive.

Extract the alkaloids by tincturing foxglove. A small dose is therapeutic, a large one, lethal.

Concentrate the alkaloids by cooking foxglove leaves; eat them, you will likely die.

Purify/isolate or *synthesize* one digitalis alkaloid; you have a drug that can be lethal.

Synthetics & Contaminants

In 1998, an amino acid supplement ($20 million annual sales) sold as a sleep aid was found to contain a contaminant associated with a potentially fatal immune system disorder (EMS). A similar contaminant in L-tryptophan supplements caused 1,500 cases of EMS and at least 38 deaths in 1989.

Synthetics: Isomers

Plants have many active ingredients/molecules; a drug has one. In pursuit of predictable remedies, science reduces complex herbs to a single active ingredient, and then synthesizes those individual molecules. Unique, chaotic, earthy herbal medicine – people's medicine – becomes standardized, simplified, sterilized synthetic medicine: Pharmaceutical Medicine.

No supplement, whether vitamin, hormone, herbal, amino acid, alkaloid, or anything else, is "nature identical," due to processing and synthesizing. Synthesis, we are told, allows us to avoid the variables inherent in crude plant medicines, and to make a remedy that is pure, measurable and repeatable.

The synthesis of drugs, including dietary supplements, gives rise to *isomers*. Isomers are both the original molecule and the synthetic rearrangement of its atoms. Sometimes the body converts a drug into an isomer.

Some isomers are optically rotated mirror images of the original. Because our cellular receptors are aligned to dextro (right-handed) or to dextro/levo (right-/left-handed) molecular shapes, and the rotated isomers are levo (left-handed) molecules, odd reactions can occur.

A slight shift in a molecule's shape can change it from helpful to deadly. And synthesis creates more than slight shifts. Some isomers are twenty times more active than normal; others less active.

For example: Naturally-occurring glutamic acid gives meat broths, miso, and tamari a rich flavor. Synthesized glutamate (monosodium glutamate/MSG) does too, but it contains "isomers that cause dangerous neurological reactions and adverse reactions in many individuals," such as weight gain, obesity, eyesight problems, less attention span, and worsening memory. The use of MSG in commercial food has doubled every decade since the 1940s.

For example: Folates – naturally found in most green plants – are the natural form of vitamin B_9. Folic acid is not. It is a synthetic compound used as a dietary supplement. Folate, available in high amounts in nourishing herbal infusions and organic liver, creates abundant health. Folic acid, found in enriched foods and multi-vitamins, is strongly linked to increased risk of prostate and colon cancer, all-cause mortality, and dementia. Worse yet, synthetic folic acid blocks the folate receptor site. (I notice my body's ability to utilize B vitamins is impaired when I eat "enriched" pasta or bread.)

"The subtle chemical differences between food-derived folate and synthetic folic acid may explain why a woman who could eat folate-rich foods without problems nearly died from an injection of it."   ScienceNews, March 1996

"Human exposure to folic acid was non-existent until its chemical synthesis in 1943, and its introduction as a mandatory food fortification in 1998."   Chris Kresser, integrative medicine specialist

"Nutraceuticals" – active ingredients isolated from foods – are clearly *pharma*ceuticals, not super nutrition, as claimed.

Women and Drugs

o Biological variations in the ways males (XY chromosomes) and females (XX) metabolize drugs can be dangerous to women, who have a greater risk of overdose, liver damage, and heart damage.
o Women metabolize drugs more slowly, and differently, than men do.
o Women's body chemistry is different than men's.
o Women wake from anesthesia faster and are three times as likely to complain of being awake during surgery.
o The vast majority of drugs on the market were never tested on women.
o Eighty percent of drugs pulled from the market were found to be more dangerous for women than for men.
o Benzodiazepines are attracted to fatty tissues, so they stay in women's bodies longer than in men's.
o Women have more active CYP3A4, a liver enzyme responsible for metabolizing many prescription drugs, than men.

Most standards, such as cholesterol levels, are based on men.

How have we come to confuse synthetic supplements with real nutrition? And to believe that drugs are good for our health?

The reductionistic scientific belief that "the whole is the same as the most active part" has brought us here. If ascorbic acid is the most active part of vitamin C, then ascorbic acid *is* vitamin C. And if foods rich in vitamin C help create abundant health, then, so this belief tells us, taking ascorbic acid will do the same thing. The evidence tells us something else, however. (See page 185.)

"Research on . . . herbal drugs is at least partly reflected by numerous references to pharmacological tests on isolated constituents."   Max Wichtl

In 2011, American doctors wrote 4 billion drug prescriptions. These properly prescribed and properly taken drugs killed 106,000 people and caused 36 million serious adverse reactions requiring hospitalization or an emergency room visit.

The Whole is the NOT the Same as Its Most Active Part

Do Drugs Cause Obesity?

Some drugs, like steroids, can activate the master receptor for fat cell development causing significant weight gain. A tin-based chemical (tributyltin) – found in vinyl plastics, antifouling marine paint, wood preservatives, disinfectants, agricultural fungicides, snail killing agents, textiles, insecticides, and house dust – activates that receptor, too. If pregnant mice are exposed to tributyltin, their offspring become obese.

"If I treat pregnant mice with a very low dose of tributyltin, their off-spring get fatter all the way out to four generations later. . . ."
Bruce Blumberg, professor of pharmacy, UC/Irvine

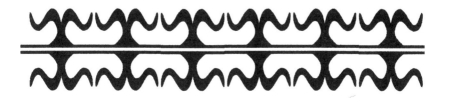

Drugs in Food

Most people are surprised by the ubiquity of drugs in food. In addition to residues of agricultural chemicals, there are preservatives, binders, fillers, flavoring, vitamins, and isolated proteins.

I grow and forage for much of what I eat. I make my own cheese and yogurt. I am a member of a local community farm (CSA). I visit nearby farmer's markets. And when I buy packaged food, I make it a point to read the label carefully, using magnifying and light aids if I need them. I look for and avoid:

 Drugs in Food
Avoid

- Artificial sweeteners
- Autolyzed, hydrolyzed additives/proteins
- Binders, fillers, gums
- Commercial tofu
- Dried eggs/whites
- Enriched foods, inc. water
- Flavors, natural/artificial
- Hydrogenated fats
- Almond, oat, soy "milk"
- Partially-hydrogenated oils
- Preservatives, propionate
- Protein powders/isolates: milk, soy, pea, whey
- Textured protein
- Thickeners, stabilizers
- Ultraprocessed foods
- Vegetable oil
- Vitamin-enriched anything
- White sugar (page 133)

Artificial sweeteners, which harm the gut microbiome, increase mood disorders, trigger weight gain, and increase cravings for processed foods.

Binders, fillers, gums, and thickeners are not food at all.

Commercial **tofu**/soy milk contain calcium supplements.

Enriched foods, fruit juices, contain synthetic vitamins.

Hydrogenated and **partially hydrogenated** fats and vegetable oils are linked to increased risk of obesity, diabetes, stroke, and heart attack.

Propionate, found in cereals, pasta, sports drinks, increases insulin levels.

Protein powders, ¾ test positive for lead, cadmium, arsenic.

Ultraprocessed foods include frozen pizza, instant soup, prepared desserts, frozen meals, and flavored snacks.

Supplements Are Drugs, not Food

It can be difficult to believe that a common, ordinary daily vitamin (and mineral) supplement is a drug. Confusion about the difference between actual nourishment as found in whole foods, and synthetic nourishment in pills and added to food, is rampant.

Step 5 remedies, including supplements, are important medicines that counter disease processes, remedy organic deficiencies, and aid those who are malnourished. Medicines. Not foods.

Those with good diets do not benefit from supplements; those with poor diets may be harmed. Step 5 is not a substitute for Step 3. Supplements are not nourishing. They are drugs, and like drugs, they are dangerous. The higher the dose, the greater the risks.

A review of 3 trials of multivitamins and 27 trials of vitamins A, C, D, folic acid, selenium, and calcium taken by nearly half a million people with no known nutritional deficiencies, found **"no clear evidence of a beneficial effect of supplements on all-cause mortality, cardiovascular disease, or cancer."** [*Annals of Internal Medicine*, 17 Dec 2013]

"Enough is enough: Stop wasting money on vitamin and mineral supplements."   Eliseo Guallar MD, Editor, *Annals of Internal Medicine*

Supplements are not just a waste of money, they can have detrimental effects as well, some that may take years to become evident. In the Selenium and Vitamin E Cancer Prevention Trial, neither supplement, alone or together, reduced prostate cancer risk. But eighteen months after the study ended, those who had taken vitamin E had a 17 percent higher rate of prostate cancer diagnosis than those who took the placebo. In men with high baseline levels of selenium, selenium supplementation doubled the risk of high-grade prostate cancer. In men with low baseline selenium, vitamin E supplementation increased the risk of all prostate cancers by 63 percent, and doubled the risk of high-grade cancer.

Supplementation of specific nutrients may be an appropriate intervention in some cases, short term, but is not suitable for daily use. Supplements fix; herbs and foods heal.

Chemistry is simple, linear, orderly, clean. Nature – and abundant health – is complex, fractal, and messy. Combining nourishing and tonifying herbs with drugs can give us the best of both.

Throw away your supplements and get your vitamins and minerals from nourishing herbal infusions and well-cooked greens, grains, and beans. A daily quart/liter of nourishing herbal infusion provides lavish amounts of vitamins, minerals, protein, and antioxidants for less than fifty cents a day.

Antioxidant supplements, especially vitamins E and C, "don't prevent disease and may even cause harm." How could that be?

A surplus of antioxidants eliminates the free radicals that are essential to the proper functioning of the immune and hormonal systems. The smaller amounts of vitamins found in foods are just right; the larger amounts in pills are too much.

o   In a study of 38,772 women (mean age 62, mostly white, 85 percent of whom were taking one or more supplements), the use of multivitamins, folic acid, iron, or magnesium supplements was associated with a 6-15 percent *increase* in risk for death; copper supplements increased all mortality risk by 45 percent. Calcium supplementation lowered mortality risk nine percent.

Vitamin A is created in the liver from thousands of carotenes and carotenoids found in brightly colored fruits and vegetables. Beta-carotene is considered the most active.

o   Taking 6,000 IU of supplemental vitamin A doubles the risk of hip fracture in postmenopausal women. Postmenopausal women with the highest blood levels of vitamin A are up to eight times more likely to have osteoporosis than those with low levels. [*Archives of Osteoporosis,* 2013]

Supplements Are Made by Drug Companies

Vitamin supplements are made by large petrochemical corporations, including Hoffmann-LaRoche, BASF, and Dupont. These drugs are sold to companies that use them to fortify food and to companies that formulate them, encapsulate them, bottle them, and affix their brand name.

"Natural" vitamins are the same synthetic drugs, but cycled through food-grade yeast or blue-green algae, before being pressed into tablets and sold.

o Beta-carotene supplements promote deficiencies of other carotenoids, especially in individuals with marginal nutritional status or severe depletions from smoking or using alcohol to excess. [*Journal of the American College of Nutrition*, 1994]

o The Beta-Carotene Efficacy Trial with 18,000 American men confirmed an earlier study of 30,000 Finnish men. Supplement takers *increased* their risk of lung cancer by 18 percent and risk of death by 8 percent. [*Science News*, Jan 1996]

o Men and women at high risk of lung cancer who took beta-carotene and vitamin A supplements for 4 years had a 28 percent *increase* in lung cancer and a 17 percent *increase* in deaths compared to those taking a placebo. [National Institutes of Health]

o In high doses Vitamin A supplements cause hair loss, nausea, liver damage, birth defects, coma, and death. [ods.od.nih.gov]

Vitamin C is a limiting nutrient, that is, one that we must get daily from food. It is highly water-soluble, easily destroyed, and impossible to keep in reserve in the body. Like all vitamins, it is a group of related substances which work synergistically together.

o Vitamin C supplements might make cancer treatments less effective; cancerous tumors "stock up on copious amounts of vitamin C." [*Cancer Research*, Sept 1999]

o However, intravenous infusions of vitamin C help chemotherapy work better. [*Cancer Cell*, 30 March 2017]

o Supplements of ascorbic acid and chromium picolinate react to create hydroxyl radicals, which are known to induce DNA damage leading to cancer.

Vitamin E is a complex group of antioxidant tocopherols and tocotrienols. They are found in fats, nuts, and whole grains. Alpha-tocopherol is considered more active than beta- or gamma-.

Most writers confuse vitamin E, which is many tocopherols packed together, with alpha-tocopherol, a single substance, or dl-alpha-tocopherol, a synthetic form of vitamin E. Consumption of large amounts of isolated or synthetic alpha-tocopherol can create highly reactive nitrogen compounds which push other tocopherols out of the system, lowering functional vitamin E.

o "Seventy-five years after its discovery we still don't understand what vitamin E does . . . [except] we need to get it from natural sources." [*Science News*, April 1997] o Among breast cancer patients, treatment failures are higher for women taking vitamin E supplements than for those not taking them – and the failure rate increases with dose. French researchers replicated these results with mice. [*Science News*, July 1995]

o Women who get the most vitamin E *from food* are 62 percent less likely to die of heart disease than those who get the least.

o Women who take vitamin E supplements have elevated LDL; women whose vitamin E comes from food have less LDL.

o A Cochrane Review of randomized, placebo-controlled clinical trials of vitamin E found no evidence that it improves cognitive function or prevents the progression of mild cognitive impairment to dementia.

o Vitamin E supplements actually foster the production of free radicals. [*Journal of Clinical Nutrition*, Feb 1997]

Omega-3 Fatty Acids

o Diets rich in omega-3 fatty acids promote brain health; supplements do not. [*JAMA*, August 25, 2015]

o Ten trials of people at high risk for, or already diagnosed with, heart disease who took 1000 mg omega-3 daily for four years found: "No significant reduction in fatal and non-fatal heart attacks and strokes in the supplement group . . . no benefit for people who had diabetes or high cholesterol." [*JAMA Cardiology*, Jan 31, 2018]

o High blood levels of omega-3 from fatty fish – two servings a week of herring, salmon, sardines, and mackerel – not from pills or fortified foods, confers a 27 percent lower risk of total mortality and less coronary heart disease. [*Tufts Health Letter*, July 2013]

Food Not Pills
Instead of supplements, eat more

Beans
Eggs
Fermented foods
Fish
Fruit: frozen, dried, cooked
Garlic and onions
Leafy greens, well-cooked
Miso, shoyu
Mushrooms, cooked
Nourishing herbal infusions
Nuts, roasted
Organic dairy products
Organic meats
Seaweed, seafood
Vegetables, well-cooked
Whole grains: rice, corn, wheat
Yogurt

o High blood levels of omega-3s from supplements is linked to atrial fibrillation and a 43 percent increased risk of prostate cancer. Eggs, bread, buttery spreads, oils, orange juice may be fortified. [*Prostaglandins, Leukotrienes, Essential Fatty Acids,* September 2013; *Journal of the National Cancer Institute,* July 2013]

Vitamin B, Vitamin D

o Long-term use (ten years or more) of high-dose **vitamin B$_6$** or B$_{12}$ supplements increases men's risk of lung cancer by 3-4 times. [*Journal of Clinical Oncology,* Oct 2017]

o There is no evidence that **vitamin D** supplementation prevents the onset or worsening of osteoarthritis or depression, reduces the incidence of type-2 diabetes, or helps prevent colorectal cancer. High doses are associated with an increased risk of falling. [*Tufts Health Letter,* April 2016; also: *Mid East Journal of Rehab;* July 2015.]

o Vitamin D confers no significant protection against upper respiratory infections. [*Clinical Infectious Disease,* 57:1384, 2013]

o Taking 1000 mg supplements of **glucosamine** daily is associated with increased intraocular pressure, a risk factor for glaucoma.

Minerals

Minerals are vital for abundant health. When we are rich in minerals our immune system is stronger, our nerves are calmer, our hormones dance well together, and our structure is sound.

Commercial foods and refined grains are short of minerals. But supplements are a risky response. Instead, I eat mineral-rich organic foods, weeds, and nourishing herbal infusions.

"Elevated intake of iron has been linked by many to an increased risk of infections . . . [and] rheumatoid arthritis. This may be due in part to iron's well known free-radical promoting effect."   Steve Austin, ND

Many minerals – including lithium, iron, selenium, and iodine – have a very narrow therapeutic range and a high risk of toxicity.

o Taking 200 micrograms of supplemental selenium daily doubles the risk of being diagnosed with type-2 diabetes. [*Journal of National Cancer Institute,* 2016]

Some minerals – such as lead, mercury, and cadmium – are heavy metals and should be avoided. (Mercury used to be considered a useful cathartic drug.)

Other minerals – including calcium, potassium, and magnesium – are rarely toxic as supplements, but do injure and degrade health. Calcium supplementation, for instance, has a boomerang effect: the more calcium we consume, the less our bodies absorb and the more they excrete. Thus calcium supplemention actually increases the risk of broken bones. Calcium supplementation also increases the risk of kidney stones and prostate cancer, and interferes with thyroid medications, corticosteroids, and tetracycline.

o Calcium supplements increase the risk of plaque build-up in the blood vessels; calcium in the diet has the opposite effect. [*Journal of the American Heart Association*, Oct 2016]

o In women with a history of stroke, taking a calcium supplement increases the risk of developing dementia within five years by a factor of seven. [*The Week*, 9 Sept 2016]

Minerals seem so simple, elemental. But simple elements, like a calcium atom, are not usable by living things. The electron cloud around the atom must be disturbed, so it can interact with another atom. When it does, it becomes a usable mineral salt.

Mineral salts of calcium include (but are not limited to) calcium lactate, calcium carbonate, calcium ascorbate, calcium citrate, calcium gluconate, calcium phosphate, calcium orotate, and calcium citrate malate. All minerals have many salt forms.

A supplement contains only one mineral salt. Real foods, including nourishing herbal infusions, contain hundreds.

o Use of 75 mg lozenges of zinc *acetate* halved cold symptom days. Less than 75 mg: no effect. No zinc acetate: less effect.

"There is no conclusive evidence that taking vitamin and mineral supplements helps prevent cardiovascular disease or cancer in people who are in generally good health."   Annals of Internal Medicine, November 2013

Get an Abundance of Minerals: 1, 2, 3 (4)

1. Drink 2-4 cups of nourishing herbal infusion daily.
2. Eat ½ cup leafy greens (cooked for at least 1 hour) daily.
3. Add seaweeds and mushrooms to your diet often.
4. Sally Fallon says: Consume more bone broth. (See page 218.)

Cosmetics

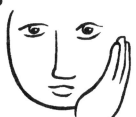

Using as few as 12 personal-care products daily puts more than 500 chemicals directly on the skin, e.g. heavy metals including lead, cadmium, aluminum, manganese, and chromium (in lipstick and lipgloss, excessive amounts even with average use), nanomaterials (in blush, sunscreen), coal-tar (in hair dye), and carcinogenic triclosan (in make-up, eye-shadow, deodorants, antiperspirants, toothpaste, cleansers, and hand sanitizers).

o **Parabens** have been detected in breast cancer cells. Found in makeup, liquid soap, deodorant, shampoo, facial cleanser, soft drinks, frozen dairy products, sauces, processed vegetables.

o **Artificial Colors** irritate the skin. FD&C Green#3 linked to tumors in bladder and testes. Yellow#5 linked to hyperactivity.

o **Fragrances** may cause allergies, immune, respiratory, and reproductive system distresses according to the Environmental Working Group. Found in deodorant, lotion, lip balm, bar soap, and shampoo. Phthalates may be added to fragrances.

o **Phthalates** cause endocrine disruption, reproductive problems, and early breast development. Linked to breast cancer. Especially dangerous for pregnant and lactating women. Found in nail polish, lotions and body washes, hair care products.

o **Formaldehyde** is a skin irritant harmful to the immune system; linked to nasal and nasopharyngeal cancers. Found in nail polish, nail hardeners, deodorants, makeup, soap and shampoos.

o **Sunscreen chemicals** can cause cellular damage/cancer. Easiliy absorbed through the skin; found in blood, breast milk, urine.

The vast majority of professional toxicologists believe that cosmetics are safe and the risks of these chemicals are overstated.

I prefer unscented **Castile soap** to wash my hair and body. I prefer unscented **shea butter**, coconut oil, or jojoba oil to moisturize my skin and hair. I prefer **yarrow tincture** as a dentifrice and mouthwash. I use **St. Joan's wort oil** as my sunscreen.

Drug Interactions

Drugs, supplements, foods, your own genetics, and your gut flora can stimulate or inhibit the production of specific liver enzymes that metabolize drugs, changing the amount of the drug in the blood, increasing side effects, and decreasing benefits. Drugs, it turns out, are not completely predictable.

"[Drug] metabolism is largely environmental: how stressed you are, what gut microbes you've got. . . . "   Lora Robosky, metabolomics researcher

Drug/Drug Interactions

Prescribed drugs interact with everything, including other prescribed drugs and over the counter (OTC) drugs. Be sure to ask your pharmacist to check interactions when you start a new drug. Or visit a website devoted to interactions.

It is almost always dangerous to mix alcohol and drugs.

Drug/Food Interactions

Some foods can interfere with drugs.

o Even 7-8 ounces of grapefruit juice can cause adverse interactions with 85 common drugs, including anti-infectives and statins.

Most drugs interfere with nutrient uptake. Suzy Cohen's *Drug Muggers* details the specific deficiencies caused by specific drugs.

o These drugs reduce vitamin B_{12} levels: methotrexate, colchicine, metformin; anti-seizure drugs (Dilantin), non-statin cholesterol-lowering drugs (Colestid), PPIs (Prevacid), H2 blockers (Zantac).

Drug/Herb Interactions

I once collected lists of possible herb-drug interactions. I pay scant attention to them now. The primary side effect of combining nutritive, adaptogenic, and tonic herbs with drugs is better health.

About 94 percent of Americans take both prescription drugs and a dietary or herbal supplement. Half those combinations could have potential interactions, but only 3-6 percent do.

"There is a relationship between the level of processing of herbal dietary supplements and the length of the DNA fragments; the more processed the

ingredients are, the more fragmented the original DNA becomes. As a result, DNA barcoding in highly processed botanical materials often results in findings indicating the absence of any DNA, or finds DNA from excipients or fillers."   American Botanic Council

Herbs in capsules are most likely to interact poorly with drugs.

In general, herbal teas, infusions, vinegars, tinctures, and honeys – but not capsules – interact with drugs in beneficial ways, countering drug side effects and helping drugs work longer and more effectively. For example:

o Drinking tea of fennel seed or raspberry leaf when you take acetaminophen counters pain longer and interferes with the formation of a problematic metabolite (NAPQI).

o Eating blueberries makes radiation therapy more effective. So does taking ginseng.

o Daily use of *Ginkgo biloba* extract plus aspirin is associated with less cognitive decline and improved executive function following stroke, compared with aspirin alone.

Antihypertensive herbs help antihypertensive drugs. Antidepressant herbs help antidepressant drugs. Herbs that improve blood sugar help drugs that influence blood sugar. Heart-healthy herbs help heart drugs.

Add a drug with a side effect of drowsiness and a soporific herb, and you are more likely to fall asleep unexpectedly, it is true. But add vitamin-K-rich leafy greens (including nettle infusion) when you are taking an anticoagulant, and you will be just fine.

Remember: The goal is to take less drugs.

For abundant health, we want to return to the other side of the Great Divide, replacing drugs first with herbs, then with lifestyle and the other elements of abundant health.

In the pages that follow, I offer you the best alternatives to prescription and OTC drugs.

"A recent [2016] review of more than two dozen studies in which patients discontinued medications (including sedatives like Valium as well as blood pressure drugs) found that people did surprisingly well when they stopped taking them. Adverse symptoms abated, and their health generally improved. "   John Schumann MD

Heart-Healthy Alternatives
These remedies can increase safety and effectiveness of cardiac drugs.

Lifestyle Medicine:

o There are many **foods** that lower/reduce cholesterol significantly. Find them in Appendix I, pages 301-302.

o Regular **exercise** reduces the risk of heart disease by 49 percent and the risk of atrial fibrillation by 60 percent, even for those who are at the greatest risk.

"Numerous studies of cholesterol lowering have failed to demonstrate a mortality benefit. . . . The Mediterranean diet has consistently lowered cardiovascular events and mortality in numerous studies though it does not typically lower cholesterol levels." Robert DuBroff and Michel de Lorgeril

Herbal Medicine (*safest first*):

o **Hawthorn** (*Crataegus* species) – 2-6 dropperfuls tincture of fresh/dried haws; 1-2 cups infusion of leaves/flowers daily – is the world's most-respected herb for maintaining heart health.

o **Linden** (*Tillia* species) – 2-4 cups infusion of dried flowers daily – dramatically and quickly lowers C-reactive protein, a measure of a kind of inflammation closely tied to heart attacks.

o **Shiitake** (*Lentinus edodes*) – 1-ounce fresh, one large dried, ½ cup infusion or 100 grams of dried powder used daily lowers blood levels of inflammatory proteins and reduces cholesterol. Shiitake's beneficial **effects on cholesterol are astonishing.**

o **Ginseng** (*Panax* sp.) – 1-4 dropperfuls tincture of fresh or dried root daily – lowers total cholesterol, LDL, and triglycerides.

o **Codonopsis** (*Codonopsis pilosula*) – 2-4 dropperfuls tincture, 3-4 times a day; 1-2 cups infusion of mature root, daily. Higher doses give better results. Counters angina pectoris, improves cardiac function, lowers blood pressure.

Of the 20,400 deaths prevented between 2000 and 2007 as a direct result of reductions in blood pressure and cholesterol, only 750 a year are linked to statin use. Other interventions, such as reducing salt and fat consumption and upping activity levels, prevent 4,600 deaths a year.   [*BMJ Open*, 22 January 2015]

Cholesterol-Lowering Drugs

More than 30 million Americans take statin drugs to lower their LDL cholesterol, and they are told this translates into less risk of a heart attack. This may not be true.

"The 4S study employed a cholesterol-lowering statin drug and reported a 30% mortality reduction. The Lyon Diet Heart Study utilized the Mediterranean diet and reported a 70% mortality reduction. Subsequent studies of the Mediterranean diet have confirmed these findings and also shown a reduced risk of cancer, diabetes, and Alzheimer's disease. Subsequent statin studies have led the United States Food and Drug Administration to issue warnings regarding the increased risk of diabetes and decreased cognition with statin drugs. Paradoxically, statins have gone on to become a multi-billion dollar industry." Robert DuBroff; Michel de Lorgeril

o **Statins** (e.g. atorvastatin/Lipitor, rosuvastatin/Crestor) inhibit the enzyme HMG-CoA reductase, which lowers cholesterol but also reduces levels of CoQ10, an enzyme needed for cognition and muscle function. Consider supplementing CoQ10 if on statins.

Among 10,000 patients, daily use of statins will cause "only" five new cases of myopathy, 5-10 hemorrhagic strokes, 50-100 new cases of type-2 diabetes, and 100 or more adverse events.

o **Cholestyramine**/Cholybar and **Colestipol**/Colestid reduce cholesterol by binding with bile acids. *Side effects* include constipation, black tarry stools, bloating, rapid weight gain/loss, abdominal pain; worse in those over 60.

o **Ezetimibe**/Zetia: Except for death from an allergic reaction to the drug, there are few side effects other than infrequent chest pain, fatigue, headache, and diarrhea.

o **Gemfibrozil**/Lopid: *Side effects* include indigestion, irregular heartbeat, chest pain, stomach ache, vomiting, diarrhea.

o **Niacin** supplements (vitamin B_3, nicotinic acid, nicotinamide) are a "natural" way to lower cholesterol; they do not decrease cardiovascular deaths. *Side effects:* dry skin, gut pain, diarrhea, flushing, headache, dizziness, tingling in hands and feet.

o **Cynarin** – up to 1500mg daily – from artichoke (*Cynara scolymus*) reduces triglycerides and total cholesterol.

Antacid Alternatives

Generally safe and effective to combine these with antacid drugs.

Lifestyle Medicine:

o *Eliminate triggers:* coffee, animal fats, alcohol, nicotine, processed food, spicy food, chocolate, refined or artificial sugars.

o **Nourishing herbal infusions** supply generous amounts of **folate**, which reduces acid reflux by 40 percent; vitamins B_2 and B_6, both known to help prevent reflux; and glutamine.

o **Glutamine** – an amino acid abundant in meat, fish, eggs, dairy, nuts, and cabbage – repairs damage from *H. pylori* infection.

o **Cabbage Cure** for those with ulcers: Grate a potato very fine and collect the juice. Do the same with a small cabbage. Alternate hourly spoonfuls of the juices until they, and your ulcer, are gone.

o Help yourself with a sip of diluted **kombucha**, **sauerkraut,** or cabbage juice, just before eating.

o **Sea salt** provides chloride to help you make enough hydrochloric acid, the main digestive juice, to prevent reflux.

Herbal Medicine (*safest first*):

o **Slippery elm** (*Ulmus fulva*) bark – taken freely as tea, tincture, or powdered and mixed with honey and formed into balls. Soothes the mouth, throat, stomach, and intestines, and, by stimulating nerve endings in the gastrointestinal tract, increases mucus to protect against ulcers and damage from excess acidity.

o **Dandelion** (*Taraxacum off.*) root, leaves, flowers, and stalks – taken just before meals. Dose is ½ glass of wine, tea, or infusion, a dropperful of tincture, or a spoonful of vinegar. Cures chronic acid reflux for most folks within a few weeks.

o **Ginger** (*Zingiber off.*) root tea – blocks excess acid and suppresses *H. pylori*. Proven to be 6-8 times more effective than lansoprazole for preventing ulcers. Steep 2-3 slices of fresh ginger root in 2 cups hot water for 25-30 minutes. Drink *before* meals.

Prescription medications that cause acid reflux: anxiety medications, antidepressants, antibiotics, blood pressure medications, nitroglycerin, osteoporosis drugs, and pain relievers.

Emergency Relief: ½-1 teaspoon **baking soda** (sodium bicarbonate) in 1 cup water neutralizes stomach acid and stops the pain.

Antacid Drugs

Acid reflux – heartburn, gastro-esophageal reflux disease (GERD), peptic ulcer disease – affects half of adult Americans. More than 16,000 medical studies show that suppressing stomach acid, as antacid drugs do, only temporarily treats the symptoms.

Side effects of suppressing or lessening the acid in your stomach:
o *Helicobacter*, the bacteria which may be causative, thrives.
o Gut flora diversity, essential for health, is diminished.
o Infections with *campylobacter, salmonella*, and *C. difficile* increase in frequency and severity, and may be fatal.
o Absorption of iron, magnesium, and vitamin B_{12} is greatly diminished. Mineral malabsorption increases bone loss.

Antacids/Tums have the fewest side effects. But 15-20 million Americans use dangerous proton-pump inhibitors (PPIs), truly warranted only for those with bleeding ulcers, endoscopy-confirmed damage to the esophagus, or the rare Zollinger-Ellison syndrome. Ordinary heartburn responds very well to botanicals.

"*60 to 70 percent of people taking these drugs [PPIs] shouldn't be on them.*" Mitchell Katz, director, San Francisco Department of Public Health

"*PPIs interfere with blood vessels' ability . . . to generate nitric oxide.*" Ghebremariam, Houston Methodist molecular biologist

"*When they [PPIs] came out, in the 1980s, we thought: 'It's a quick fix and they're very safe.' But in actuality . . . simple home remedies work as well.*" Anonymous family practice MD

o **H_2 blockers**/histamine$_2$ receptor antagonists (e.g. ranitidine/Zantac, famotidine/Pepsid). *Side effects:* increases risk of pneumonia (22 percent).
o **PPIs** (e.g. omeprazole/Prilosec, esomeprazole/Nexium, lansoprazole/Prevacid). *Side effects:* increases risk of dementia/Alzheimer's (44 percent), ischemic stroke (21-94 percent), pneumonia (27 percent), bone loss, hip fractures, infection with *C. diff.*, kidney disease, heart attack (16-21 percent); B_{12} and magnesium deficiencies. *Addictive, severe withdrawal symptoms.* Dandelion facilitates a slow withdrawal and transition to slippery elm and, if needed, H_2 blockers or antacids.

Pain-relief Alternatives
These herbs may be used with pain-relief drugs with care.

Serenity Medicine: Meditation alters brain regions that process pain.

Mind Medicine: o Acupuncture releases endorphins.

   o Alexander Technique is more effective than massage or exercise in relieving low-back pain.

Lifestyle Medicine: o Regular exercise counters chronic pain.

Alternative Medicine: o Reflexology releases endorphins.

   o A cold plunge alters pain perceptions, counters chronic pain.

   Herbal Medicine (*safest first*):

   o **High CBD** (*Cannabis*) – up to five drops of tincture of the fresh flowering plant, taken as often as every fifteen minutes – is my favorite non-addictive pain reliever. Often, a single dose will do. There will be some THC in the tincture, as all plants contain a mix of cannabinols, but this does not, in my experience and the experience of many students and friends, make you "high." First choice as an ally for transitioning off opiates/opioids.

   o **Skullcap** (*Scutellaria lateriflora*) – 5 drops of tincture of the fresh flowering plant, taken as often as needed – is my favorite pain relief, especially when I need to sleep.

   o **Kava kava** (*Piper methysticum*) – sips of the lightly-fermented infusion or dropperful doses of root tincture – offer fast, effective relief of musculo-skeletal pain, traumatic pain, chronic pain from injuries, heartache. Less likely to put you to sleep, too.

   o **Willow** (*Salix alba*) – 1-2 dropperfuls of tincture as needed – is as effective as aspirin and contains the same active ingredient. So does **meadowsweet** (*Filipendula ulmaria*).

   o **Wild lettuce** (*Lactuca virosa*) – tincture of the fresh sap taken by the spoonful – may be as pain-relieving as poppy juice.

   o **Valerian** – up to a teaspoonful of root tincture – counters chronic pain, puts you out, leaves you hung-over and groggy.

   o **Poppy** (*Papaver somniferum*) is the source of opium, heroin, opiates, and poppy seeds. Opiates are addictive; poppy seeds aren't. A tea of the fresh poppy seed heads entices the brain to make natural opiates (endorphins). *Do not combine with drugs or alcohol.*

See page 220: **Drugs that Cause Pain.**

Pain-relief Drugs

Ancient peoples used opium for pain relief. About a hundred years ago, we figured out how to make heroin and morphine, opiate drugs. Today, we have sophisticated synthetic opioids. As always, when we move from plant to lab, from many constituents to one active ingredient, and from concentration to synthesis, the risk of side effects, including death, increases.

Injured rodents given morphine become more sensitive to pain.

From mid-2016 to mid-2017, there were 150,000 emergency room visits and 65,000 deaths (180 a day) from opioid overdose. In the past twenty years, a quarter million Americans died from unintentional opioid overdoses. Opioids accounted for more than two-thirds of all overdose deaths in 2016.

Side effects of pain-relief drugs:

o **Non-steroidal-anti-inflammatory-drugs**/NSAIDs (e.g. acetaminophen/Tylenol, aspirin, ibuprofen/Motrin, Advil): *Non-addictive*. Stomach problems, ulcers, gut damage in 20 percent of daily users; kidney problems, sensitivity to sun, sunburn increased; heart attack/stroke (10-50 percent increase in risk); hearing loss (10 percent increase in risk). **Acetaminophen** accounts for more than 100,000 calls to poison control centers, more than 50,000 emergency room visits, and at least 450 deaths annually. Regular users double their risk of kidney cancer.

o **Opiates** (e.g. morphine, heroin): *Addictive; rarely deadly.*

o **Opioids** (e.g. Oxycodone, Codeine, Fentanyl): *Addictive; deadly.* Dizziness, falls, heart attack, sleepiness, abdominal pain, nightmares, hallucinations, confusion, dry mouth, urinary distress, constipation, nausea, weakness, headache, restlessness, sexual dysfunction, respiratory depression, hypo- and hyperglycemia, high risk of deadly accidental overdose. Opiates/opioids are most lethal when combined with alcohol, sedatives, sleeping pills, tranquilizers.

o **Tramadol:** *Addictive and deadly.* Seizures, difficulty breathing, double the risk of hypoglycemia compared to codeine.

". . . daily use of strong opioid pain medications is a lousy option for most patients with chronic pain. These drugs become less effective at controlling pain over time, and ultimately may even make people more sensitive to pain." Andrew Kolodny, opioid-addiction expert

Sedatives, Tranquilizers, Sleepy Alternatives
Non-addicting. Strong enough to work alone.
Mild enough to be combined with sleepy drugs if needed.

Lifestyle Medicine:
- o **Warm milk,** hot chocolate, warm bath: all encourage sleep.
- o So does a **cold bedroom.**

Alternative Medicine/Herbal Medicine (*safest first*):
- o **Cognitive Behavorial Therapy** is the most effective non-drug treatment for those with insomnia. [www.sleepio.com]
- o **Skullcap** herb in flower (*Scutellaria lateriflora*) – 5-50 drops of tincture – strengthens the nervous system, deepens rest, clears the mind, and eases all pains. No hangover, no dependence.
- o **Passionflower** (*Passiflora incarnata*) – 50 drops of tincture – is official in Germany, and found in 40 British sedatives. As effective as benzodiazepines. No side effects, even in repeated doses.
- o **Lemon balm** herb (*Melissa off.*) – one cup tea or 10-20 drops tincture – official remedy in Germany for "difficulty falling asleep."
- o **Catnip** herb (*Nepeta cataria*) – one cup tea or 10-20 drops tincture – "significantly increases sleep duration." Exceptional ally for children, but some get stimulated, so use small doses.
- o **California poppy** (*Eschscholzia*) – 1-3 cups tea or 30-90 drops tincture – "cools the heat of the mind" and eases pain, spasm, and inflammation in muscles and joints. Used against bedwetting.
- o **Rhodiola** root (*Rhodiola rosacea*) – one cup infusion or 50-100 drops tincture – is a hypnotic sedative in high doses.
- o **Hops** flower (*Humulus lupulus*)– one cup of the bitter tea or 20-40 drops tincture – is so effective I have seen folks nod off as they sip it. Also used as a sleep pillow. Plays well with others.
- o **Valerian** root (*Valeriana off.*) – 1 cup tea or a teaspoon of tincture – shortens time needed to fall asleep and reduces nighttime waking, unless it agitates you. Valerian is easy to grow.
- o **Ashwagandha** root (*Withania somniflora*) – "sleep flower"– a teaspoon/6g of powder in warm milk for those who are running on empty, burned-out, debilitated, stressed out, agitated, deeply distressed.
- o **Wild lettuce** (*Lactuca virosa*) – 50-75 drops of fresh plant tincture several times a day – is "one of the best sleep aids known," especially for those with chronic insomnia. Like poppy for children.

Sedatives, Tranquilizers, Sleepy Drugs

About 50-70 million Americans have trouble sleeping. Four percent of those over 20 use a sleeping aid at least once a month.

These drugs are quickly addictive, and mind-altering, with a high like being tipsy. Long-term use worsens anxiety and depression. Overdose leads to coma and death.

More than 100,000 people a year are diagnosed with "poisoning" from tranquilizers and antidepressants.

Alcohol, even a small amount, can cause unexpectedly severe intoxication when combined with tranquilizers.

Side effects of **all** sedatives, tranquilizers, sleep-inducing drugs: dizziness, drowsiness, clumsiness, breathing difficulties, anxiety, paranoia, 53 percent increased risk of a broken bone, reduction of circulating levels of vitamins B, C, and D.

o **Benzodiazepines** (e.g. Valium, Xanax, Rohypnol): *Addictive and deadly. Side effects*: compromises all cognitive functions, impairs memory, judgment, and coordination, impairs driving ability, reduces mobility, increases risk of falling, increases paranoia, irritability, agitation and aggression, and increases Alzheimer's risk (51 percent increase if used at any time in the previous six years). Up to a third of all deaths from pharmaceutical agents are due to benzodiazepines, with three-quarters of those being unintentional overdoses. *Severe withdrawal symptoms.*

Recent estimates find at least 16,000 of the 217,000 auto crashes that cause injury each year to elders are attributable to benzodiazepines and tricyclic antidepressants. *Both are overprescribed, especially to those over 65.*

o **Z-drugs or Hypnotics** (e.g. zolpidem/Ambien, zaleplon/Sonata): *Additional side effects*: strongly linked to delirium, psychosis, hallucinations, imbalance, falls, inappropriate drowsiness, driving accidents, bizarre behavior.

o **Barbituates** (e.g. secobarbital/Seconal, downers): *Easily addictive. Additional side effects*: clumsiness, headache, nightmares, depression, breathing difficulty, coma. *Withdrawal may be deadly.*

Antibiotic Alternatives
Effective and safe to use with antibiotic drugs.

Serenity Medicine:
Do not delay; treat signs of infection promptly.

Alternative Medicine/Herbal Medicine (*safest first*):

o **Echinacea** (*Echinacea augustifolia* or *E. purpurea*) – A drop-perful for each 50 pounds of body weight, taken 3-20 times a day, depending on the severity of the infection. Dried *E. augustifolia* tinctured in 100-proof vodka for a year is a highly effective anti-infective. Active ingredients tingle the tongue. Works well with poke tincture. (Tincture *E. purpurea* from fresh roots only.)

o **Honey** – the darker the better – alone or with herbal tea, or applied directly, counters infections in wounds and throats.

o **Reishi** extract – kills bacteria better than most antibiotics.

o **Yarrow** (*Achillea millefolium*) – 10-25 drops of tincture of the fresh flowering plant, as needed, is effective against virtually all bacteria. It is especially loved for clearing infections in the bladder, uterus, vagina, gums, teeth, and throat.

o **Berberine** – dropperful doses of tincture of the root of *Berberis* (barberry), *Mahonia* (Oregon grape), *Coptis,* and *Hydrastis canadensis* (golden seal) are highly active against a wide range of respiratory (sinus, mouth, throat, lung) and gut infections. Effective against MRSA and *C. diff.* infections.

o **Garlic** or **ginger,** fresh or dried, as a tea, resolves infections from staph, strep, *E. coli, Pseudomonas aeruginosa,* and *Serratia marcescens.* "Cost-effective, and no drug-resistance problems."

o **Usnea** (*Usnea barbarata*) – 25 drops of tincture of the whole plant, fresh or dried, as needed. Medicinal tinctures are orange. Usnea goes deep against bone infections, post-surgical infections, joint-replacement infections, tooth abscesses, lung infections.

o **Poke** (*Phytolacca americana*) – 1-4 drops, fresh root tincture, against chronic sinus, ear, throat, and lung infections. *Caution.*

o **Phages** – destroy antibiotic-resistant bacteria. *See* page 276.

"Give the body a synthetic magic bullet, and it has no menu, no choice. Give the body . . . echinacea and you are giving it a menu of useful phyto-chemicals, including probably more than a dozen different immune-stimulating compounds."   James Duke, *CRC Handbook of Medicinal Herbs*

Antibiotic Drugs

Antibiotic overuse leads to death by increasing antibiotic-resistant bacteria. In the first nine months of 2017, the CDC identified 221 new antibiotic-resistant bacteria.

o   About half a million Americans are diagnosed with antibiotic-resistant *Clostridium difficile* each year; 29,000 die within 30 days.

o   Data from 4 million office visits in 2016 found 93 percent of antibiotic prescriptions were written for too long (over ten days) and 20 percent were for antibiotics that doctors are advised not to use due to concerns about resistance. [*NEJM*, March 2018]

o   In 2017, nearly half of all seniors with non-bacterial infections were prescribed antibiotics, which treat bacterial infections only.

o   Global human consumption of antibiotics increased 39 percent from 2000 to 2015. [*National Academy of Sciences*, March 2018]

o   In 2015, a 6-month study at a costly day care center found the majority of the children on antibiotics. "One was on five different antibiotics. Another, on triple antibiotic therapy, wasn't even sick." In April, 2018, *JAMA Pediatrics* reported: "Antibiotic use in childhood is tied to increased risk for food allergies and asthma."

"Taking the full course of antibiotics unnecessarily wastes medicine, and ... [creates] drug-resistant genes which transfer to bad bugs. Wiping out drug-susceptible bacteria in infections too quickly makes it easier for drug-resistant bacteria to compete over a host's resources."
Brad Spellberg, LA Biomedical Research Institute

Combining herbs and antibiotics allows us to take less antibiotic, for a shorter time, with complete effectiveness, and far more long-term health. Unlike most antibiotics, which only counter infection, herbs counter *and* prevent infection.

Side effects of **All**: gut flora changes, nausea, stomach pain, dehydration, antibiotic-resistant diarrhea, aplastic anemia, hepatic necrosis; depletion of B vitamins, calcium, magnesium, iron.

Side effects of **Bactrim**: elevated potassium.

Side effects of fluoroquinolone (e.g. **Cipro**): increased risk of Achilles tendon rupture, aneurysms, heart arrhythmias (especially if combined with thiazide diuretics) leading to seizure, death.

Side effects of **Doxycycline**: increased sensitivity to the sun, increased risk of sunburn.

Anti-Hypertension Alternatives
Generally safe, effective when combined with anti-hypertension drugs.

Serenity Medicine:
  o Extra sleep lowers blood pressure.
  o Meditation for five or more minutes lowers BP 20 points.

Story Medicine: Achieving a number or creating abundant health?

Lifestyle Medicines reduce blood pressure as well as drugs do, without side effects, for about three-quarters of all people, and are *safe to use alone, for up to six months, before trying any drug.*
  o Repeat after me: Stop smoking. Eat less salt. Walk more. Drink less alcohol. Eat more vegetables. Monitor your weight.
  o One ounce of **dark chocolate** a day lowers blood pressure as well as any drug. Tastes a lot better too.
  o Eight ounces of **beet juice** (cooked or raw) daily is as fast and as effective as drugs. Beets' nitrates turn into nitric oxide, which widens blood vessels and increases blood flow.
  o Half a cup, twice a day, of **purple potatoes** or **blueberries** is as effective as taking an ACE inhibitor.
  o **Sesame oil** in food compares favorably with drugs in studies.
  o **Flaxseed** – 2-3 tablespoons daily, ground and cooked – lowers heart attack risk by 30 percent, stroke risk by 50 percent within six months.

Alternative Medicine/Herbal Medicine (*safest first*):
  o Potassium-rich **dandelion** root tincture and stinging **nettle** infusion lower BP by increasing kidney health.
  o **Hibiscus** (*Hibiscus sabdariffa*) – 1-2 cups of dried flower tea – acts like a combination of lisinopril and hydrochlorothiazide.
  o **Hawthorn** (*Crataegus* species) – the flowers, leaves, and haws taken as tea or tincture, 1-3 times a day, is a superb heart tonic that is wonderful for elders and safe to use daily for long periods of time.
  o **Motherwort** (*Leonorus cardiaca*) – fresh flowering top tinctured and taken in doses of 1-3 dropperfuls, 2-3 times a day – the lion-hearted herb works its magic in 6-8 weeks; especially for those who have had a stroke, those who are anxious.
  o **Passionflower** (*Passiflora incarnata*) – tea or tincture as desired – perfect for lowering blood pressure. Warms and opens hard hearts. Strengthens the spiritual heart.

Anti-Hypertension Drugs

"*Americans spend more than ten billion dollars a year on drugs to lower blood pressure and billions more on medications to mask the side effects of anti-hypertensive drugs and to treat the heart attacks and strokes associated with these drugs.*"   JAMA editorial, 2010

While blood pressure drugs certainly save some lives, they harm many more. There were 164 million ACE inhibitor prescriptions and 86 million ARB prescriptions written in 2011.

A rigorous review of 33 high-quality trials comparing single drugs against an ACE inhibitor combined with another drug found that combination therapy did not reduce the chance of dying, including deaths from cardiovascular disease, but it did increase the risk of dangerously high potassium levels (by 55 percent), of low blood pressure (by 66 percent), and of kidney failure (by 41 percent).

Side effects of **All**: gastrointestinal distress, diarrhea, weakness; low blood pressure leading to dizziness, falls, fractures; depression, mental-health problems; dry mouth, edema.

o **ACE inhibitors** (e.g. enalapril/Vasotec, lisinopril/Prinivil) *Additional side effects*: 20 percent chance of nagging cough, potassium-overload arrhythmias, angioedema, kidney failure.

o **ARBs** (angiotensin receptor blocker) (e.g. losartan/Cozaar, valsartan/Diovan) – *Additional side effeects*: headache, high cost.

o **Beta blockers** – (e.g. propranolol/Inderal, metoprolol/Lopressor) – block the hormones adrenaline and noradrenaline. *Additional side effeects*: cold hands and feet, weight gain, fatigue.

o **Calcium channel blockers** (e.g. diltiazem/Cardizem, nifedipine/Procardia): *Additional side effects*: acid reflux, headache.

o **Diuretics** (e.g. Lasix): *Additional side effeects*: greatly increased urination, hearing loss from lack of potassium, especially when combined with Advil or Celebrex; increased sensitivity to sun, sunburn; worsens gout and erectile dysfunction.

o **Thiazide diuretics** (e.g. Esidrix, Microzide, Thalitone) and **loop diuretics** lower potassium, so a supplement is prescibed at the same time. *Additional side effeects*: magnesium depletion, confusion, muscle pain, cramps.

Combines poorly with: NSAIDs, decongestants, amphetamines.

Antidepressant Alternatives
Generally safe to combine these herbs with antidepressant drugs.
Non-addictive; few side effects.

Serenity Medicine:
o Sleep deprivation reduces depression in half of all people.

Mind Medicine:
o Antidepressant drugs are often no better than placebos.

Lifestyle Medicine:
o **Exercise.** Go outside. Walk. Be in the sun. Laugh.
o **Low-fat yogurt** consumers are four times less likely to be depressed than those who never eat yogurt.

"Clinical guidelines from the American College of Physicians suggest that St. John's wort can be considered an option along with antidepressant medications for short-term treatment of mild depression."
Charles F. Glassman MD, 2017

Herbal Medicine (*safest first*):
o **St. John's/St. Joan's wort** (*Hypericum perforatum*) – tincture of fresh flowering plants, 2-10 dropperfuls a day. Most studies use dried, encapsulated herb with great results, but side effects, especially drug interactions. Get the same great results, without side effects or interactions, with tincture. **Avoid capsules**.
o **Lemon balm** (*Melissa officinalis*) – dropperful doses of tincture or sips of the tea have a gradual antidepressant effect.
o **Rhodiola** (*Rhodiola rosea*) – root tincture, 1-3 dropperfuls a day – counters mild depression, writer's block, ennui.
o **Cannabis** (*Cannabis indica*) – female flower buds smoked or tinctured, 3-10 drop doses – interferes with sad/bad memories.
o **Saffron** (*Crocus sativus*) – 15 mg twice a day for 8 weeks – as much improvement in mood as those taking Prozac or Tofranil.

Pharmaceutical Medicine: (*May not be safe with other drugs.*)
o **SAMe** – 400-3,000mg/day – as effective as tricyclics.
o **DHA** – 500-1000mg/day with standard drugs for bipolar disorder – counters depression, decreases number of episodes.
o **5-HTP** (Precursor to serotonin) – 50-3000mg/day for 2-4 weeks – as beneficial as standard antidepressant therapy.
o **GABA** – 100-250mg three times/day – effectively inhibits mood-regulating neurotransmitters.

Antidepressant Drugs
It takes at least 6 weeks to determine if these drugs work for you.

Depression affects 11 percent of those 18-25 and 8 percent of those 25-44, but only 5 percent of those over 50. Twice as many women as men are affected. Fifteen million Americans use antidepressants. One-third are over sixty; they have the most severe side effects, including death. Severe withdrawal symptoms prolong the time spent on antidepressants from months to years.

Side effects of **All**: *Mental*: confusion, delirium, short-term memory problems, disorientation, impaired attention; increased risk of suicide, especially in teens. *Addiction/dependence likely.*

Physical: Most antidepressant drugs are anticholinergic, sedative, and hypotensive. They may cause weight gain, sleep disturbances, nervousness, tremors, nausea, dry mouth, constipation, bone loss, manic reactions, blurred vision, sexual dysfunction, anorgasmia, dizziness, changes in heart rhythm, heart attacks, strokes, and falls. *Seniors on antidepressants have more than twice as many hip fractures compared with unmedicated peers.* [Medscape, 2 Jan 2019]

Withdrawal symptoms: headache, nausea, agitation, dizziness.

o **SSRIs/**Selective serotonin reuptake inhibitors (e.g. fluoxetine/Prozac, sertraline/Zoloft). *Extra side effects*: disrupted sodium levels.

o **SSNRIs** and **NRIs/**Serotonin and norepinephrine reuptake inhibitors (e.g. atromoxetine/Strattera, duloxetine/Cymbalta, venlafaxine/Effexor). *Extra side effects*: drowsiness, deep fatigue, liver damage, weight loss, anxiety.

o **Tricyclics** (e.g. imipramine/Trofanil, trimipramine/Surmontil). *Extra side effects*: urine retention, sensitivity to sun, sunburn, fatigue, irregular heart rate, seizures; fatal in excessive doses.

o **MAOIs/**Monoamine oxidase inhibitors (e.g. isocarboxazid/Marplan, selegiline/Emsam). *Extra side effects*: dangerously high blood pressure; can be fatal. Transdermal patches are safest.

Drugs that can **cause depression:** Antivirals, hormonal birth control, statins, corticosteroids, antihypertensives, barbiturates, tranquilizers, reserpine, beta-blockers, heart-rhythm drugs, ulcer drugs, Levodopa, anticonvulsants, antibiotics (especially ciprofloxacin/Cipro and metronidazole/Flagyl), painkillers, arthritis drugs, ibuprofen, Accutane, metrizamide, and Antabuse.

Anti-Anxiety Alternatives
Generally safe and effective to combine these with anti-anxiety drugs.

Story Medicine:
   o Write down your anxious thoughts. Once you have done so, you can read them anytime, but not think them at all. Ahhh.
   o *Fear and excitement feel the same. I choose excitement!*

Lifestyle Medicine:
   o Exercise relieves anxiety. If you feel like running away, run!
   o Caffeine makes anxiety worse; alcohol and sugar do, too.

Herbal Medicine (*safest first*):
   o **Motherwort** (*Leonorus cardiaca*) – tincture of fresh flowering tops by the dropperful, as needed – is my top choice for both immediate and long-term relief of anxiety. Or use **Lemon balm** (*Melissa off.*) the same way; it grows very easily.
   o **Passionflower** (*Passiflora incarnata*) – proven as effective as anti-anxiety drugs, without side effects. Wonderful for children.
   o **Schisandra** (*Schisandra chinensis*) – tincture or infusion of dried berries, used lavishly – is known as "Chinese Prozac."
   o **Skullcap** (*Scutellaria lateriflora*) – tincture of fresh flowering plants, in tiny 5-10 drop doses – relieves nervous fears without causing drowsiness. I do not find tincture from dried plants useful.
   o **Chamomile** or **lavender** – flowers in teas, baths, or hydrosols – soothes tense nerves, calms irritability, and brings peace.
   o **California poppy** (*Eschscholzia*) – 1-3 cups tea or 30-90 drops tincture of the fresh flowering plant – quickly eases tension.
   o **High CBD** cannabis – 3-5 drops tincture or oil of fresh herb.
   o A review of studies found the most successful anti-anxiety herbs: chamomile, skullcap, echinacea, milk thistle, ginkgo, kava kava, ashwagandha, and rhodiola; plus sage, lemon balm, passionflower, gotu kola, or bitter orange for those with dementia, too.

   "Existing preclinical evidence strongly supports CBD as a treatment for generalized anxiety, panic disorder, social anxiety disorder, obsessive-compulsive disorder, and post-traumatic stress disorder." Michael Backes

Pharmaceutical Medicine:
   o **Omega-3 supplements**, 3 grams daily, for 6 months, lessen anxiety, especially in those withdrawing from drugs.

Anti-Anxiety Drugs

More than a dozen drugs, and at least as many soft drugs, are marketed to relieve panic and the jitters. But since we don't know what causes anxiety, we don't know what will reliably relieve it.

Side effects of **All:** dry mouth, leading to increased tooth decay and periodontal problems; drowsiness and dizziness, leading to bone-breaking falls and traffic accidents; headache, nausea.

o **Benzodiazepine tranquilizers** *Addictive.* About 10 percent of all people older than 65 take a benzodiazepine drug – like Xanax, Ativan, or Valium – to counter anxiety. One-third of them are long-term users. Even doctors agree that this is overdoing it.

o **Beta-Adrenergic Blocking Agents**

o **Buspirone**/BuSpar. *Side effects*: restlessness, nightmares.

o **Haloperidol**/Haldol. *Side effects*: very high fever, rapid pulse, confusion, jerky and involuntary movements, spasms, tremors, seizures, muscle rigidity and inflexibility.

o **Phenothiazines** (e.g. Thorazine). *Same side effects as above.*

o **Thiothixene** (e.g. Navane). *Same side effects as haloperidol.*

o **Hydroxyzine** (e.g. Atarax). *Side effects*: blurred vision, agitation, fainting, appetite loss.

o **Loxapine** (e.g. Loxitane). *Side effects*: very dry mouth, difficulty swallowing, tremors, constipation, blurred vision, loss of sex drive.

o **Meprobamate** (e.g. Miltown). *Side effects*: rashes, weakness, addiction, death.

o **Barbiturates.** See page 201.

o **SSRI, SNRI, Tricyclic antidepressants.** See page 207.

"Nearly 80 percent of subjects with both anxiety and depression experienced heightened anxiety when one eye was covered and lessened anxiety when the other eye [alone] was covered."
Harvard Medical School, 2010

Deep Medicine: Psilocybin can help those with serious anxiety, depression, and post traumatic stress disorder (PTSD).

Anti-Inflammatory Alternatives
Generally safe and effective combined with anti-inflammatory drugs.

Lifestyle Medicine:

o   Although some herbal traditions think of pepper as helpful, it is inflammatory to many. **Eliminate all pepper** and peppery foods, like curries, Thai, Mexican, and Indian food, from your diet for six weeks and decide for yourself.

Alternative Medicine/Herbal Medicine (*safest first*):

o   **Linden** (*Tillia* species) – as a tea or infusion of the flowers, freely, with or without honey – is soothing to throat, guts, nerves, skin, bladder, blood vessels, and lungs. A million times better than turmeric. Tastes divine. Safe enough for infants.

o   **Marshmallow** (*Althea officinalis*) – as tea, infusion, or tincture of the dried root, freely, sweetened with honey – is a classic, safe, soothing anti-inflammatory for the digestive and respiratory organs. A bath/poultice of hot marshmallow tea eases aching joints.

o   **Slippery elm** (*Ulmus fulva*) – bark, as a tea, tincture, or powdered and mixed with honey into lozenges – restores intestinal strength, closes gaps in the mucus lining, heals ulcers, quiets irritability, nourishes robust health, quells auto-immune reactions.

o   **Plantain** (*Plantago* species) – Seeds in tea or cooked in food, taken freely, soothe the gut. Leaves, infused in oil, or as a spit poultice, soothe skin distresses. Plantain overcomes all itches.

o   **Arnica** oil (fresh herb in flower) and homeopathic arnica gel are necessary first-aid items for tending all closed skin injuries: contusions, bumps, bruises, sprains, overexertions, and overuse. I apply immediately and often; swelling disappears before my eyes.

o   **Comfrey** (*Symphytum* hybrids) – infusion of the leaf and stalk internally; infused oil, externally – soothes immediately, then works to create flexible strength in the skin, ligaments, tendons, bones, muscles, joints, and the mucus surfaces of the digestive, respiratory, and reproductive systems.

o   **Aspirin-like herbs** are powerful against musculo-skeletal inflammation. They generally lack aspirin's side effects. Tinctures, teas, decoctions, infused oils, and vinegars of **willow** (*Salix*) bark and buds, **wintergreen** (*Gaultheria procumbens*) leaves, and **meadowsweet** (*Filipendula ulmaria*) flowering herb, are useful.

Anti-Inflammatory Drugs

Steroids and **corticosteroid** drugs – including cortisone, hydrocortisone, and prednisone – are the primary anti-inflammatory drugs used to treat allergies, asthma, bronchitis, COPD, hay fever, rashes, reactions to radiation and chemotherapy, eczema, ulcerative colitis, and auto-immune diseases like lupus, IBS, Crohn's and rheumatoid arthritis. Anti-inflammatory agents cause an estimated 7,000 deaths annually and 70,000 hospitalizations. Corticosteroids suppress inflammation by mimicking the effects of natural adrenal hormones.

o **Oral** steroids (tablets, capsules, syrups) – e.g. Cortef, Medrol, Prelone – have the worst side effects because they are systemic.

Short-term use side effects: blood clots (triple risk in first 30 days), thin skin which wounds, bruises, gets infected and is slow to heal (5 times greater risk of sepsis), glaucoma, leg swelling, hypertension, mood, memory, and behavior problems, weight gain, fatty deposits on abdomen/face.

Long-term use side effects: cataracts, hyperglycemia, diabetes, osteoporosis, fractures, suppression of adrenals, lowered immunity.

o **Inhaled** steroids – e.g. Ventolin, Flonase, Qvar, Pulmicort, Asmanex, Flovent – allow a smaller dose for fewer side effects, less hoarseness, fewer oral fungal infections. *Rinse mouth well after use.* Requires 1-3 months of daily use before improvement is seen.

o **Topical** steroids – e.g. Aclovate, Aristocort, Cyclocort, Vanos – *Side effects*: skin thinning/reddening, skin lesions, acne.

o **Injected** steroids – e.g. Kenalog, Clinacort, generics. *Side effects with chronic use*: Skin thinning, loss of skin pigment at injection site, facial flushing, insomnia, high blood sugar, bone loss, immune suppression, glaucoma, cataracts. Injections – often combined with lidocaine – damage the skin and underlying tissues. Injected cortisone can clump and crystalize in the joint, increasing pain. Tiny amounts of the injected cortisone enter the blood stream and breast milk and have systemic hormone-like effects. **Steroid shots double the rate of cartilage loss compared to placebo.**

Steroids are *weakly addictive* and dosage needs to be reduced gradually to avoid painful withdrawal effects.

Antihistamine Alternatives

Generally safe and effective used with antihistamine drugs.

Serenity Medicine:
 o Relaxation techniques are antihistamine wonders for many.

Lifestyle Medicine:
 Calm down histamine response with these natural antihistamines:
 o **Flavonoids** from carrots, sweet potatoes, blueberries, tomatoes.
 o **Omega-3s** from salmon, walnuts, grass-fed meat, flax.
 o **Quercetin** from onions, apples, citrus, broccoli, berries, garlic, tea, grapes, or **fennel** seed tea, sipped 2-3 times per day.
 o **Vitamin C** from pineapple, citrus, wild salads, sauerkraut.

Alternative Medicine:
 o **Acupuncture** has reduced symptoms in several studies.

 Herbal Medicine (*safest first*):
 o **Reishi** (*Ganoderma lucidum*) tea, tincture, or in food, inhibits release of histamine; strengthens adrenal function; moderates reactions to allergens.
 o **Jewelweed** (*Impatiens pallida*) is my favorite natural antihistamine. I boil the entire plant, root and all, in either water (for internal use, freely, against joint pain, allergies) or witch hazel (for external use against poison ivy/oak rash, heat rash, hives).
 o **Ragweed** (*Ambrosia ambrosioides*) – dropperful doses of the tincture of the flowering plant, taken as often as needed.
 o **Echinacea** (*E. augustifolia*) – is a natural antihistamine.
 o **Fennel** seed/root supplies the strong antihistamine quercetin.
 o **Osha** (*Ligusticum porterii*) – 3-7 drops of the dried or fresh root tincture – is a powerful herbal antihistamine. I have seen it counter allergy symptoms, even anaphylactic shock, in seconds.
 o **Oregano** (*Origanum vulgare*) has 7 different antihistamines.
 o **Ephedra** (*Ephedra sinica*) – tea as needed – contains pseudoephedrine, which has the opposite effects of histamine.
 o **Papaya** (*Carica papaya*) – juiced or frozen – inhibits histamine release internally and topically.
 o **Nettle** (*Urtica dioica*) – freeze-dried, daily for 3-6 weeks – 58 percent said allergic symptoms were relieved; 69 percent found it better than the placebo. I prefer nettle infusion; it may take a year or two to completely eliminate allergies though.

Antihistamine Drugs

Histamine is an organic nitrogenous compound produced by connective tissue cells. It is involved in 23 different physiological functions, including regulation of blood pressure, sleep-wake cycle, mood, and sexual function.

Antihistamines are drugs that inhibit the action of histamine in the body by blocking the histamine receptors. They are considered by the medical profession to be "drugs used against the immune system."

Antihistamines are used to treat hay fever, allergies, conjunctivitis, stuffy and runny noses, coughs, chicken pox, chronic fatigue, motion sickness, dermatitis, hives, eczema, *Molluscum contagiosum* (water warts), and more. They are easily available and widely used. Combining several antihistamines in one pill, a current practice, increases risk of side effects..

"The efficacy, tolerance, and safety [of antihistamines] in humans has been widely established and hence they make up one of the largest groups of pharmaceutical agents used worldwide." F. E. Simmons, immunologist

Side effects include: drowsiness, lightheadedness, blurry vision, change in ability to think clearly, dry mouth, nose, or throat, thickening of mucus, gastrointestinal upset, stomach pain, nausea, increased appetite/weight gain, premature presbyopia (farsightedness).

First-generation antihistamines – e.g. Dimetane, Benadryl, Tavist, Drixoral, Triaminic – cause severe drowsiness, leading to falls and auto accidents.

Consumer Reports Antihistamine Best Buys
Based on convenience, cost, effectiveness, safety

o cetirizine/Zyrtec
o fexofenadine/Allegra
o loratadine/Claritin

Second-generation antihistamines – e.g. Claritin, Alavert, Allegra, Zyrtec, Xyzal, Clarinex – are formulated to be less sedating, but are often much more expensive.

"I started with Claritin and it worked good for two years then quit. I went to Flonase [a steroid]; that worked for at least a year. I was fine for a couple years. Then my allergies came back with a vengeance. Allegra worked great for two years. Now I am back on Flonase." Alex, biker, 58

Antiviral Alternatives
Generally safe and effective to use with antiviral drugs.

Story Medicine:
   o   Read *Herbal Antivirals* by Stephen Buhner.

Lifestyle Medicine:
   o   **Sauerkraut** is validated as one of the best ways to prevent and deal with flu viruses. A tablespoon or two of lacto-fermented kraut daily keeps one abundantly well. If infection threatens, double or triple the amount.

Alternative Medicine/Herbal Medicine (*safest first*):
   o   **Elder** (*Sambucus nigra* and other species) – in dropperful doses of tincture of fresh or dried berries, taken as needed – is directly virucidal and protects against viral infections too. Effective against flu (including H1N1), HIV, FIV (feline AIDS), herpes, and strep, staph, salmonella. If it isn't already, this lovely plant will become a favorite once you give it a try. It is easy to make enough tincture to take it every day of the winter.
   o   **St. John's/St. Joan's wort** (*Hypericum perforatum*) – 1-10 dropperfuls daily of **tincture** of the fresh flowering plant internally; infused oil externally. My first choice when nerves are involved. Reliably clears shingles, herpes, cold sores; strong activity against HIV. Frequent doses prevent colds and the flu when I am traveling or at high risk of infection. **Do not take in capsules or as a tea.**
   o   **Chinese skullcap** (*Scutellaria baicalensis*) – a dose of 2-4 dropperfuls of root tincture 3 times a day – used alone or in combination with licorice is an active antiviral and antibacterial agent against flu (including H1N1), pneumonia, SARS, polio, viral encephalitis or meningitis, Lyme, hepatitis, and measles. Herbalist and author, Stephen Buhner, believes the root of American skullcap (*S. lateriflora*) can be used the same way.
   o   Two antiviral compounds – oleanolic and ursolic acids – are found in rosemary, tulsi, and apple peels. This trio would make a lovely tea, but be sure to use organic apple peels.
   o   **Poke** (*Phytolacca americana*) – in doses of 1-100 drops of the fresh root tincture – activates the entire immune system to counter viral infections. The fresh root contains a tremendously potent antiviral compound that, in its purified form, can inactivate HIV.

Antiviral Drugs

Antiviral drugs need to be very specific, as there is a bewildering array of different types of viral particles and viral diseases. There are antiviral drugs that counter flu, others to counter herpes, and different ones to help those infected with HIV.

o **Flu antivirals** (e.g. oseltamivir/Tamiflu, zanamivir/Relenza, peramivir/Rapivab) Many strains of flu, including H1N1, are now resisant to rimantadine/Flumadine and amantadine/Symadine.
Side effects: headache, dizziness, insomnia.
Extra side effects of Tamiflu and Relenza: cough, fever, rash, swelling, back pain, heartburn.

Flu antivirals are not much better than a placebo, and nowhere near as effective as elderberry and sauerkraut. A review of 20 studies found Tamiflu reduced flu symptoms by only 17 hours. Relenza, in 26 studies, reduced flu symptoms from 6.6 days to 6 days but did not prevent pneumonia, ear infections, or sinusitis.

o **Herpes antivirals** (e.g. acyclovir/Zovirax, famciclovir/Famvir) *Side effects*: headache, nausea, dizziness, fatigue, diarrhea; hard on the kidneys.

Herpes antivirals are erratic in their curative abilities in my experience. I find applications of *Hypericum* oil directly on the site and large doses of the tincture internally successful against shingles in a few days and against cold sores/genital sores in even less time.

o **AIDS antivirals** include nucleotide reverse transcriptase inhibitors (e.g. TDF, AZT, abacavir), non-nucleotide reverse transcriptase inhibitors (e.g. EFV, NVP), protease inhibitors (e.g. ATV), fusion inhibitors, CCR5 antagonists, integrase inhibitors, and post-attachment inhibitors (e.g. ibalizumab). Each drug has its own side effects. For instance, AZT causes tingling, burning, numbness in feet, headache and digestive problems.

Hypericum contains an active alkaloid that is highly effective against HIV. I know several people who take it right along with their other AIDs antivirals, without problems.

When drugs are needed, herbal allies help quell side effects, minimize cellular damage, and protect vital organs.

Pharmaceutical Business

"It is a myth that legal drugs have been proven safe."
Thomas J. Moore, Institute for Safe Medicine Practices

Nine out of ten senior citizens and 58 percent of non-seniors regularly rely on a prescribed drug, according to the Agency for Healthcare Research and Quality. More than a million Ritalin prescriptions are written yearly in the US; use increased 83 percent between 2006 and 2010.

Top drugs by function (pharmacytimes.com, 2017)
- Gastrointestinal: PPIs, H2 antagonists, anti-nausea, laxatives
- Musculoskeletal: pain relief, NSAIDs, opiates, opioids
- Respiratory: corticosteroids, anti-inflammatories
- Immune: antibiotics, anti-virals, antifungals
- Neurological: amphetamines, lithium, SSRIs
- Cardiac: statins, beta-blockers, ACE inhibitors, potassium
- Endocrine: insulin, testosterone, estradiol, progestins, anti-histamines, alpha blockers

Most prescribed drugs by class (2010)
- Lipid regulators, mostly statins (e.g. Crestor)
- Antidepressants, fastest growing class (e.g. Prozac)
- Narcotic analgesics (e.g. Oxycodone)
- Beta-blockers (e.g. Inderal)
- ACE (angiotensin-converting enzyme) inhibitors (e.g. Lotensin)

Most commonly prescribed drugs (2014): *per month*
- Synthroid (synthetic thyroid hormone) 21.5 million
- Crestor (statin) 21.4 million
- Ventolin (steroid inhaler) 18.2 million
- Nexium (PPI) 15.2 million
- Advair (corticosteroid) 13.7 million
- Lantus (insulin)10.9 million
- Vyvanse (stimulant, ADHA) 10.4 million
- Lyrica (anti-convulsant) 10 million

Best-selling drugs (2014)
- Humira (interleukin inhibitor; against joint pain)
- Abilify (depression, schizophrenia, bipolar, autism spectrum)
- Sovaldi (antiviral; against hepatitis C)

Step 5: Pharmaceutical Medicine References & Resources

Drugs in General

"Adverse Drug Reactions Cause Over 100,000 Deaths Among Hospitalized Patients Each Year." *JAMA*, 15 April 1998.

Consumer Reports Complete Drug Reference. Consumer Reports, 2000.

Eaton, Joe. "Black Market Meds." *AARP*, May 2016.

Escohotado, Antonio. *A Brief History of Drugs, From the Stone Age to the Stoned Age.* Park Street Press, 1999.

Fried, Stephen. *Bitter Pills: Hazardous Legal Drugs.* Bantam, 1998.

Griffith, Winter MD. *Complete Guide to Prescription & Nonprescription Drugs.* Perigee, 2015.

Goldacre, Ben. *Bad Pharma.* Fourth Estate, 2012.

"How to Save When Your Drug Isn't Generic." *Consumer Reports on Health,* June 2107.

"Impact of Heart Drugs is Different in Men and Women." *Duke Medicine HealthNews.* September 2017.

Inlander, Charles et al. *The Over-the-Counter Doctor.* People's Medical Society, 1998.

Marsa, Linda. "When Good Drugs Do Harm." *LA Times.* Jan 8, 2001. [articles.latimes.com/2001/jan/08/health/he-9609]

Moore, Thomas J. *Prescription for Disaster.* Simon & Schuster, 1998.

"Pay Less for Your Meds." *Consumer Reports,* May 2018.

Physician's Desk Reference: all the FDA-approved package inserts.

Starfield, Barbara. "Is US health really the best in the world?" *JAMA.* 26 July 2000.

Weil, Andrew. *From Chocolate to Morphine.* Houghton Mifflin, 2011.

Wolfe, Sidney. *Worst Pills, Best Pills: A Consumer's Guide To Avoiding Drug-Induced Death or Illness.* Simon & Schuster, 2005.

Zuger, Abigail. "Careful meta-analyses cast doubts on flu drugs." *NEJM Journal Watch.* 15 May 2014.

- www.worstpills.org
- www.lowestmed.com
- www.iodine.com
- www.GoodRx
- www.consumerreports.org
- www.WellRx
- www.nih.gov
- www.drugs.com
- www.ncbi.nlm.nih.gov

- www.medicalnewstoday.com
- www.nlm.nih.gov/medline/

Food Drugs

Blaylock, Russell MD. *Excitotoxins: Tastes that Kill.* Health Press, 1996.

"Ultraprocessed Foods Linked to Cancer." *Tufts Health & Nutrition Letter.* April 2018.

"Propionate activated . . . insulin resistance and weight gain." *Science Translational Medicine.* 24 April 2019.

- https://spinet.org/eating-healthy/chemical-cuisine
- https://wisetraditions.org

"Drug companies . . . have produced some of the most amazing innovations of the past fifty years, saving lives on an epic scale. But that does not allow them to hide data, mislead doctors, and harm patients." [Yet they do.]

Ben Goldacre, Centre for Evidence-Based Medicine, Oxford

Chronotherapy

It makes a difference when you take a drug. Both side effects and efficacy vary by time.

☞ Take blood thinners at night, prevent a.m. strokes.

☞ Take asthma medications late in the day. A single dose of inhaled steroid at 5:30pm is as effective as four doses spread across the day.

☞ Evening chemotherapy improves the odds of success, shrinks tumors more rapidly, and reduces toxic side effects.

[Wright, Kenneth. "Timing is Everything." *Bottom Line Health.* July 2018.]

Supplements

Barrett, S. MD. *The Vitamin Pushers.* Prometheus, 1994.

DeCava, Judith. *The Real Truth about Vitamins.* Printery, 1997.

Fallon, Sally. *Nourishing Broth.* Grand Central, 2014.

Khan S. U. et al. *Annals of Intern Med.* 9 Jul 2019. [Meta-analysis of 16 nutritional supplements and 8 dietary interventions finds minimal cardiovascular benefit and some risks.]

Kresser, Chris. "The little known (but crucial) difference between folate and folic acid." 9 March 2012. (www.chriskresser.com)

"Most Multivitamins Don't Add Up." *Tufts Nutrition Letter.* Feb 2010.

"Should you still take that multi?" *UCB Wellness Letter.* May 2014.

"Vitamin supplements no help. . . ." *Harvard HeartLetter.* March 2014.

"Vitamin Supplements: Hope vs Hype." *Tufts Nutrition.* Aug 2011.

"What Doctors Tell Their Friends About Vitamins." *Reader's Digest.* Aug 2013.

Interactions

"A Grapefruit a Day." *Nutrition Action*, April 2018.

"Blueberries battle cancer cells." *Bottom Line Health*, April 2018.

Cohen, Suzy. *Drug Muggers*. Rodale Press, 2011.

Environmental Nutrition's Guide to Drug-Herb Interactions, January 1999. Available from EN, 52 Riverside Dr, NY, NY 10024.

Fraedon, Joe and Teresa. *The People's Guide to Deadly Drug/Drug, Drug/Food, Drug/Vitamin Combinations*. St. Martin's, 1998.

———. *The People's Pharmacy*. St. Martin's Press, 1989.

Alan Gaby MD. *A-Z Guide to Drug-Herb-Vitamin Interactions* 2nd ed). Harmony, 2006.

McGuffin, Michael, Christopher Hobbs, Roy Upton, Alicia Goldberg. *Botanical Safety Handbook*. CRC Press, 1997.

Penga, CC et al. "Incidence/severity of potential drug-dietary supplement interactions in primary care." *Archives of Internal Medicine*. 22;164(6):630.

Treasure, Jonathan and Mitch Stargrove ND. *Herb, Nutrient, and Drug Interactions*. Elsevier/Mosby Medical, 2017.

• drugs.com/drug_interactions.html
• medlineplus.gov/druginformation.html

Cholesterol

The Cholesterol Myth. www.PeterAttiaMD.com

DuBroff, Robert. "Cholesterol confusion and statin controversy." July 2015. www.ncbi.nim.nih.gov

"Extended-Release Niacin (Niaspan): Do Not Use." *Worst Pills, Best Pills News*. April 2018.

"Top Five Lifestyle Choices to Improve Your Cholesterol." Mayo Clinic. 2017.

"Two years ago, my doctor, who is a dear friend, told me I had to take a statin to lower my cholesterol, which was dangerously high despite a healthy diet and regular exercise. Instead I drank a quart of oatstraw infusion daily for a few weeks, then rotated with nettle every other week. Three months later, after another test, my physician texted me: 'Holy sh*t! Your cholesterol is GREAT. You got your bad (LDL) down from 201 to 117 without taking a statin. And your good cholesterol (HDL) went up. How!?!'

"I still drink my nourishing herbal infusion daily, and my cholesterol is still low."　　　　　　　　Marc, punk rocker, parent, 49

Acid Reflux

"Acid-Suppressing Drugs Associated with Serious Infectious Diarrhea." *Worst Pills, Best Pills.* July 2017.
"Acid Reflux Drugs Overused." *Worst Pills, Best Pills.* Sept 2013.
"Proteon Pump Inhibitors: Increasingly Linked with Stroke, Serious Conditions." *HealthNews,* June 2017.

"PPIs interfere with the ability of blood vessels to relax [by about 30 percent] by reducing their ability to generate nitric oxide."
Gebremariam, Houston Methodist molecular biologist

Pain-Releif

Aliaga, Luis MD. "The Secrets of Pain Relief." Skyhorse, 2016.
"CBD Oil: What's the Evidence?" *Self Healing.* Jan 2018.
"Empire of Pain." *New Yorker.* 30 Oct 2017.
Gill, Lisa. "New Hope for Pain Relief." *Consumer Reports.* Oct 2018.
Ortner, Nick. *The Tapping Solution for Pain Relief.* Hay House, 2015.
"Unexpected Alternative for Pain Relief." *Health News.* Oct 2018.

Drugs that Cause Pain

Chemotherapeutic drugs cause pain in three-quarters of those taking them. Statin users are four times more likely to have nerve pain. Antibiotics, especially Macrobid, Cipro, Levaquin, and Avelox, cause a variety of pains.

Sleep/Sedatives

McIntyre, Anne. "California poppy." (online at positivehealth.com)
Hobbs, Chris. "Herbs, Natural Remedies for Insomnia." (online)
Tannenbaum, Cara MD. "The Dangers of 'Feel Good' Sedatives." *Bottom Line Health.* May 2018.

Antibiotics

Buhner, Stephen Harrod. *Herbal Antibiotics, Natural Alternatives for Drug-Resistant Bacteria.* Storey, 2012.
Hadhazy, Adam. "Stop taking antibiotics when you feel better?" *Discover.* Oct 2014.

"Antimicrobials or antibiotics given early in life can have significant implications upon obesity, diabetes, and the propensity for other diseases."
Jack Gilbert, Microbiome Center, 2018

Hypertension

"Further evidence confirms danger of blood pressure drugs used together." *Worst Pills, Best Pills.* April 2015.

"Which hypertension drug is right for you?" *Men's Health Advisor.* Dec 2015.

"Blood pressure drugs linked to depression and other mental-health disorders." *Washington Post.* 17 October 2016.

"Initial treatment of hypertension." *NEJM,* April 2018.

Drugs that Raise Blood Pressure
NSAIDs, antidepressants, hormonal birth control, deconges-tants, cyclosporine, cocaine, amphetamines, anabolic steroids.

More than 11 million Americans take too much statin, aspirin, and blood pressure medications due to outdated data used to cal-culate risk and dose. [*Annals of Internal Medicine,* 5 June 2018]

Depression

"Use of Common Drugs with Depression as a Side-effect Increas-ing." *NEJM.* June 2018. (up to 61 percent of these using gabapentin or cyclobenzaprine)

"Sleep Deprivation Effective Anti-depressant for Nearly Half of Depressed Patients." *University of Pennsylvania School of Medicine.* 19 September 2017.

Depression Can Be Triggered by: Cancer of the pancreas, bowel, brain, or lymph nodes; viral pneumonia; hepatitis; stroke; Parkinson's; Alzheimer's; hypothyroidism.

Anxiety

Overcoming Depression. Massachusetts General Hospital. 2018.

"Plant-based medicines for anxiety disorders: Review of clinical studies." *CNS Drugs,* 27(4):301-19.

Antivirals

Buhner, Stephen Harrod. *Herbal Antivirals.* Storey, 2013.

Evans, Sanford. *Herbal Antibiotics and Antivirals.* (online)

• www.bbc.co.uk (Why can't we beat viruses)

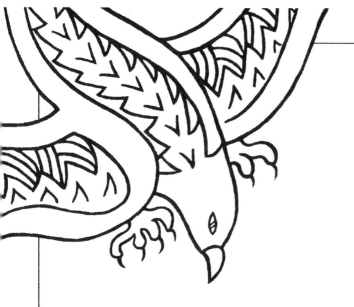

Be Ready

Be ready for inevitable talons
that grip you up through hot green summer grass
and carry your flailing little mouse self
into a sunblinded sky.

If you would be food for gods
if you would offer up your spirit to the Source
then let go of all that pitying nonsense
let go your cherubic candy visions
of any enlightenment less fierce   less absolute
than the hawk's blazing yellow eye.

Miriam Dyak
9 March 2011

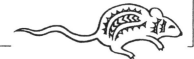

Step Six

Break 6 & Enter

Deep Medicine

"To become wise, one must wish to have certain experiences and run, as it were, into their gaping jaws. This, of course, is very dangerous; many a wise guy has been swallowed."
                                Nietzsche

Break & Enter

- o Bloodletting, self-induced vomiting, enemas, colonics
- o Psychoactive plants ingested by the patient
- o Ultrasound, sonogram
- o Drilling /filling a tooth, root canal, tooth extraction, braces, bone implant, plates
- o Needles: blood draw, IV, epidural, transfusion, liposuction, injections, lumbar puncture, bone marrow transplant
- o IVs: chemotherapy, chelation, saline, drugs, vitamin C drips
- o X-rays: mammogram, angiogram, CT scan
- o Shaving, dermabrasion, chemical peels, skin grafts
- o Laser surgery: face, nose, eyes, vagina
- o Catheterization, conization, cauterization, cryosurgery
- o Body piercing, tattoos, enhancements/reductions
- o Violence, bullying, rape, enslavement
- o Implants: breast, cochlear, birth control, pacemaker
- o Mesh slings for hernias, incontinence, prolapses
- o Electroshock, electroconvulsive therapy, transcranial magnetic stimulation, vagus nerve stimulation
- o Spinal cord stimulation; deep brain stimulation, infrared irradiation; radio-frequency nerve ablation
- o Surgery: open, laparoscopic; biopsy, reattachment, bypass, amputation, stents, transplants
- o Endoscopies: sigmoidoscopy, arthroscopy, laparoscopy, bronchoscopy, colposcopy, colonoscopy
- o D & C abortion, endometrial biopsy, laser ablation
- o Radiation treatments, ingestion of radioactive materials
- o Magnetic Resonance Imagery (MRI)
- o Positron Emission Tomography (PET)

Tap sharply on that which is stuck. Penetrate the boundary. Go in with sharp edges, points, barbs, saws, tools, lasers, streams of atoms, microwaves, radiation, sound. Shape a hole for the holy/whole/healthy self to grow in. Go to the edge of the realm of death. Poison yourself. Enter the deepest mystery. Take the last step. Surrender. Expand. Be rendered, reshaped, remade.

Benefits of Deep Medicine

o Creates miracles
o Saves/extends lives
o Works immediately
o Permanent results
o Last-chance hope

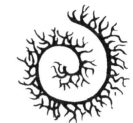

Deep Medicine is the last choice. It is violent, dangerous, out-of-the-ordinary, and often miraculous. When all else has failed, it is time to pull out all the stops and cease being nice, time to drop the bomb, poison the ground, and massacre without regard to innocent bystanders. It is time to do whatever it takes to stay alive.

Sometimes we are thrust into Step 6, unconscious, unaware, bleeding, not breathing. Sometimes we have tried all the Medicines and now come to the last one. Sometimes we stumble into Step 6 deceived into thinking it is preventive, or because we think we must go there, or simply to satisfy our curiosity about what's inside. Deep Medicine is awesome, terrible, thrilling, risky.

Deep Medicine can cause irreparable harm, permanent disability, severe injury, and death, in unplanned and unexpected ways. When faced with a fatal illness, a severe trauma, or unrelenting pain, we accept these dangers. When our problem is too large, too frightening, too invasive for moderate measures, we turn to Deep Medicine. We allow ourselves to be wounded, burned, and poisoned. Deep Medicine makes sense as the last choice.

Step 6 pushes, breaks, cuts, punctures, burns, and violates personal and social norms. At its best, Deep Medicine wrenches us out of unhealthy patterns and creates an opening for wholeness. Surgery, chemotherapy, radiation therapy, or any other Step 6 treatment, can be mythologized, ritualized, understood as a metaphor, and used as a wellspring of energy and gratitude.

"[During chemo] The boundaries of our bodies break. Everything we were supposed to keep inside us now seems to fall out. Blood drips. . . . We emit foul odors. We throw up. . . . Our urine is full of toxins. . . ."
Anne Boyer, *New Yorker*, 15 April 2019

Grandmother Growth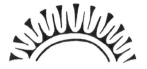

You are standing on a high headland looking down at a torrent of water foaming over jagged rocks. Dark purple lights flicker along the water's surface, prickling the hairs along your arms. You aren't entirely sure you are awake. The strangeness of your previous dream journey lingers. You are trembling.

Grandmother lays a comforting hand on your arm. Her touch eases your tension.

"Be at peace."

You sigh, then laugh as your nervous anxiety subsides.

"But be alert," she warns. "Be aware. The stakes are high: Life. Or. Death. What will you win? What will you lose? What are you gambling with? What are you gambling on? Proceed slowly, carefully, cautiously."

She draws you to her side. Your breath deepens, slows. You feel safer now. But a slight thread of nervous energy still hums in your nerves.

As if reading your mind, Grandmother turns you softly toward her so she can look into your eyes.

"We are here to push the edge, to break through, to be torn apart and sewn together, to be destroyed and reborn. We are here to learn about making sacrifices. We are here to reach into our depths and find our power. We are here to give birth to ourselves and consume ourselves and make love to ourselves and lose ourselves and find ourselves all over again."

You feel the tears brimming up, sliding down, as the wise woman weighs your soul with her eyes.

"Few come here willingly, on their own. They arrive desperate, fearful, and anxious to be accepted. They feel threatened, coerced, bullied, pushed, given no choice. So I give you the gift of knowing that you can choose how to handle being broken: You can despair or you can go down the rabbit hole and see what you can find."

Once again, you are alone, facing your own fears. But you notice that her smile lingers in the air, and in your heart.

Dive Into Deep Medicine

Break the boundary: cut and puncture the skin, push past the sphincters, break the coils of DNA, vibrate until the cell membranes open, wear away the sense of self until it disintegrates, disrupt all that offered protection. Expand your consciousness; taste the colors of the wind.

Release blood, lymph, waste, vomitus, tears, words, secrets, visions, dreams, emotions. Push the reset button.

The only remedies left are violent ones. All else has failed. Rage, mourn, and fight for all you are worth. Fling yourself into the jaws of death; demand rebirth.

Dive into Deep Medicine. Offer yourself up, hang upside down from the Tree of Life, be turned inside out and shaken deeply. Go down the rabbit hole and into the underworld. Sacrifice yourself.

Deep Medicines work at the deepest physical and emotional levels, at the blood and guts levels, cutting and burning, piercing and peering into the depths. For abundant health, integrated medicine reminds us to engage symbolically as well as surgically, psychically as well as physically. Numerous allies, detailed in this chapter, help us take care of our health while medical professionals save our lives, seemingly without regard for our well-being.

The Scientific Tradition of Healing relies heavily on Step 6. If we choose it for diagnosis or treatment, we can best protect ourselves by understanding the real risks, setting strict time limits, and actively working to be our own expert on being healthy.

The Heroic Tradition also relies on Step 6, medically, symbolically, and emotionally: long fasts, flagellation, pilgrimages on bloody knees, penances, hair shirts, sacred mutilations. When we feel guilty about our problem, it seems only right to suffer before we are allowed to regain health.

Choosing Deep Medicine can be a strong choice for life. The risks and the pain can open portals of wholeness, can reveal our personal death, can help us integrate the strong experiences of trauma, and show us how to nourish ourselves to our depths.

Step 6 As Metaphor

Step 6 raises the stakes. Where is safety when we invite a knife to cut into us, radiation to burn us, drugs to poison us? Can that which is divided be rejoined? Can what is broken be mended? Can Deep Medicine nourish wholeness? Can we be whole after parts of us are removed?

The answers, like the questions, are metaphorical. In Korea, witches say the personality must be fractured to permit the guiding spirits to enter. In ancient shamanic healing rituals, the patient is cut off from family, deprived of any personal history, freed from a particular past to create space for the new, healthy person.

(◉) "My **vasectomy** was a ritual initiation. I wish the scars were more obvious."

(◉) "My 10½ pound baby is the great size of our love. The **C-section** opened me to her."

(◉) "I was **Radiant Woman** for the duration of my radiation treatments."

When we peer into our skull with high-tech imagery and slice open our skin with scalpels, we also symbolically alter our mind and create new edges. In Deep Medicine, we pull ourselves apart, crack ourselves up, break ourselves down, get reduced to the nub, and face our own death and dissolution. Without blame. Without shame.

Deep Medicine *dis*-members us; to become whole, we *re*-member and reunite. Deep Medicine forces open the doors and windows of our innermost being, widening us into greater health/wholeness/holiness. Deep Medicine joins with Serenity and invites us into the Void.

"... torn apart ... when you find out that you have cancer. The tearing apart of yourself, along with your loved ones, is visiting hell and coming back alive – at least for now."   Ana Smulian, 38, mother

Be aware of the **hierarchy of harm** in Step 6. Blood draws are safer than spinal taps, which are safer than surgery with a local, which is safer than a bone marrow transplant.

Deep Medicine: Scientific Tradition

Deep Medicine is the glory of the Scientific Tradition. High-tech tests and surgery save countless lives. But screening tests beget mental, physical, and emotional distress. Even necessary tests actively harm. Hospitals, doctors, and treatments can kill you.

The complementary integrated medical revolution helps you protect yourself against over-testing, radiation from necessary tests and treatments, dangerous hospitals, and scary surgery.

Screening Tests

High-tech screening tests subject healthy people to harm in the hopes of finding disease, especially cancer, early. This small harm prevents greater harm, so the thinking goes. This desire is more hope than reality, however. Screening tests do direct and indirect damage to our health while doing little to increase our longevity.

"The claim that a screening test saves lives is almost always based on disease-specific mortality and not overall deaths." Vinay Prasad, oncologist

The physical, financial, and emotional harm done by a Step 6 *diagnostic* test may be justified by the information it provides. But the harm done by a Step 6 *screening* test is rarely justified.

The U.S. Preventive Services Task Force (USPSTF) is an independent expert panel that advises the government and medical organizations about preventive health care. They say too many people are screened too frequently, at the wrong age, with tests that are inaccurate, and too few are getting the tests they do need.

All high-tech screening tests have risks. When those risks are downplayed, we need a revolution, a complementary integrated medical revolution. Go back to Steps 0 and 1 to find safer ways to get information about your health.

". . . a lot of tests seem like they would help, but aren't backed by data and actually open up a whole set of harms." Alex Krist MD, USPSTF

The U.S. Preventive Services Task Force Guidelines for High-Tech Screening Tests

Recommended:

o   One-time **osteoporosis** screening for women over 65
o   Yearly or every-other year **Pap smear** with HPV screening is highly recommended for women 21-65.

Not recommended except for those at very high risk:

o   **Mammogram** (*Biennial screening for women aged 50-74*). No study has shown a decrease in overall mortality for women of any age. An independent meta-analysis of 600,000 women who had regular mammograms found no overall benefit. False alarms, experienced by 50-61 percent of US women who get regular mammograms, cause substantial emotional, physical, and financial distress, including vastly increased insurance premiums. *Instead:* Be in touch with your breasts. Literally.

o   **PSA** test. No decrease in overall mortality for men of any age. Screened groups have much higher rates of impotence and incontinence from biopsies, surgeries, radiation, and chemotherapy. Diaper manufacturers sponsor PSA screening drives. Enough said. *Instead:* Eat pumpkin seeds.

o   **Colonoscopy.** (*Every 10 years after 50*) Does not reduce overall deaths. Serious complications occur in 1 of every 220 tests. Internal bleeding occurs in most tests. "Screening colonoscopy maximizes profits for hospitals and highly paid subspecialists – a result of . . . the profit driven monstrosity that is the US health system." *Instead:* Fecal occult blood test and or sigmoidoscopy, yearly; reduces overall deaths by 2.5 percent.

o   **CT scan** for lung cancer. High risk of serious complications from unnecessary follow-up procedures.

o   **Coronary/carotid artery calcium screening**. CAC and CCTA scans. "Ill-advised." *JAMA Internal Medicine* says carotid screening is "one of the most over-used procedures."

"Clearing a clogged carotid artery could be a solution in search of a problem. The vast majority of people with a blocked carotid artery will die with it, not because of it."   Laura Beil, *Science News*

Some harms are caused by inaccurate tests. **False positives** send hundreds of thousands of people into unneeded surgery. False security from screening tests leads us to believe that every problem will be found by tests early enough to save our lives. Mammograms fail to find 1 in 5 breast cancers. [American Cancer Society, 2015]

Exposing ourselves to radiation is neither safe nor healthy. Even yearly dental x-rays add up over a lifetime (chart, page 273). It is safe to refuse most screening tests. To counter the climate of fear and misinformation around screening tests, ask yourself: "Will this help me create abundant health?" Deep Medicine is too dangerous to be used casually.

Screening tests are not preventive medicine.

The watchdog group Association for the Advancement of Retired Persons (AARP) warns: "Screening tests generate billions of dollars a year, and there's no shortage of hospitals, clinics, and doctors willing to use our fears about cancer and heart disease to recommend and profit by them."

Direct-to-consumer screenings are projected to bring in $350 million a year from: mobile screening with useful EKGs, non-useful carotid artery scans, online and walk-in labs for blood and urine tests, at-home genetic tests, and full-body CT scans. Buyer beware.

Instead, have your eyes examined.

"My chronic, nauseating headaches consistently defy diagnosis. Since I can't be defined by a CT scan, an MRI, or an x-ray, they say it's 'all in my head!' It is, but not the way they mean it." Martina, 33, entrepreneur

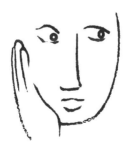

Before Any Step 6 Procedure or Test Ask:

o   Why are we doing this?
o   How will I benefit from it?
o   What are the risks?
o   Might it make my problem worse?
o   Do I need to do this?
o   Are there alternatives?
o   What could happen if I don't do it?

An **eye exam** is an excellent non-invasive screening test. Your retina vasculature can show changes associated with cardiovascular disease, hypertension, multiple sclerosis, rheumatoid arthritis, complications from diabetes, leukemia, and eye lymphoma.

[27 April, 2018; www.uchicagomedicine.org]

Step 6 for Diagnosis

Using Step 6 for diagnosis is hard to resist. Everybody does it. High-tech diagnosis helps medical professionals of all kinds:

o   Provide a standard of care
o   Protect themselves if there is a malpractice claim
o   Take home a bigger paycheck
o   Provide for patients who insist on them

Curiosity can kill us. High-tech diagnosis facilitates disconnection from our corpus, our body. The machine's view is limited; it both magnifies and distorts our human view. We become isolated pieces to be treated by separate specialists.

We need to disconnect just to endure the MRI, the CT scan, the prying and poking of x-rays and blood tests. We need to disconnect to endure waiting for results, wondering if we are measuring up, wondering if the news is good or bad. And the test results are often grounds for further Step 6 tests and interventions.

Once we cross the Great Divide, high-tech diagnosis can save or extend our lives, but at a cost: the loss of our health, the destruction of our mental ease, and sometimes the loss of life itself.

Go back to Step 1 and consider other means of diagnosis. If Step 6 diagnosis is the best choice, protect yourself. Be responsible for maintaining and nurturing your health whenever you venture into Deep Medicine.

Caesarean rates rise when fetal monitor use is commonplace.

"I knew the monitor was broken, but they wouldn't believe me. They insisted that my baby was dying, and did an emergency C-section. It was unnecessary as my baby was never in danger." Corelle, mother of three

Radiation Tests and Therapies

X-rays, Mammograms, DEXA, CT, PET, Tracers

"The medical profession is avidly pursuing better ways to use radiation to increase the benefits to risks ratio."

Louis Wagner, diagnostic physicist

Radiation is invisible. Although it does not cause direct pain, it damages DNA and kills cells, both as a big blast and in small amounts which accumulate over a lifetime or a course of therapy.

Radiation is hot. Its intense heat breaks open and ultimately kills cells. Even if a cell survives, radiation breaks and changes its orderly DNA, making cancer more likely 20-30 years later.

Despite its known ability to initiate and spread cancer, radiation is used in more and more tests and therapies ranging from dental x-rays to CT scans, from the insertion of radioactive materials (pellets) into the body to the use of finely focused and directed radioactive rays to destroy tissues.

We are cautioned to protect ourselves against radiation from the sun to prevent skin cancer. Yet we are told we must expose our breasts and our mouths to radiation as preventive care.

Ninety percent of the total ionizing radiation received by most people comes from x-rays such as mammograms, dental panoramas, and CT scans. Angiograms and DEXA scans are x-rays, too.

Radioactive medical waste and the mildly radioactive excretions (feces, urine, and vomitus) of those treated with radiation now contaminate our environment and are in our food, seeding cancer in generations to come.

The complementary integrated approach partners Deep Medicine professionals – whose focus is saving lives even at the expense of health – with you, the consumer, the patient, for active creation of abundant health using the Seven Medicines.

CT/CAT-scans

Only 5 percent of medical examinations that use radiation are CT scans, but CT scans constitute 35 percent of all medical radiation exposure.

"CT uses truly scary x-rays. Abdominal CT scans cause 12.5 cancer deaths per 10,000 persons exposed to a single examination, comparable to the yearly smoking-induced deaths of 12 per 10,000 smokers . . . that's 2,600 [extra] cancer deaths . . . per year."   Everett Lautin MD

More than 85 million CT scans are done yearly in the US. The National Cancer Institute estimates that 29,000 of the 1.7 million cancers diagnosed in 2007 were **caused** by CT scans. Risks increase with repeated exposures.

"Researchers estimate, in fact, that at least 2 percent of all future cancers in the U.S. – about 29,000 cases and 15,000 deaths each year – are likely to come from CT scans alone. The threat is greatest in children. . . ."
Orly Avitzur MD, *Consumer Reports*

PET and SPECT

These scans capture views of photons released by radioactive isotopes which have been injected into, inhaled by, or swallowed by the patient. PET tests are **the major contributor to low-level radioactive waste pollution.**

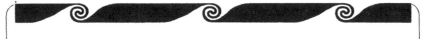

Say "No" to a CT Scan for

o   Severe headaches, back pain [MRI is better]
o   Head injuries in children [unless accompanied by confusion, weakness, loss of hearing or vision]
o   Sinus pain/infections [nasal smear is better]
o   Lung cancer screening [unless you are between the ages of 55-80 and have smoked a pack or more a day for 30 years]
o   Calcification in coronary blood vessels [see page 230, bottom]
o   Pain in side or flank [ultrasound is better first choice]
o   Bowel pain [colonoscopy slightly safer; no radiation]
o   Any reason not having to do with your health and well-being: e.g. if your doctor is worried about malpractice suits or has a financial incentive to order scans

Protect Yourself From Radiation Damage

Radiation causes inflammation. Radiation increases free-radical production. Radiation initiates new, and spreads old, cancer cells.

Compelling scientific evidence confirms plants' effectiveness in protecting against the long-term negative effects of radiation, including the initiation of secondary cancers and the spread of existing cancer. When used before, during, and for 6-24 months after radiation therapy, herbal allies can prevent damage to cells and their DNA, and support healing. Daily use for years is considered safe. Most work best taken before exposure, but some (*) are effective if used afterward. Even one ally will help; more help more.

o   Anti-inflammatory foods: health.harvard.edu
o   Anti-inflammatory herbs: nchi.nim.nih.gov
o   A light film of *Hypericum* oil* – applied an hour before and after radiation therapy, to all skin exposed to radiation – protects normal cells from radiation damage. Also heals radiation burns.

o   **Soy*** activates genes involved in DNA repair and prevents radiation-induced skin cell death. Soy's radioprotective enzyme inhibitors survive processing into **tofu, miso, soy milk**, and **shoyu**. The US military relies on soy supplements to protect personnel "in case of nuclear threat."

o   A dropperful of **Panax ginseng*** tincture – taken an hour before and after each session – sustains energy, reduces damage to both cells and DNA, and supports cellular repair/regeneration. In human cell studies ginseng protected white blood cells from DNA damage for up to 90 minutes after radiation exposure.

o   **Vitamin A,** not in a pill, but from foods like carrot juice, well-cooked carrots, sweet potatoes, winter squash, frozen or dehydrated papaya or mango ameliorates radiation side effects, prevents radiation-induced death of healthy cells, and enhances cancer cell die-off from radiation. **Carrots** contain the water-soluble anti-cancer compound **falcarinol**. To retain it, cook carrots whole and uncut in an inch of water until tender.

o   **Seaweeds,*** like kelp, wakame, and kombu, especially when cooked, absorb radioactivity and carry it out of the body in the feces. This is true even if the seaweed is high in radioactivity.

o   Polyphenol-rich **nourishing herbal infusions**, especially nettle, drunk before exposure to radiation, build healthy blood.

o   **Exercise** speeds recovery from radiation damage. Walk as much as you can, especially when exhausted or in pain.

o   A handful of **nuts** or a spoonful of **nut butter** provides vitamin E, which enhances the effects of radiation on cancer cells while protecting normal cells. **Almonds** protect against cancer.

o   Simmering a tablespoon of powdered **turmeric** in a cup of full-fat milk for a few minutes releases the active ingredient, **cucurmin**. Drinking this golden beverage, with or without the addition of cocoa powder, protects normal cells and up-regulates genes that trigger cell death in cancer, thus enhancing the tumor-destructive powers of radiation therapy.

o   **Ginkgo*** tincture, by the dropperful, can ameliorate radiation damage, even after exposure.

o   **Garlic** – cooked, roasted, raw, powdered – in any amount, is especially effective at protecting red blood cells from radiation damage. It also down-regulates radiation-induced inflammation.

o   Also: avocado, applesauce, beets, broccoli, coconut, cooked greens, grapes/juice/wine, green tea, lemon, sauerkraut.

Adaptogens Aid Radiation Therapy and Chemotherapy

Adaptogenic herbs enhance the cancer-killing effects of chemoradiation, while protecting healthy cells, both during and after therapy. Daily use of 1 cup of infusion, or 25-100 drops of tincture of American ginseng (*Panax*), amla (*Phyllanthus emblica*), and/or Siberian ginseng (*Eleutherococcus senticosus*) during and for a year or more after treatment dependably:

o   Increases survival time and reduces mortality
o   Reduces the inflammatory response
o   Reduces all short- and long-term radiation side effects
o   Reduces pain and fatigue
o   Shields healthy cells from radiation damage
o   Inhibits mutations of genes sensitive to radiation damage
o   Protects the thyroid, heart, and lungs from damage
o   Protects the genome from epigenetic damage
o   Prevents radiation fibrosis
o   Protects lipids from radiation-induced peroxidation

Non-Radiation Tests
Sonograms/Ultrasound, Thermography, Stress Test, MRI, Blood Tests

Sonograms/Ultrasound

Used as a medical diagnostic tool since 1942, ultrasound sends high frequency sound waves into the body, like sonar. A frequency too high/fast to be heard is projected into the body from a small vibrating crystal. The echos from different surfaces are correlated in a computer to create a real-time, moving, grainy, flat, black-and-white image of solid, reflecting surfaces, such as kidney stones, gall stones, aneurysms, uterine masses, ovarian cysts, brain tumors, beating hearts, and developing fetuses.

"[Ultrasound's] interaction with biological tissues is known to induce a wide variety of nonthermal effects ranging from hemorrhage and necrosis to more delicate manipulations of cells and their membranes such as permeability enhancement, angiogenesis induction, and increased gene transfection."   Michael Plaskin, Society for NeuroScience

Ultrasound treatments are used to counter prostate cancer, increase cerebral blood flow, break up stones in the kidneys and gall bladder, and destroy unwanted tissues. In the hierarchy of harm, these treatments are safer than laparoscopic or open surgery.

Diagnostic sonograms are also fairly benign, especially as compared to PET and CT scans. Routine, repeated exposure to ultrasound is not safe for adults however, and any ultrasound may be detrimental to a developing fetus.

". . . routine [fetal] ultrasound [should] be avoided. Only if there are exceptional medical indications should ultrasound be allowed, and at minimum intensity. Sessions should be very brief, no more than 3 minutes, 5 minutes at most. Multiple sessions should be avoided because hazards are cumulative. Human studies had found sensitive organs damaged at 1 minute exposure." Ruo Feng, *Chinese Journal of Ultrasound in Medicine*

Is there a link between ultrasound and autism?
[*JAMA Pediatrics*, 12 Feb 2018]

Routine sonograms do not make babies healthier, nor do they improve pregnancy or birth outcomes. In 2014, the Food and Drug Administration issued a *caution on ultrasound during pregnancy.* Ultrasound is at its most dangerous when used for screening. The U.S. Preventative Services Task Force (USPSTF) recommends a one-time ultrasound to check for aneurysms in men 65-75 who currently or formerly smoked commercial cigarettes. They recommend against this test for nonsmoking women 65-75.

Ultrasound screenings looking for thyroid cancer send thousands to surgery to remove thyroids with nonaggressive, extremely slow-growing thyroid cancer, necessitating life-long dependence on pharmaceutical thyroid hormone. Overtreatment is one of the worst harms of high-tech screening.

Ultrasound screening for ovarian cancer has a high frequency of false-positives. This leads to unnecessary removal of the ovaries, which compromises a woman's health for the rest of her life, increasing her risk of heart disease, cancer, dementia, and premature death. [*Science Daily*, Feb 2017]

Thermography

Thermal images made by an infrared camera reveal heat patterns and blood flow in body tissues, without radiation, compression, or risk, but you are likely to be over- or undertreated: *Thermograms have very high false-positive and false-negative rates.*

Thermograms see heat. Cancer cells and their blood vessels are warm, but warmth can be caused by many things. Biopsies, scans, and surgery following a false positive thermogram damage health directly and indirectly. Thermography doesn't detect breast cancer. A study of over 10,000 women found 72 percent of those correctly diagnosed with breast cancer had normal thermograms.

Cardiac Stress Test

No major medical organization recommends cardiac stress tests – usually an EKG done while exercising hard – for healthy individuals. These low-risk tests are more harmful when combined with drugs and radioactive tracers. Inaccurate results lead to unnecessary angiograms (heart x-rays) and angioplasties (placing a stent in an artery using x-ray guidance).

MRI, Magnetic Resonance Imaging

An MRI scan is loud and tedious, but safe, with the possible exception of contrast dyes. Nonradioactive, but potentially kidney-damaging, **contrast agents** – such as the metal *gadolinium*, which can linger in the brain, skin, and bones for years – are used to improve MRI images of soft tissues. Eating burdock root and/or kelp both before and after the scan helps those dyes move on.

A narrow tube of strong magnets (with you squeezed inside) is used to create a strong field that orients the atoms in your body. Then, a short radio wave burst disorients them.

Your atoms realign themselves as soon as they can, and as they do, they give off tiny radio signals which are computer-analyzed and displayed as three-dimensional images. An MRI can visualize tissues and cells right down to the details of bone marrow.

The visual maps that MRIs provide help with diagnosis, and are used to track the progress of some diseases/treatments.

Blood Tests

A blood draw is Step 6, but low risk, with sterile procedures. Cholesterol levels, kidney and liver function, white and red blood cell counts, inflammatory status, presence of bacteria and viral particles (like hepatitis), vitamin and mineral levels, blood sugar, and antigens produced in the presence of cancer are some of the many diagnostic factors that can be seen in blood.

Overtreatment is the biggest problem. Once a number is established, treatment becomes focused on changing the number, usually with Step 5 drugs and supplements, and actual health is not addressed.

Unless there is a reason to believe it is needed, a complete blood screen is generally not helpful. The USPSTF recommends neither for nor against a complete blood screen for healthy people.

A **fecal occult blood test** is not a blood draw, but a way to look for blood in the stool. It is quite safe, unless you panic over a false positive result and wind up injured by Step 6 procedures.

"It is estimated that over the span of a decade the results of 50-61 percent of mammograms, 10-12 percent of PSA tests, and about 23 percent of regular fecal occult blood tests will be false positive."
Berkeley School of Public Health, August 2018

Surgery

*"Any time you go under the knife, there is a potential for life-threat-
ening complications. Even in the best of circumstances, bad things
can happen."* Lawrence Schlachter, neurosurgeon

Odds of having a successful surgical outcome are improved if
we start with a conscious decision which has come from deep
thought, clear goals, and loving support.

All surgery, no matter how safe the surgeon claims it is, can
lead to unexpected death and disability. A 2015 review of 2.3 million surgeries done in the US revealed 63,000 patients who suffered serious injury and 3,405 who died. A third of those hospitalized get worse or die due to medical errors and hospital-acquired
infections.

Before you agree to surgery: Collect information. Get a second opinion. Investigate alternatives. Comparison shop. Seek non-
surgical, non-drug options. Push back.

A study of 200 people with a meniscus tear in a knee found 100
percent of those who had surgery developed arthritis within a year,
compared with 59 percent of those who didn't have surgery.

Protect yourself when you venture into Deep Medicine by con-
tinuing to ask questions. Reach out to knowledgeable friends. Find
an advocate: a trusted person who ideally accompanies you to all
doctor visits and to the hospital for all treatments. Share your
thoughts and feelings with your advocate. Listen to your advocate.

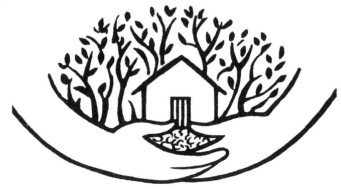

With your advocate or by yourself: make a plan to increase your personal health before surgery, decide which treatments suit you best, choose a surgeon, pick a hospital, select an anesthesiologist, and read the consent form before signing it.

Increase Your Personal Health

Surgery is as dangerous as white water rafting or climbing a 20,000-foot peak. To survive and benefit, you must be well prepared. Your resiliency, fitness, and mental state before and after surgery are as important to the outcome as the skill and knowledge of the surgeon and anesthesiologist.

Every bit helps, even a few days, even small changes.

o **Sleep** more.

o **Relax**/meditate and you will heal faster.

o **Exercise**. 84 percent of surgical/chemo patients who did aerobic and resistance exercises before treatment recovered faster.

o Do simple **breathing** exercises to lower risk of pneumonia and other respiratory infections. Inhale for 3-5 seconds, hold for 3-5 seconds, exhale like blowing out a candle for 6-10 seconds.

o Eat more **phosphate**-rich foods, such as cheese, yogurt, shrimp, fish, pumpkin seeds, meat, lentils to prevent infections.

o Eat more **zinc**-rich foods, like spinach, nuts, chocolate, beans, meat, and seafood to increase your immune power.

o Eat more **protein**: Reduce post-op complications 50 percent.

o Increase the amount of **iron** in your blood to guard against blood loss, fatigue, and infections. Molasses, nettle infusion, and yellow dock root tincture are good sources of iron.

o Donate your blood, just in case it is needed.

o **Prehab** instead of/in addition to rehab. STAR programs (oncologyrehabpartners.org) and Strong for Surgery (strongfor surgery.org) offer help. Specific moves – such as shoulder stretches for women facing breast removal – can help you heal faster.

o Engage in yoga, Tai chi, or Qi Gong to calm the mind, center the body, and access universal healing energy.

o Cut back on/eliminate cigarettes, alcohol, refined and artificial sugars, supplements, aspirin, and encapsulated herbs.

Is it Time for Step 6?

When life and death seem to hang in the balance, we agree too readily to Deep Medicine. Take your time. Use Serenity Medicine as an aid to decision making. If pressed to decide, ask for time to think it over. Deep Medicine draws one in, deeper and deeper. One scan begets the next; one surgery makes the next more likely. When fear calls the shots, we often shoot ourselves in the foot.

If you agree to Deep Medicine, set a time limit for leaving Steps 5 and 6. Join the Complementary Integrated Medicial Revolution and be healthy even as Deep Medicine tears you open. Imagine yourself in abundant health in a specific season. Increase nourishment and tonification. Collect information before and throughout your treatment to protect your health.

Your Advocate

stays with you – overnight too, when possible – so they can:
- ♥ Prevent nurses from waking you up
- ♥ Insist all medical personnel wash their hands
- ♥ Be sure you are given the correct meds at the proper times
- ♥ Oversee sterile procedures for blood draws, catheters
- ♥ Sanitize surfaces in your room with alcohol/bleach wipes
- ♥ Get copies of your labs, tests, scans, meds, all reports, doctors comments, everything that is available
- ♥ Provide you with hydration
- ♥ Rub arnica gel on your feet (not on the surgical site)
- ♥ Orient you during emergence
- ♥ Focus love on you throughout your stay
- ♥ Be with you at these times:
  - ♥ When you sign anything
  - ♥ Before and after any procedure
  - ♥ Before and after surgery
  - ♥ When you are moved
  - ♥ When the doctor does rounds
  - ♥ When you are given medication
  - ♥ When you are discharged

Choose the Best Surgeon

Do not assume that the surgeon who recommended the surgery is the best. Treat the search for a surgeon as though your life depended on it. It does. Mortality among patients of top surgeons rarely exceeds 3 percent, for poorly-rated surgeons, it is 11 percent: nearly four times as many deaths.

Stanford University researchers found 1 percent of doctors account for 32 percent of paid-out malpractice claims.

- o Confirm state credentials at Federation of State Medical Boards using their Consumer Resources. (fsmb.org)
- o Confirm surgical certification with certificationmatters.org
- o Uncover reprimands at fsmb.org/policy/contracts
- o Confirm that s/he has "recent and significant" experience
- o Check ratings, number of procedures performed, and complication rates of 50,000 doctors at SurgeonRatings.org.

Interview potential surgeons

Ask: Is this your specialty?

Ask: How do you handle complications?

Ask: Are you yourself going to do the entire procedure?

You can write the full name and title of your chosen surgeon on the consent form with a statement that you consent only to that person doing the actual surgery. Initial it.

Ask: What else will you be doing while you are operating on me? *Some surgeons do two surgeries at the same time.*

Ask: How can I help myself?

Ask: Is minimally-invasive surgery (laparoscopic) or open surgery better for me? Surgeons push the less invasive surgery, but overall survival is often better with open surgery.

Two studies published in the New England Journal of Medicine found that laparoscopic or robot-assisted radical hysterectomy was associated with better surgical outcomes but poorer survival rates compared to open surgery. Minimally-invasive surgery was also associated with significantly *higher* mortality (9 percent) compared to open surgery (4 percent).

Choose the Best Hospital
Hospitals Can Kill You

"When I tell people that my children were born at home, they often ask: 'Weren't you afraid?' 'Oh, yes, I was scared to death – of hospitals!' I would reply."   Eve G., mother, accountant

Hospitals are dangerous places. According to Johns Hopkins School of Medicine, more than 250,000 Americans die each year from medical blunders and safety lapses **in hospitals**. A fifth of the hospitals ranked best on social media were the worst in terms of infections and readmissions.

"Among patients undergoing surgery to remove cancer . . . 17.3 percent of patients at low-volume hospitals died within a month, compared with just 3.4 percent of those treated at the highest-volume centers."
Damaris Christensen [*J Nat Can Inst*, 20 Aug 2003]

Greater transparency and accountability create better outcomes.
o   CR.org/hospital-ratings offers info on incidence of five types of infections and other measures of patient safety.
o   Qualitycheck.org tells you if the hospital is accredited.
o   Teaching hospitals have lower complication rates.
o   Intensivists, who are specially trained to manage the complex care of those requiring intensive care (ICU) reduce critical care deaths by 40 percent. Is there one available?
o   What kind of prehabilitation/rehabilitation is offered?
o   What criteria have to be met for your discharge?

"Each year an estimated 400,000 people die from medical error."
Leslie Michelson, Private Health Management

"The Harvard Medical Practice Study, published in 1991 in The New England Journal of Medicine, found that nearly four percent of hospital patients suffered complications from treatment which prolonged their hospital stay or resulted in disability or death, and two-thirds of such complications were due to errors in care. It was estimated that, nationwide, 120,000 patients die each year . . . as a result of errors in care."
Atul Gawande MD, public health researcher, Harvard

The Consent Form

Get a copy of the consent form as soon as you agree to surgery. Do not read it for the first time on the day of your surgery. Read it carefully, every word.

Ask questions. You do not have to consent to anything you do not fully understand.

On some forms you can cross out and initial any items you do not consent to. On others, your surgeon must add your exemptions, such as no blood products, no general anesthesia. You are *not* required to agree to allow the surgeon to do "whatever is deemed necessary."

o   Talk with your surgeon about your wishes before the day of the surgery.

o   Be clear on the consent form about what tests you want done on excised materials.

o   If you want to maintain possession of any parts of yourself that are removed, say so, and write it on the consent form.

"Overwhelming data show that when patients actively participate in their own care, they have better outcomes." Peter Pronovost MD

o   Radio frequency chipped sponges are far less likely to be left behind. Does this surgeon use them?

o   Be clear about the costs. Ask your surgeon to make sure everyone involved – anesthesiologist, surgical staff, pathologist and radiologist – is in your network. Ask the hospital too.

o   Make your advocate your health-care proxy.

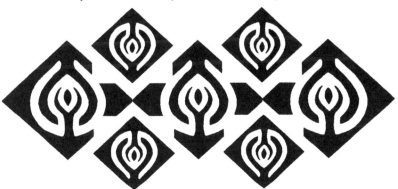

Anesthesia

" We have four goals: to see that you have no pain, that you're drowsy or unconscious, that your body is still so the surgeon can work on it, and that you aren't left with bad memories of the procedure."

Kristen Schreiber, MD, anesthesiologist

Anesthesia, from the Greek *anaisthetos,* "without sensation," affects pain sensing, ability to move, memory, breathing, blood pressure, blood flow, and heart rate/rhythm during and after surgery.

Anesthesias have very different effects on cells with XX genes (female) and those with XY genes (male). If you present yourself or wish to be seen as different from your true genetic sex, it is vital that you let the anesthesiologist know the truth of your cells.

To protect yourself against overuse of anesthesia, which can cause long-term damage, use the least you can during your procedure.

One can ask for (insist on, demand) local, regional, or neuraxial anesthesia even if the standard is sedation or general anesthesia.

Combine a regional block or epidural with general anesthesia to reduce the amount of general anesthesia needed, reduce side effects and after effects, and reduce the amount of narcotic painkillers needed.

One can even refuse local anesthesia. At the dentist's, some find the pain of drilling more tolerable than the injection pain, the hours of pain afterwards, and the lingering numbness.

Local anesthetics – e.g. novocaine, lidocaine – are injected or applied dermally to numb a small area, like the gum around a tooth. You remain awake. *Side effects* such as dizziness and tremors are minimal unless epinephrine is also used; persistent numbness, fatal allergic reactions, heart attacks can occur, but are rare.

Local is the safest choice. If you can lie still, remain calm, and tolerate the sensation of pressure, choose local anesthesia, even when sedation is the norm, for abundant health.

Caution: Local anesthesia is not deliverd via an IV. If you and your doctor have agreed to use only local anesthesia, you have the right to *refuse the insertion of an IV line before the surgery.* You may have to be very firm about your wishes.

Regional anesthesias – e.g. bupivacaine – are injected into a nerve cluster to block nerve impulse transmission between the brain and an area of the body; often combined with hypnotics. You remain awake. *Side effects:* numbness, tingling, tremors, abnormal heart rhythms, anxiety, apprehension, back pain, blurred vision, cardiac arrest.

Neuraxial anesthesias, or **peripheral nerve blocks**, numb large areas; useful for hernia repair, stent placement, and C-sections. Epidural, caudal, and spinal blocks remove sensation to the entire abdomen and lower body. When used with general anesthesia, the need for post-operative pain-killers is reduced. *Side effects:* Headache, sudden drop in blood pressure, death.

Sedation (*dissociative anesthesia* or *twilight anesthesia*) suppresses central nervous system activity less than general anesthesia, so consciousness is maintained. Sedation provides hypnotic, sedative, anxiolytic, amnesic, anticonvulsant, and muscle-relaxing effects; it inhibits anxiety and helps prevent traumatic memory formation. *Benefits:* No tracheal intubation or mechanical ventilation required; less effect on the cardiovascular system. *Side effects:* Muscle control and coordination may be adversely affected.

General anesthesia is a mix of intravenous and inhaled drugs that suppress central nervous system activity, cause loss of consciousness, prevent memory formation, relax muscles, and minimize pain. The drugs are safe, however, they interfere with the ability to breathe so much that intubation is the standard during a procedure requiring general anesthesia. *Side effects* of general anesthesia include nausea/vomiting, headache, sore throat, chills, impairment to bowel and bladder functions, heart problems/attack, pneumonia, pulmonary embolism, delirium, persistent memory problems/cognitive dysfunction, death.

Patients under general anesthesia must undergo continuous physiological monitoring to ensure safety. In the U.S., monitoring includes electrocardiogram (ECG), heart rate, blood pressure, inspired and expired gases, oxygen saturation of the blood, and temperature. In the UK, monitoring may also include urine output, central venous pressure, pulmonary artery pressure, cardiac output, cerebral activity, and neuromuscular function.

A quarter of us dream during general anesthesia and 1 or 2 of us per 1000 are left "aware but unable to move or communicate."

Allies for Those Choosing Surgery

Complementary integrated medicine uses Mind, Lifestyle, and Herbal Medicines before, during and after surgery to prevent and offset the problems it causes – including blood clots, mental diminishment, scars, adhesions, contractures, chronic pain, disability, and nerve, heart and lung damage – some of which may occur right after surgery, some not until years later, and some never.

 ## Close to Surgery Allies

o   Request the earliest day of the week and the earliest **time** of day available. Cuts and burns that are suffered during the day heal 60 percent faster than those incurred at night.

o   **Say "No" to tests** before the surgery. Seven medical societies of specialists advise against pre-op stress tests. Unless specific to the surgery, x-rays and blood tests are also unnecessary.

o   Stop taking vitamins, aspirin, and herbs in capsules 3-7 days before your surgery. Nourishing herbal infusions and tinctures of tonifying and adaptogenic herbs count as foods, not drugs.

o   If you haven't already, meet and talk to your anesthesiologist. By phone is fine. A 5-10 minute talk with the anesthesiologist was more calming to 200 patients awaiting surgery than a sedative. Ask about the anesthesia/s. Would s/he would be willing to play a tape of affirmations for you during surgery?

o   Guided imagery, **affirmations**, or visualization before and after surgery helps you heal faster, sleep better, need less pain medication, and feel safer.

o   Positive conversation just before surgery is more relaxing than drugs are.

o   Being scared, nervous, or upset before any invasive test or procedure doubles your risk of an adverse after-effect. A 5-10 drop dose of **motherwort** tincture under the tongue safely relieves pre-surgical jitters.

Right Before & During Surgery Allies

"Patients who heard positive affirmations on a tape played while they were under anesthesia required 50 percent less postoperative medication than a control group."   Andrew Weil MD

o   NPO, that's *non per os*, Latin for "nothing by mouth," after midnight before surgery is the standard advice, but it is not good for your health. If your surgery is delayed or scheduled for later in the day, going 8-12 hours without a drink will leave you dehydrated, and at risk for complications.

You need good blood sugar levels to endure and recover from anesthesia and surgery. That's difficult if you fast for more than eight hours. Surgical patients allowed to drink feel better overall, experience less anxiety, require less IV fluids, maintain a better metabolic rate when under anesthesia, and recover faster.

o   Let nourishing **oatstraw** infusion build your electrolytes and calm your nerves. Avoid milk, alcohol.

o   Ask those who love you to focus **loving kindness** toward you and the surgical team on the day of your surgery. You'll feel it.

♥   Arrange for your pillow, nightgown, music, pictures of nature, and your pain remedies to be in your recovery room.

♥   Pack your own toiletries, tissues, and toilet paper.

♥   Be sure homemade healing foods can be brought to you.

♥   Ask if a pet can visit you.

♥   Get up as soon as you can. Patients who get out of bed get out of the hospital up to two days earlier.

o   Dr. Andrew Weil urges your surgeon to authorize high doses of **vitamin C in an IV drip** – 20 grams over a 24-hour period – during the entire time you are in surgery. *Note:* Even if the surgeon is willing, this may not be allowed, or covered.

o   Surgeons who work with the **music** of their choice in the background have been found to be more accurate and efficient.

o   Patients who listen to music beforehand are less anxious going into surgery and request less pain medication afterward.

Immediately After Surgery Allies

Emergence from general anesthesia or sedation requires careful monitoring. Common complications include hypothermia, shivering, nausea, and confusion.

"Recovery from anesthesia is not simply the result of the anesthetic 'wearing off,' but also of the brain finding its way back through a maze of possible activity states to those that allow conscious experience. Put simply, the brain reboots itself."   Andrew Hudson, professor of anesthesiology

o   Be especially kind to yourself after surgery.

o   Find a way to say "Please forgive me" to your body. You have allowed it to be pierced with needles and cut with sharp knives.

o   Receive **Reiki** or energy work while in the hospital.

o   Hasten healing and avoid complications with drinkable protein: nourishing herbal infusion, miso soup, bone broth.

o   Stretch. Roll over. Sit up. Swing your legs. Stand. **Movement** decreases your risk of pneumonia and hastens recovery.

o   But don't go to the toilet alone. About 15 percent of patients fall in the bathroom, resulting in serious injury a third of the time.

Nausea

The most common side effect of anesthesia is nausea/retching/vomiting, experienced by about a third of all patients.

o   **Ginger** is the world's best anti-nauseant; better than drugs. It warms deeply, too. Chew on candied ginger or sip ginger tea.

o   **Slippery elm** balls – I mix the powdered bark with honey or maple syrup and roll it into balls – dissolve in the mouth to stop vomiting and nausea, soothe the throat, and hasten the clearance of anesthesia from body. So does **marshmallow** root infusion.

Pain

All postsurgical patients experience pain. Meditation, herbs, and drugs can relieve it. Pain relief helps the immune system, decreases the risk of infection, hastens healing, and decreases the risk of blood clots. Avoid opiate and opioid drugs when possible.

Persistent pain can sensitize the nerves and turn into chronic pain. The standard is to give pain-killers "before any pain is felt." This almost always results in overuse, with larger doses taken closer and closer together, and loss of abundant health.

Pain is a dynamic process that can also be changed with relaxation, meditation, affirmation, and herbs. Because these medicines change your perception of pain, not the pain, they become more effective the more often you use them. Use less pain-killing drugs by combining them with Mind Medicine and Herbal Medicine.

o **Nature**. A window, a painting, even a photo of a "green view" shortens stays after surgery, reduces the amount of pain-killers needed, and lowers the number of complications.

o **Arnica** gel applied liberally and frequently to the soles of the feet counters postsurgical pain, prevents bruising, and discourages swelling and inflammation. So does homeopathic arnica.

o **CBD** oil or tincture (*Cannabis*), taken in small (3-10 drop) doses, as often as needed, even hourly, quickly eliminates most pain, is non-psychoactive, and is reliably non-addictive.

o **Kava kava** (*Piper methysticum*) root infusion, by the cup, or 25-50 drops of the tincture, several times a day, helps prevent chronic pain, reduces muscle soreness, and calms fears.

o **Skullcap** tincture (best from fresh flowering plant), taken in 10-25 drop doses, as needed, also works immediately to mute pain. I like to alternate doses of skullcap and CBD tincture.

o **St. John's/Joan's wort** (*Hypericum perforatum*) tincture of fresh flowering plants, taken in 25-30 drop doses as often as needed, eases musculo-skeletal pain, soothes and counters nerve pain, prevents chronic pain, reduces stiffness and soreness, nourishes rapid healing of nerves, acts as a potent anti-viral, and prevents postoperative depression. *Do not use capsules, tea, or dried plant tincture.* Homeopathic preparations of *Hypericum* work the same way.

As long as these herbal remedies are **not taken in capsules**, *it is considered safe to use them with pain-relieving drugs.*

Stroke

From 1-10 percent of patients have a stroke during or after surgery, often from a blood clot. Nettle infusion may help prevent that.

Cognitive problems

Anesthesia muddles our ability to think and focus. The immediate post-anesthesia confusion (emergence delirium) dissipates very rapidly. But when diminished cognitive function lingers, it can slowly and subtly deteriorate into long-term cognitive dysfunction.

Mineral-rich nourishing herbal infusions protect the brain and help keep neural pathways clear.

Post-operative cognitive dysfunction (POCD) occurs mostly after cardiac surgeries. Older age is a strong risk factor.

Pneumonia

Half of the 2 percent of patients who develop pneumonia after surgery die of it. Keep your lungs strong and free from infection with preventive doses of **elecampane** (*Inula helenium*), **mullein** (*Verbascum thapsus*), and **echinacea**, alone or together. They are generally considered safe to take with antibiotic drugs.

o   Tincture of the fresh or dried root of elecampane, 10-25 drops, taken frequently, scares infection away.

o   Infusion of dried mullein leaves, hot with milk and honey, or tincture of the fresh leaves, in doses of 25-50 drops several times a day, restores health to the lungs as if by magic, and protects the lungs, but does not counter infection.

o   Doses of 50-100 drops of *Echinacea augustifolia* root tincture, taken every 1-4 hours, gets my vote as best herbal antibiotic.

Also

o   Engage the power of art to heal the psychic wound.

o   Ask for nurses to do a bedside shift change so your up-to-date health information is shared in your presence.

o   Keep a log, or have your advocate do it. Include all doctor visits, the meds you are given, everything.

o   Do not leave the hospital until your follow-up appointment is scheduled. It is the "single most effective strategy to reduce your chance of readmission."

o   A third of adults experience medication-related problems within eight weeks of discharge after surgery. Nearly 80 percent require treatment; some die. [*British Journal of Clinical Pharmacology*, 23 May 2018]

Deep Medicine: Fear as an Ally

Fear may join us anywhere along the path of the Six Steps of Healing, but it lives at Step 6. Fear drives us to it and fear haunts us when we are there. We fear the harm we invite; we fear more that we will die unless we do that harm.

Fear makes the breath shallow, which brings less oxygen to the brain, interfering with thinking. We may suffer a paralysis of will, a kind of depression where our distorted thinking tells us that since we are going to die we might as well try anything that could work.

Faced with a diagnosis that implies death if we don't try Step 6, we are bound to feel afraid. It seems easiest and best to turn our health over to the experts and to trust that what they do is for the best. Fear can make us distrust ourselves and our bodies.

Fear can derail our healing efforts. It is a useful emotion; it protects us. But it is difficult to discern whether the dangers it points out are true dangers, and whether they are as large and gruesome as they seem to our imagination. Waiting too long to have a cancerous tumor removed can have extremely adverse effects on quality and quantity of life, but so can doing it too fast, without emotional backup and personal preparation.

When we stop struggling against fear, it becomes an ally. When we use all Six Steps of Healing, we allow fear its due, but avoid giving ourselves to its compulsions. We use it to fire our curiosity and to hone our wits in difficult situations. We use it to protect our wholeness. We use fear to reach our goal when we must enter into the realm of death itself to claim our wholeness. Only the foolish enter there without fear as fuel for the return.

We fear the needle and dread the knife, but our desire for life, for healing, for wholeness pushes us over the edge, into the deep.

Deep Medicine: Heroic Tradition

Humoral Theory
Balance and Detoxification

"Balance is the opposite of life. Cleansing damages and destroys."
                                                    Grandmother Growth

The Humoral Theory – that balance of the four humors is the key to good health, and that the humors must be detoxified to achieve health – defines the Heroic Tradition.

If you have been told to drink after a massage, or that some herbs are blood cleansing, or that sweating will remove toxins, you have encountered the Humoral Theory.

For good health, or to reverse disease, the humors – red blood, yellow bile, black bile, and white phlegm – must be balanced by cleansing away toxins with six "Hygienic Purification Methods."

1. Derivation – Drawing out toxins through the skin
2. Diaphoresis – Cleansing toxins out by sweating
3. Diuresis – Increasing urination to void toxins
4. Emesis/*Puking* – Vomiting to throw up bile toxins.
5. Purgation/*Purging* – Purging with laxatives, cathartics, enemas, and colonics to eliminate bowel toxins.
6. Venesection/*Poking* – Bloodletting to remove toxins from the blood. Cupping is a Step 4 way to "let" the blood.

Liver cleanses are a modern addition to the classic purification methods. They can be quite damaging to the liver and gall bladder. Nothing can cleanse the liver, and it isn't dirty. It can be nourished with dandelion or chicory to do a better job however.

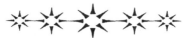

Poking, purging, and puking are all Step 6 methods and carry high risks, despite protestations to the contrary by practitioners. Beware. You are not toxic. The best way to "detoxify" is to strengthen and nourish the organs of elimination: the liver, the skin, and the kidneys.

Poking: Bloodletting

"[Aggressive bloodletting and vigorous purging with mercury] . . . strangles a fever . . . imparts strength to the body . . . renders the bowels, when costive, more easily moved by purging physic . . . removes or lessens pain in every part of the body. . . ."
Dr Benjamin Rush MD (1745–1813)

Blood is dangerous. It is the stuff of life, and death. The other humors are expelled regularly by the natural body processes of defecation, urination, sweating, crying, coughing, and blowing the nose. Only blood has no "spontaneous" exit; it must be "let."

Menstrual blood is toxic in the Humoral Theory. How toxic? Pliny the Elder (23-79 CE) says:

"If a woman strips herself naked while she is menstruating, and walks around a field of wheat, the caterpillars, worms, beetles, and other vermin will fall off the ears of corn."

Bloodletting began at least 3000 years ago in Egypt and spread to the Greeks, Romans, and Arabs. In Europe in the Middle Ages, it was the standard treatment for most complaints. In America, its medical popularity peaked in the nineteenth century and has waned ever since.

"The membrane between medicine and myth is thinner than we suppose, and blood is continually circulating back and forth across it."
Jerome Groopman, "Pumped" [Reviewing *Nine Pints*]

Famous Bleedings

Charles II (1630–1685) was treated for a seizure by the letting of 16 ounces of blood directly from his left arm and another 8 ounces cupped out. This was followed by emetics, enemas, purgatives, mustard plasters, and bloodletting from the jugular until he died.

George Washington (1732–1799) was treated for fever and respiratory distress with bloodlettings, blisterings, emetics, and laxatives. He died from the side effects of the treatments, which, even then, aroused controversy.

Bloodletting is done by venesection, arteriotomy, scarification with cupping, and by leeching. Venesection, the most common procedure, uses special knives called lancets and fleams. The premier medical journal in England today is still called *The Lancet.*

"Different blood vessels serve different purposes. Bleeding the veins between the eyebrows is good for long-stand headache, cutting the veins under the tongue . . . is useful for angina. . . . Opening the sciatic vein relieves elephantiasis; menstrual problems are alleviated by cutting the saphenous vein."   Avicenna, Persian physician (980-1037)

Leeching is the most common form of bloodletting used in modern medicine, though in steep decline from its glory years. In the 1830s, 5 to 6 million leeches a year were used in Paris alone.

There are more than 600 leech species. Medicinal leeches are freshwater, multi-segmented annelid worms. They have ten stomachs, thirty-two brains, nine pairs of testicles, and hundreds of teeth. The bite causes far less trauma than a cut with a scalpel, and the leech injects a natural anesthetic, so there is no pain. Leeches are used medically today to help control and stop hematomas after micro-surgery and reimplantation surgery. They secrete biologically active substances helpful in healing such as hyaluronidase, fibrinase, proteinase inhibitors, and hirudin, an anticoagulant. A "mechanical leech" was created at the University of Wisconsin.

Bloodletting therapy is used in modern medicine to treat blood diseases such as hemochromatosis.

"We may wonder why the practice of bloodletting persisted for so long . . . [and] be tempted to laugh at such methods of therapy. But what will physicians think of our current medical practices 100 years from now? They may be astonished at our overuse of antibiotics, our tendency to polypharmacy, and the bluntness of treatments like radiation and chemotherapy."
  Gerry Greenstone MD, *History of Bloodletting*

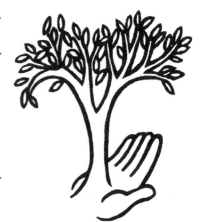

Puking: Therapeutic Vomiting

While expectorants like cayenne are used to reduce the phlegm humor, the favored technique is **emesis,** that is, therapeutic vomiting. Because this activates the gastropulmonary reflex, it was one of the best ways, in the days before antibiotic drugs, to clear the lungs of fluids and improve the outcome for those with pneumonia, chronic bronchitis, and lung congestion. Lobelia (*Lobelia inflata*), also known as puke weed, is a favorite in the Heroic Tradition.

Vomiting puts stomach acid in the mouth where it can cause cavities as it erodes tooth enamel. If done regularly, it can turn into an eating disorder. At the worst, it can cause death from blood chemistry changes leading to cardiac arrest.

"I was vomiting from my soul, getting rid of pain, of an evil that had been destroying me. . . . I could be rid of the rapist . . . he would be outside and no longer a part of me."   Ashheena, 28, teacher

Purging: Colonics, Enemas, Implants

While bleeding and puking are no longer common practices, cleansing the colon is still in vogue. The colon was mistakenly believed to be the cause of illness because it is filled with feces, which harbor many bacteria, and bacteria can cause illness.

We now know that gut bacteria are helpful and healthy, and that colonics wipe them out. Nonetheless, traditions as diverse as Ayurveda and Anthroposophy, Naturopathy and Chiropractic, Massage and Functional Medicine, teach that a clean colon is a necessity for health. Nothing could be further from the truth.

All colon cleanses, whether herbal laxatives and cathartics (like senna and cascara sagrada), enemas, or colonics deeply disturb and destroy healthy gut flora. Because colon bacteria are natural detoxifiers, their loss leaves us with more toxins, not less.

Colon cleanses remove electrolytes, too. Rapid change in electrolyte balance can kill, especially those with kidney or heart disease. Colon cleanses and colonics can critically dehydrate all cells and leave one feeling a lot worse from the inevitable side effects:

cramping, bloating, nausea, vomiting, diarrhea, excessive urination, infections, rectal tears, and (rarely) perforation of the bowel.
If you complain, you will be told (falsely) that your distress, whether
physical or emotional, is due to the elimination of toxins.

A meta-analysis found **colon cleansing** to have a host of dangerous side effects, including death, with **no known health benefits of any kind.** [*Journal of Family Practice.* Aug 2011]

A colonic is an extreme form of colon cleansing, sometimes
called a "high enema." A colonic hygienist/hydrotherapist pumps
up to 16 gallons of water, herbal brew, or coffee into your large
intestines at various temperatures and pressures using a machine
or gravity. Afterwards, raw juices or herbal brews may be im-
planted/injected into the clean colon.

The idea that toxins can get stuck in the folds of the gut and
cause a host of health problems falls into and out of favor. Colonics
were popular in the early 1900s in the U.S. By 1919, when science
failed to find them safe or effective, they were shunned. Now, a
century later, celebrities and a major marketing campaign have
caused a comeback of this dangerous practice. Beware.

I asked over 5000 surgeons and surgical nurses if they ever
saw anything stuck to the intestines. The more polite said "No."
The less polite laughed in my face. The digestive tract is lined with
slick mucus cells which prevent anything from getting stuck. These
cells are replaced daily. Notice how quickly wounds in the mouth
heal. Notice that chemotherapy (which kills rapidly-reproducing
cells) is destructive to the gut; so are laxatives, enemas, colonics.

Colonics, like enemas, are *habit-forming.* The food moves
through the intestines as a result of *peristalsis.* Peristalsis, like swallowing, is a complicated, finely-tuned, precisely-timed interaction
of muscles, nerves, and hormones. Introducing liquids into the
large intestine disrupts peristalsis, resulting in short-term bowel
irregularities and long-term habituation as injuries multiply.

Keep your colon healthy with **fiber.** Whole grains, beans, well-
cooked greens, frozen fruit, roots, and herbs such as plantain seed
and marshmallow root are excellent sources of fiber. Fiber brushes
the colon and feeds helpful flora which eliminate unwanted substances like cholesterol. Fiber increases peristalsis naturally, in-
suring regularity.

Deep Medicine: Body Modification
Internalized Violence

It is understandable to do violence in pursuit of healing. Deep Medicine deliberately injures, introduces infection, maims, causes future cancers, breaks bones, and risks addiction in an effort to prolong and save lives.

But how are we to understand the violence we do to ourselves to comply with social norms? We are on the far side of the Gap, deep in Step 6, every time we remove hair (shave, wax, use chemicals/lasers), add or subtract to our form with lifts, injected fillers, peels, liposuction, tattoos, scarification, piercings, tooth modification, microderm-abrasion, foot binding, tummy tucks, genital mutilation (circumcision, infibulation, clitorectomy, castration, sex-assignment surgery, vaginoplasty, labioplasty, penis enlargement), binge dieting, fasting, vomiting, anorexia, bulimia, body sculpting with ultrasound, infrared light, vacuums, extreme cold, and injected drugs.

"The images that bombard us daily, in magazines, advertising, television, and movies are insidious, encroaching on the way we see ourselves. . . . Gradually our so-called inner reality grows so estranged from our outward appearance that only a surgeon can reconcile the two, carving our flesh to make it conform to the images in our minds. Our bodies have betrayed us, we think, not recognizing that it is we who have betrayed them, by moving out." Holly Brubach, *A Dedicated Follower of Fashion*

A trapped animal may chew off a limb. A distressed bird may preen off its feathers. Humans have cut off the clitorises of and broken the feet of young girls, jabbed themselves with dye-filled needles, filed their teeth, and circumcised baby boys. Self-mutilation is not self-destruction, it is self-preservation. Humans mutilate themselves to belong, to be part of the group, to fit in.

"The complexity of this web of denial . . . demonstrates women's ability to embody, embrace, and reinforce patriarchal power. . . . [It] made me realize how deeply fossilized these customs and traditions are in women's psyches, and that even if there were legislation against female genital mutilation, it would not disappear overnight." Alice Walker, *Warrior Marks*

The definition of beauty and desirability varies from culture to culture, but frequently requires the use of Deep Medicine to achieve its ideal: wasp-waists, lotus feet, pneumatic breasts, unlined faces.

"The death rate for cosmetic surgery is estimated by the industry itself as one in 30,000. An industry survey of 100,000 patients put it at one in 10,000. No one knows for sure."
                           Naomi Wolf, *Keep Them Implanted and Ignorant*

Three million cosmetic procedures were performed in the U.S. in 1998; 17.5 million in 2017. [www.plasticsurgery.org]
    In 1999, Americans spent $9 billion on hair and skin care and $20 billion on diet products. In 2017, we spent $20 billion on manicures/pedicures/haircuts and $60 billion on diet products.

"Vaginal laser has been aggressively marketed to menopausal women with symptomatic genital atrophy. I will continue to not recommend [it]. It can cause [burns, scars, recurring/chronic pain, inability to enjoy intercourse]. . . . "   Andrew Kaunitz MD, editor *NEJM*

Cultural body preferences are taught, and can be caught. Anorexia, first documented in Japan in the 1960s, now affects one in 100 Japanese women (and ten in 100 American women). Three years after television came to Fiji, fifteen percent of young women were anorexic or bulimic, illnesses previously unknown there.

"I gained self-confidence as I lost physical presence in the world, as if self-sacrifice was the heart of self-esteem. [I saw] the erasure of my body as my salvation, the only goal I could achieve in life." Patricia Foster, anorexic

As with all Deep Medicine, body modification ritualizes trauma, somatizes change, makes our internal process external, and allows us to change ourselves. A tattoo can commemorate the death of a beloved and give grief visible form. A piercing can create an opening for expanded consciousness. Hikers, lost in a cave and thought dead, shaved their heads in a public ceremony of gratitude after being rescued.
    What is your story? How will you express it?

Deep Medicine: Wise Woman Tradition
Change Your Mind
Power Plants

In the Wise Woman Tradition, the archetypal Deep Medicine is psychoactive, psychotropic, psychedelic mind-altering plants. These are the plants that awakened music, art, and culture in early humans and nourish wholeness today.

Mind-altering plants, mushrooms, and cacti are used everywhere on this planet as Deep Medicine. They are:

o A part of sacred rites and spiritual observances
o A means of communicating with ancestors and nature
o A way to perceive universal patterns and be part of them
o An accurate way to diagnose and a highly effective way to treat disruptions to mental and spiritual health
o An adjunct to diagnosing and treating physical problems
o A way to prepare for actual or symbolic death/initiation
o A means of retrieving lost souls and restoring those souls damaged by trauma

"The most important thing to know about humans is that they have souls, and that everybody starts out with more than one soul or else they wouldn't be human."   Robert Moss, *Dreamways of the Iroquois*

Modern science validates psychoactive plants as the safest and least invasive of all Deep Medicines. In most instances, one experience with a mind-altering plant is deeply helpful for those:

o Who have a terminal diagnosis
o Who experience cancer-related anxiety and depression
o Who have survived cancer treatment and feel unwhole
o Whose depression is chronic and drug-resistant
o Who seek a boost to creativity, want a breakthrough
o Who want to increase cognitive functioning
o Who seek a spiritual epiphany, a life-changing experience
o Who desire increased personal awareness

**Aboriginal people say psychoactive plants are
"Gifts of the Gods."**

Psychedelic Agent Dosage Guide

A high dose opens spiritual gates, connecting you to All.

A moderate dose lays bare the heart, facilitating deep emotional work.

A low dose improves cognitive functioning, revealing the answer outside the box.

A microdose is an "all-chakra enhancer, where everything's just a little bit better. . . . People behave better, are happier, are more tolerant; not necessarily more creative, but more in the flow," according to respected psychedelic expert James Fadiman.

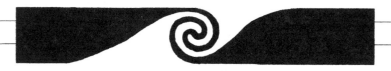

How Safe Are Psychedelics?

"[Smoking] Tobacco causes approximately 400,000 deaths a year. Alcohol about 125,000 deaths per year. Peanuts about 100 deaths. Psychedelics aren't even on the list."   James Fadiman, *The Psychedelic Experience*

A study of 22,000 individuals reporting on lifetime use of psychedelics found a *lower* rate of mental health problems in users.

"Psychedelics are very safe when used in controlled environments and administered by skilled clinicians . . . more than 2,000 doses of psilocybin administered – and zero adverse events."   Stephen Ross MD

In 2014, 1.2 million Americans said they had used a hallucinogen in the past month.

"If you handle LSD with care, it isn't any more dangerous than other therapies."   Dr Peter Gasser, Swiss LSD psychiatrist

"Of 20 drugs ranked according to individual and societal harm, LSD was third to last, approximately 1/10th as harmful as alcohol. The most significant adverse effect was impairment of mental functioning."   David Nutt, neuropsychopharmacologist

By activating serotonin receptors, the Deep Medicine of psychoactive plants opens us to mystical, spiritual experiences. Seventy percent of those given psilocybin in a recent study said it was one of the most significant experiences of their lives.

Wise use of "power plants/drugs" – tobacco, psilocybin, peyote, mescaline, LSD, ayahuasca, cannabis, or any of hundreds of others – requires: 1. Respect for the power of the plant. 2. Respect for your own power. 3. A ritual which defines and limits use.

It is wise to approach psychedelics with the same care we use for approaching surgery or any Deep Medicine: 1. An intention for an outcome. 2. An appropriate setting, such as a sterile field in a well-equipped hospital/a cozy nest/a safe place in nature. 3. A skilled, experienced surgeon/an experienced guide/a trusted ally.

"Breaking the habitual experience of the world can help patients caught in an ego-centered problem cycle to escape from their fixation and isolation."
Christian Ratsch, *Encyclopedia of Psychoactive Plants*

Psychoactive plants have been shown to have enormous psychotherapeutic value in the treatment of those with:

- o Anorexia nervosa
- o Chronic anxiety attacks
- o Chronic, severe depression
- o Addictions to alcohol, cocaine
- o Cluster headaches
- o OCD
- o PTSD

"A paye's [shaman's] soul should illuminate, it should shine with a strong inner light rendering visible all that is . . . hidden from ordinary knowledge and reasoning." G. Reichel-Dolmatoff, *The Shaman and the Jaguar*

When a healer/helper consumes a power plant, we have Story Medicine; there is little or no risk. When you yourself ingest a power plant, that's Deep Medicine, which is inherently risky.

Deep Medicine reveals our flaws and faults, our fears and our foibles. Usually, Deep Medicine cuts us so we can heal into wholeness, but it may break us. Latent psychosis can be triggered, especially in adolescence but even in adults, by the use of power plants.

". . . employed for prophecy, divination, sorcery, and medicinal purposes . . . so deeply rooted in native mythology and philosophy that there can be no doubt of its great age as part of aboriginal life." R.E. Schultes

Psilocybin (*Psilocybe* species)/Psilocybine (a tryptamine)
Danger Level: Nonexistent to extremely low
Addiction Risk: None
Animal totem: Hummingbird
Side effects: Subtle visual, auditory, and proprioceptive hallucinations, inner knowing, peace; nausea, muscle weakness, confusion, dis-coordination, panic, paranoia.
One dose: 20-30 grams of fresh mushroom, or 1-2.5 grams of dried powder; peak effects in 1-2 hours, lasting for 6-8 hours.
One microdose: .3 gram dry psilocybin once every four days.
   "The sacred mushroom takes me by the hand and brings me to the world where everything is known."   María Sabina, Mazatec shaman

The Little Flowers of the Gods, psilocybin mushrooms, are one of the safest and surest psychoactive allies. Hundreds of stone effigies of psilocybin, some dated to 1000 BCE, have been found in Guatemala, El Salvador, Honduras, and Mexico.

In one of the largest trials of Deep Medicine, 80 percent of cancer patients showed major reductions in psychological stress, anxiety, and depression for seven months or longer after taking psilocybin once.

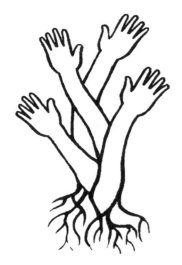

   In a trial of those with drug-resistant chronic depression, all participants reported a lifting of their depression, sustained for up to three months, after one dose of psilocybin.

   Psilocybin helps the brain repair damaged cells; it improves cognition and stimulates hippocampal neurogenesis. The hippocampus is responsible for learning as well as converting short-term memory into long-term memories.

   ". . . psychedelics and entactogens have demonstrated rapid and long-lasting antidepressant and anxiolytic effects . . . after a single dose."
      Juan R. Sanchez-Ramos, brain researcher [ncbi.nlm.nih.gov]

Peyote (*Lophophora willamsii*)/Mescaline (synthetic peyote)
Danger Level: Medium to extremely low
Addiction Risk: None
Animal totem: Deer
Side effects: Colorful visual hallucinations, inner knowing, heightened healing abilities; nausea, vomiting, anxiety, emotional instability, dizziness, increased blood pressure, heart rate, and respiration. Mescaline can cause birth defects.
One dose: 200 milligrams of mescaline or two or more peyote buttons, defuzzed and boiled into a thick tea.

"*. . . they formed as large a circle of men and women as could occupy the space that had been swept off for this purpose. One after the other, they went dancing in a ring or marking time with their feet, keeping in the middle the musician and choir-master, and singing in the same unmusical tune that he set them. They would dance all night, from five in the evening to seven in the morning, without stopping nor leaving the circle.*"
Spanish missionary at a peyote ceremony, 1650

Peyote is a cactus that has been used sacramentally in North America for more than seven thousand years. It is legal only when used in Native American religious ceremonies.

The traditional peyote ceremony I took part in lasted from sundown until sunrise, during which time we consumed peyote, sang individually, and journeyed the Peyote Road together. It was magical. I was deeply nourished. The Native American Church ceremony my sweetheart participated in was based on shaming, blaming Christian ideas of sin and punishment. Despite being told Mescalito would devour him if he ventured beyond the circle, he left, to save his soul.

Peyote is revelatory. It shows the seeker what is lost. It ensures safety from betrayal. Peyote opens the doors of perception and allows the wonder of life to take up residence. Scientific studies support the use of peyote to help those dealing with addictions.

"*The Huichol say Peyote is very delicate. . . .*" Schultes, ethnobotanist

Mescaline improves creative problem solving after a single dose (200mg); the effects last for weeks. It has a strong effect on serotonin levels and relieves depression.

Ergot (*Claviceps purpurea*)/Lysergic acid (**LSD-25**)
Danger Level: Ergot can be lethal; LSD is safe.
Addiction Risk: None
LSD Totem: Flowers
LSD Side effects: Sweeping transformation of the psyche with greatly heightened sensory experiences, synesthesia, oneness; anxiety, paranoia, delusions, panic.
One dose: 500 micrograms of LSD-25 for an 8-hour trip and a lifetime of benefits. Microdose: 10 micrograms every fourth day.

"Ergot poisoning [took] thousands of lives and caused untold agony . . . convulsions, epileptic seizures, gangrene, atrophy, mummification, loss of extremities . . . delirium, hallucinations. . . ."   Richard Evans Schultes

Albert Hofmann, experimenting with the alkaloids of ergot, happened upon the safe psychedelic LSD on his 25th trial. It was approved for psychiatric uses, but eventually demonized and banned. Nonetheless, an entire generation used LSD-25 to create an outpouring of psychedelic music, art, lifestyles and politics.

Ram Dass, Timothy Leary, Aldous Huxley, Huston Smith, Francis Crick, Steve Jobs, and James Fadiman are psychedelic-taking psychonauts who have changed our collective consciousness and our view of ourselves. The founding mothers and fathers of the Herbal Renaissance of the 1960s and '70s were introduced to plant spirits by LSD, psilocybin, and peyote, changing how plant medicine was perceived and used.

"I didn't have many friends and didn't feel comfortable in my own skin. . . . I took a hit of LSD and didn't feel alone any more. It helped me to see myself differently, increased my self-confidence, and just feel at one with the world. I lost my desire to drink or smoke. I haven't touched alcohol or cigarettes since that day in 1995 and am much happier than before."
Sadie, 49, waitress

Psychiatrist John Halpern MD, of Harvard Medical School, draws our attention to the fact that most of the 53 people he studied who had cluster headaches and who took LSD or psilocybin (illegally) obtained long-term relief from their intolerable pain. He believes that *"LSD is a potentially very valuable substance for human health and happiness."*

Ayahuasca (*Banisteriopsis caapi* + *Psychotria viridis*)/DMT and harmine
Danger Level: Medium, best if used no more than 3 times
Addiction Risk: None
Animal totem: Jaguar
Side effects: Vomiting, diarrhea, visual/auditory hallucinations

"Ayahuasca . . . a psychic blowtorch, with the capacity to cut through and reduce to cinders what does not work." Chris Kilham, *Ayahuasca*

The Vine of the Soul, ayahuasca, is not one plant, but a combination of two (or more) plants, which aren't psychoactive on their own, but become so when brought together.

Ayahuasca has a profound effect on one's feelings of self worth. It can crush us with guilt and terror or compel us to face and work with our own demons, our hardness, our denial.

Taken too frequently, ayahuasca can consume the soul. An apprentice who took it in Peru as often as twice a week for a year, is still lost in her mind. And a dear friend who joined a church that uses ayahuasca as a weekly sacrament is also lost.

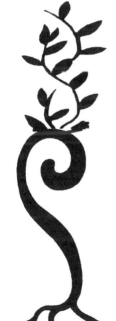

"Raising a cup of ayahuasca to the lips is a practice of transubstantiation. Within the thick, bitter fluid . . . is the taste of the salvific power of . . . evolution itself." Robert Tindall, *The Jaguar that Roams the Mind*

Ayahuasca studies show short-term benefits for those dealing with intractable depression, PTSD, or addictions.

"I discovered the impossible. The severe depression that had ruled my life since childhood had miraculously vanished." Kira Salak, 54, on her ayahuasca experience

Claims that ayahuasca cures cancer are just that: claims. Ayahuasca may show you how to change cancer cells in your body, but ayahuasca itself does not impact cancer.

It *is* a creative ally. Ayahuasca-inspired artworks – beaded and painted pieces – are valued for their complexity, intensity, saturated colors, and sinuous forms.

Witch's Garden: The Nightshades

Solanaceae: *Hyoscyamus niger, Atropa belladonna, Brugmansia* sp.,
Datura stramonium, Mandragora off., Solanum nigrum
Tropane alkaloids: hyoscyamine, atropine, solanine, scopolamine.
Danger Level: Medium to Very High
Addiction Risk: Low
Side effects: Headache, visual and temporal hallucinations, dis-
orientation, coma, death, initiation.

*"Three-twentieths of an ounce in weight is given, if the patient is to
become merely sportive and to think himself a fine fellow; twice this dose if
he is to go mad outright and have delusions; thrice the dose, if he is to be
permanently insane; . . . four times the dose is given if the man is to be
killed."*   Paracelsus (1493-1541), *Datura*

Since nightshades grow in most parts of the world, and since so
many contain outright hallucinogens, nightshades are often used,
despite their clear, and deadly, dangers.

Daturas are used during initiations in parts of Africa and as part
of puberty rites in the desert Southwest of North America. Wise
women throughout Old Europe used henbane, belladonna, and
mandrake in rituals and in flying ointments.

The active alkaloids cause the user to believe in what they hal-
lucinate, leading to grievous errors. Tropanes also distort, or eat
time, which seems to pass far too quickly after ingestion. Dulling
or muting of the senses, which can continue for days and weeks
following use of tropanes, is common.

*"The ears become deaf, the eyes almost blind; they see in a haze only the
bulk of objects, whose contours are blurred. The sufferer is slowly cut off
from the outside world and sinks irretrievably into himself and his own
inner world."* Gustav Schenk, inhaling the smoke of burning henbane seeds

Like Hippocrates, Hildegard of Bingen believed mandrake was
a cure for depression and lovesickness.

According to Dale Pendell: "... *in Ecuador, guanto* [Brugmansia]
*is drunk once or twice in a lifetime, at an important crossroad of change or
decision. The drinker first builds a small shelter in the forest, and then
makes arrangements with friends/relatives to take turns watching over
him, so that he won't injure himself. The ordeal may last several days."*

And, this nightshade:

Tobacco (*Nicotiana tabacum*)/Nicotine
Danger Level: Quite High
Addiction Risk: Quite High-Absolute
Side effects: Lessening of appetite, mucosa irritation, nausea, mild headache, blurred vision, dizziness, nervousness, pounding in the ears, fast or irregular heartbeat, hives, itching, rash.

"Only the revered cigarette, like last words and the Holy Cross, is privileged to share the last rites of the condemned."　　　Dale Pendell

Tobacco is used as Deep Medicine by numerous indigenous peoples in North and South America.

"The Indians say that this smoke is very wholesome for clearing and consuming superfluous humors of the brain."　André Thevet (1502-1590)

"Tobacco is the muscle. Maybe the mushrooms . . . will give you the seeing, but you need tobacco for the muscle. . . ."　South American shaman

"In some tribes, a woman may acquire extensive knowledge of plants; and occasionally she capitalizes on this knowledge, becoming fearsome, particularly amongst the young who believe that she is able to hex people through the power of her powdered tobacco and toxic plants which, accompanied by magical incantations, she blows over a patient's body."
Richard Evans Schultes, *Vine of the Soul*

Less than fifty years – from the early 1920s to the late 1960s – separate ads featuring MDs encouraging those with lung problems to smoke from scientific proclamations that tobacco in any form – smoked, vaped, or chewed – causes lethal diseases, like lung cancer, liver cancer and emphysema.

Tobacco is said to be more addictive than heroin.

"The Tibetans call tobacco the poisonous dakini killer. They say that tobacco smoke, like the smoke from burning flesh, attracts the wrong spirits, that it grows where menstrual blood drops."　quoted by Dale Pendell

"Smoking is a dying art."　　Graffito

Poppy (*Papaver somniferum*)/Opium, morphine, heroin, codeine
Danger Level: Quite High
Addiction Risk: Quite High-Absolute
Side effects: Lessening of pain, full-body orgasm, loss of appetite, digestive disturbances, constipation, sleepiness, cough suppression, increase of creative impulse, decrease of creative energy. Withdrawal, especially from synthetic opioids, can be fatal.

"Among the remedies which it has pleased Almighty God to give to [wo]man to relieve suffering, none is so universal and so efficacious as opium." Thomas Sydenham (1624-1689), *Observationes Medical*

Poppy/opium – the best painkiller – has dominated medicine for 6000 years. Unfortunately, poppy is uniformly and deeply addictive.

"Everything one does in life, even love, occurs in an express train racing toward death. To smoke opium is to get out of the train while it is still moving. It is to concern oneself with something other than life or death." Jean Cocteau (1889-1963), *La Machine Infernale*

According to the Greek physician Galen (129-216 CE), opium cures venomous bites, chronic headache, vertigo, deafness, epilepsy, apoplexy, leprosy, and all women's troubles. Indeed, by the late 1800s, opium, in the form of laudanum, was an ingredient in nearly all herbal remedies used for women's complaints.

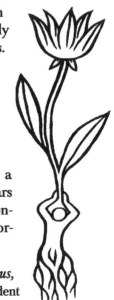

"Opium is used mainly as a painkiller or medicine. But heroin helps you run away from the truth, from the facts. Youth wants something that helps us run away from the reality of everyday life, and that's heroin." Fariboorz Koocheki, 29, Tehran

The modern-day use of syringes began as a method for delivering morphine. In 1897, Sears Roebuck sold – for $1.50 – a hypodermic kit consisting of a syringe, two needles, a vial of morphine, a vial of cocaine, and a carrying case.

"Intravenous usage of drugs is extremely dangerous, but it is also extremely pleasurable." K. Filan, 22, student

Mistletoe (*Viscum album*)/Lectins, viscotoxins, terpenes
 Danger Level: Extremely low
 Addiction Risk: None
 Animal totem: Squirrel
 Side effects: Visual disturbances, nausea, stomach pain, diarrhea, rarely death.

Mistletoe viscotoxins, small proteins that kill cells, and lectins, complex molecules that can bind to the outside of cells and induce biochemical changes in them, combine with polysaccharides to create a "botanical biological response modifier" against cancer. Mistletoe therapy has been used since the 1920s and is now used by up to half of those dancing with cancer in Germany, Israel, and Holland. It is safe and effective integrated with chemotherapy, radiation, hormones, and cytokines. It can be used alone.

Mistletoe extracts (**Iscador** or **Helixor**) vary, depending on the host tree (oak, birch, ash, elm, apple, pine), season of harvest, and preparation. An anthroposophic MD takes you and your cancer into consideration when creating a mistletoe regime for you.

Mistletoe is usually given by injection: under the skin (subcutaneously), into a vein (IV), into the pleural cavity, or directly into the tumor. Treatment generally lasts for at least two years.

A review of all controlled clinical studies of mistletoe found consistent improvement in quality of life. [*Integrated Cancer Therapies* 2010]

Mistletoe, before and after chemo/radiation, has been shown to:
 o   Improve disease-free survival
 o   Interfere with protein synthesis in cancer cells
 o   Induce apoptosis (cell death) in cancer cells
 o   Increase immune system activity against cancer cells
 o   Stabilize the DNA in damaged white blood cells
 o   Increase the number and activity of white blood cells
 o   Increase immune system enhancing cytokines, such as interleukin-1, interleukin-6, and tumor necrosis factor
 o   Decrease adverse chemo/radiation symptoms: less pain, less weight loss, better energy/less fatigue, better digestion, less nausea/vomiting, better mental focus, less depression

"Mistletoe enhances the philosophical and spiritual aspects of the being, bringing gradual, lasting, change."   Ana Lups, anthroposophic MD

Step 6: Deep Medicine
References & Resources

Step 6: Metaphor
Bolen, Jean S. *Close to the Bone: Life-Threatening Illness as a Soul Journey* (revised). Shambhala, 2019.
Turner, Kelly PhD. *Radical Remission: Surviving Cancer Against All Odds.* HarperOne, 2015.

Screening Tests
"Cancer Screening." *Health After 50.* Aug 2018.
Carr, Teresa. "Medical Tests." *Consumer Reports.* Jan 2019.
"Diagnostic Heart Tests: Are They Good or Bad for Your Health?" *Health After 50.* Oct 2015.
Lenzer, Jeanne. "Should I Get Tested?" *AARP Bulletin.* Nov 2019.
Rebar, RW MD. "Ovarian Cancer Screening: No Effect on Mortality." *JWatch.org.* 1 Jan 2012.
Rodriguez, Fatima MD. "Is Measuring Lipoprotein(a) Clinically Useful in Women?" *NEJM.* July 2018.
"Screening Test You Probably Don't Need." *Harvard Women's Health Watch.* Jan 2017.
Swartzberg, John MD. "Guidelines Galore." *UC Berkeley Wellness Letter.* Feb 2019.
"Your Eyes Are Windows to Your Overall Health." *Men's Health Advisor.* Jan 2016.
• www.choosingwisely.org
• www.medconsumers.wordpress.com

Step 6: Diagnosis
Lautin, Everett MD. Letter to *Discover,* Aug 1999.
"Overexposed: Radiation Risks." *Consumer Reports.* March 2015.
   "Most people can actually go 24-36 months between bitewings and up to 10 years between full-mouth series [of dental x-rays]."

Mammograms
"A new study reveals mammograms may not be doing much good." *Time.* 24 Feb 2014.

Cowley, Goretti. "Comparing mammography and thermography."
MedicalNewsToday. 22 July 2019.

Dillner, Luisa. "Should I have a mammogram?" *The Guardian.*
16 Feb 2014.

"Do you need mammograms?" *Harvard Women's Health Watch.*
June 2012.

"Mammography Wars Reignite." *Discover.* Jan 2015.

Schwartz, Lisa. "Making informed decisions about mammograms."
Science News. 13 Feb 2010.

CT Scans

"Do You Really Need a Scan?" *CR on Health.* March 2015.

"Questions to Ask Before You Have a Scan." *Health.* Dec 2014.

A 2012 study of 180,000 British children linked CT scans to higher rates of leukemia and brain cancer.

Ultrasound

Brogan, Kelly MD. "Human Studies Condemn Ultrasound." 2015.
(www.kellybroganmd.com)

Lombardo, Jackie. "Ultrasound: It's Not Safe or Painless for Your Developing Child." *Pathways to Family Wellness.* Issue 48.

How Much Radiation?

100 millirems = 1 mSv

Background radiation = 3 mSv per year, in small doses, daily.
Dental x-ray, panoramic = .01-.1 mSv
Each mammographic image = .5-1 mSv
Coronary artery calcium scan = 1 mSv
CT angiogram = 2-7 mSv
  10 mSv is more radiation than most residents of Fukushima, Japan absorbed after the nuclear power plant incident of 2011.
Nuclear stress test = 4-10 mSv
Abdominal CT = 10 mSv
CT angiography (heart) = 12 mSv
Full body CT scan = 12 mSv
PET + CT = 25 mSv

- www.eneuro.org/content/3/3/ENEURO.0136-15.2016
- https://sarahbuckley.com/ultrasound-scans-cause-for-concern/

"A majority of women with early breast cancers continue to undergo radiation treatment despite evidence that it doesn't lower recurrence rates, but can increase the risk of rib fracture, heart and coronary artery damage, and cancer."   *Cancer* online 2 Dec 2014

MRI

Woodcock, Janet MD. "FDA Warning on MRI Dye." *Bottom Line Health.* May 2018.
- https://www.radiologyinfo.org/en/info.cfm?pg=safety-contrast
- http://www.howtosurvivelifeinthesuburbs.com/2010/06/how-to-survive-mri-html
- https://multiplesclerosisnewstoday.com/ms-in-moderation-a-column-by -tamara-sellman/2017/02/22/how-survive-mri-claustrophobic/
- http://glendalemri.com/top-3-situations-where-mri-is-the-best-solution/

Surgery

Aguilera-Hellweg, Max. *The Sacred Heart: An Atlas of the Body Seen Through Invasive Surgery.* Bullfinch Press, 1997.

Avitzur, Orly MD. "4 Questions to Ask About Surgery." *Consumer Reports On Health.* May 2017.

Beil, Laura. "Surgery That Can Give You a Stroke." *Reader's Digest.* April 2013.

Carter. Gari. *Healing Myself: A Hero's Primer for Recovery from Tragedy.* Hampton Roads (Norfolk, VA), 1993.

"Cognitive decline after non-cardiac surgery." *Lancet,* 15 Aug 2019.

Huddleston, Peggy. *Prepare for Surgery, Heal Faster.* Angel River Press, 1996.

Inlander, Charles & Ed Weiner. *Take This Book to the Hospital with You.* (A People's Medical Society Book). Rodale Press, 1985.

Marsa, Linda. "Pick the Right Surgeon." *AARP Bulletin.* Sept 2017.

Morris, Kit & Smulian, Ana (contributing artists). *Art.Rage.Us.: Art and Writing by Women with Breast Cancer.* Chronicle Books, 1998.

Naparstek, Belleruth. *Meditations to Promote Successful Surgery: Guided Imagery, Healing Words, and Soothing Music.* Health Journeys. 1996.

"Recover Faster After Surgery." *CR on Health.* March 2015.

Weil, Andrew MD. "Ten Steps to Successful Surgery." *Weil's Self Healing.* Sept 1997.

Wright, Kenneth. "Timing is Everything." *Bottom Line.* July 2018.

Youngson, Robert MD. *The Surgery Book: An Illustrated Guide to 73 of the Most Common Operations.* St. Martin's Press, 1993.

"The surgery was a success but while under anesthesia, I suffered a stroke, then went into a coma. After that, I suffered seizures, went into congestive heart failure, contracted pneumonia and MRSA. I was at death's door. However, I survived. . . . I cannot express my appreciation and thankfulness enough." Thomas T., letter, *Daily News,* 2 April 2019

Hospitals

Crouch, Michelle. "Secrets Hospitals Won't Tell You." *Reader's Digest.* Feb 2016.

Gawande, Atul. "When Drs Make Mistakes." *New Yorker.* Feb 1999.

Health Services Research, Sept 2018.

Makary, Marty MD. *Unaccountable: What Hospitals Won't Tell You; How Transparency Can Revolutionize Health Care.* Bloomsbury, 2013.

Surgery Harms

"Kidney Disease More Common After Premenopausal Oophorectomy." *CJASN.* Nov 2018. [42% increased risk in women <46]

"Minimally Invasive Surgery Tied to Worse Outcomes in Cervical Cancer." https://www.nejm.org/doi/full/10.1056/NEJMoa1806395

"Reoperation After Midurethral Mesh Sling Placement." *JAMA,* Oct 2018. [Within a decade, 1 in 15 undergo additional surgery.]

"To Protect the Brain, Look to the Ovaries." *JAMA Neurol.* Oct 2018. [Oophorectomy leads to temporal lobe degeneration that may precede dementia.]

Bloodletting

Seigworth GS. "Bloodletting Over the Centuries." *New York State Journal of Medicine.* Dec 1980.

George, Rose. *Nine Pints.* Metropolitan, 2019.

Harder, Ben. "Creepy-Crawly Care: Maggots Move into Mainstream Medicine." *Science News.* 23 Oct 2004.

• https://www.bcmj.org/premise/history-bloodletting

Colonics
- www.mayoclinic.org/healthy-lifestyle/consumer-health/
  expert-answers/colon-cleansing/faq-20058435
- www.mdedge.com/jfponline/article/64413/gastroenterology/
  dangers-colon-cleansing
- www.activebeat.co/your-health/the-dangers-of-colonics/

Body Modification
Brubach, Holly. "Beauty Under the Knife." *Atlantic Monthly.* 2000.
Cameron, Loren. *Body Alchemy, Transsexual Portraits.* Cleis, 1996.
Chernin, Kim. *Obsession: Tyranny of Slenderness.* HarperRow, 1981.
———. *The Hungry Self: Women, Eating, and Identity.* Times Books, 1985.
Dean, Carolyn MD. *Death by Modern Medicine.* Matrix Verite, 2005.
Walker, Alice & Pratibha Parmar. *Warrior Marks: Female Genital Mutilation; the Sexual Blinding of Women.* Harcourt Brace, 1993.

". . . study of 32 children's hospitals across the country showed admissions for suicidal behavior and serious self-harm among 5-to-17-year-olds more than doubled between 2008 and 2015." Susanna Schrobsdorff, *Time*

Phage Therapy

Antibiotic-resitant infections kill 23,000 Americans yearly, and injure 2 million more who survive. Bacteriophages – tiny viruses found in water, soil, and our own digestive tracts – cure these infections quickly. Bacteriophage therapy is available through **phagetherapycenter.com** (Tbilisi, Georgia). The process is simple: submit a bacterial sample; if your infection can be treated, you receive a package (usual cost around $800) in the mail with phages to be applied topically or taken orally.

Psychoactive Plants
Adamson, Sophia. *Through the Gateway of the Heart: Accounts of Experiences with MDMA and Other Empathogens.* Four Trees, 1985.
Estrada, Alvaro. *María Sabina, Her Chants.* Ross-Erikson, 1981.
Arthur, JD. *Salvia Divinorum.* Park Street Press, 2010.
Buhner, Stephen H. *Sacred and Herbal Healing Beers.* Siris, 1998.
Escohotado, Antonia. *A Brief History of Drugs: From the Stone Age to the Stoned Age.* Park Street Press, 1999 (trans. from Spanish).
Eisner, Bruce. *The MDMA Story.* Ronin, 1993.

Fadiman, James. *The Psychedelic Explorer's Guide: Safe, Therapeutic, and Sacred Journeys.* Park Street Press, 2011.

Forte, Robert (ed). *Entheogens and the Future of Religion.* Simon and Schuster, 2012.

Griffiths, Roland R, et al. "Psilocybin produces substantial and sustained decreases in depression and anxiety in patients with life-threatening cancer." *Journal of Psychopharmacology,* Nov 2016.

Heaven, Ross. *Shamanic Quest for the Spirit of Salvia.* Park St., 2013.

Hofmann, Albert. *LSD: My Problem Child.* McGraw Hill, 1980.

——. *LSD and the Divine Scientist.* Park Street Press, 2011.

Horgan, J. and J. Tzar. "Peyote on the Brain." *Discover.* Feb 2003.

Julien, Robert MD. *A Primer of Drug Action: Psychoactive Drugs.* W. H. Freeman & Co, 1998.

Kilham, Chris. *Ayahuasca: Test Pilot's Handbook.* Evolver, 2014.

McKenna, Terence. *Food of the Gods.* Bantam, 1992.

Moss, Robert. *Dreamways of the Iroquois.* Destiny Books, 2005.

Ott, J. *Hallucinogenic Plants of North America.* Wingbow, 1976.

Palmer, Cynthia and Michael Horowitz, eds. *Shaman Woman, Mainline Lady.* William Morrow, 1982.

Pendell, Dale. *Pharmako/Poeia.* Mercury House, 1995.

——. *Pharmako Gnosis.* Mercury House, 2005.

Plante, Stephie Grob. "LSD microdoses make people feel sharper. . . . " *The Verge.* 24 April 2017.

Pollan, Michael. *How to Change Your Mind: What the New Science of Psychedelics Teaches Us About Consciousness, Dying, Addiction.* Penguin Press, 2018.

Ratsch, Christian. *Encyclopedia of Psychoactive Plants.* Park St., 2005.

Roberts, Thomas B. *The Psychedelic Future of the Mind: How Entheogens Are Enhancing Cognition, Boosting Intelligence.* Park St. Press, 2013.

Ross, Stephen MD. "Psychedelic! Hallucinogens May Soon Go Mainstream as Medicine." *Bottom Line.* 12 Sept 2016.

Schultes, Richard E. *Hallucinogenic Plants.* Golden Guide, 1976.

Schultes R. E., A. Hofmann & C. Ratsch. *Plants of the Gods: Their Sacred, Healing, and Hallucinogenic Powers.* Healing Arts, 1992.

Schultes, R. E. & Robert Raffauf. *Vine of the Soul.* Synergetic, 1992.

Shroder, Tom. *Acid Test.* Plume, 2014.

Waldman, Ayelet. *A Really Good Day: Microdosing.* Knopf, 2017.

Weil, Andrew & Winifred Rosen. *Chocolate to Morphine: Mind-Active Drugs.* Mariner Books, 2004.

> 1 gram dried psilocybin = 6mg of active ingredient
> 3.5 grams dry mushroom = 21mg, the "sweet spot" for
> most people weighing 150 pounds

- www.consciouslifestylemag.com/psychedelic-trip-safely-explore/
- https://entheonation.com/blog/microdosing-magic-mush-rooms-health-benefits-psilocybin-mushrooms-microdoses/
- http://journals.sagepub.com/home/jop
- http://naturalsociety.com/research-suggests-psychedelic-mushrooms-offer-valuable-brain-treatments/
- www.nbcnews.com/id/25464338/ns/health-health_care/t/magic-mushrooms-have-long-lasting-benefits/
- www.npr.org/sections/health-shots/2012/01/24/145731952/your-brain-on-psilocybin-might-be-less-depressed
- www.soul-herbs.com

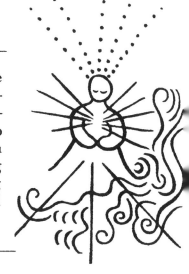

Psilocybin mushrooms activate brain receptors for serotonin, countering depletion in those who are chronically depressed. Nineteen patients who had not responded to drugs were given 10mg of psilocybin, followed by 25mg a week later. Twelve showed lasting benefit. "It rebooted my brain," said one. [*Scientific Reports*, 13 Oct 2017]

"I feel my mind crack, and in the fissures, I see the bottomless arrogance of my presuppositions."　　Jeremy Narby, after ingesting ayahuasca

Mistletoe Injections

My thanks to PDQ® Integrative, Alternative, and Complementary Therapies Editorial Board. Bethesda, MD: National Cancer Institute.

Beuth J, et al. "Impact of complementary treatment of breast cancer patients with standardized mistletoe extract during aftercare: a controlled multicenter comparative epidemiological cohort study." *Anticancer Research,* 2008. [pbmd = PUBMED Abstract]

Bar-Sela G, et al. "Mistletoe as complementary treatment in patients with advanced non-small-cell lung cancer treated with carboplatin-based combinations: a randomised phase II study." *European Journal of Cancer,* 2013. [pbmd]

Friedel W.E., et al. "Systematic evaluation of the clinical effects of supportive mistletoe treatment within chemo- and/or radiotherapy protocols and long-term mistletoe application in nonmetastatic colorectal carcinoma: multicenter, controlled, observational cohort study." *Journal Soc Integrative Oncology,* 2009. [pbmd]

Kaegi E. "Unconventional therapies for cancer: 3. Iscador. Task Force on Alternative Therapies of the Canadian Breast Cancer Research Initiative." *CMAJ,* 1998. [pbmd]

Kienle G. S., H. Kiene. "Complementary cancer therapy: a systematic review of prospective clinical trials on anthroposophic mistletoe extracts." *European Journal Med Res,* 2007. [pbmd]

———. "Influence of Viscum album L (European mistletoe) extracts on quality of life in cancer patients: a systematic review of controlled clinical studies." *Integrative Cancer Ther,* 2010.

Kim, K. C., et al. "Quality of life, immunomodulation and safety of adjuvant mistletoe treatment in patients with gastric carcinoma." *BMC Complementary Alternative Medicine,* 2012. [pbmd]

McGhee, Karen. *The Amazing Healing Powers of Nature.* Readers Digest, 2013

"Viscum album." Homoeopathic Pharmacopoeia of the United States. Washington, DC: 2002, Monograph 9444 Visc.

- NCCIH and the NIH National Library of Medicine present CAM on PubMed, a free and easy-to-use search tool for finding more than 230,000 references and abstracts on alternatives.
- https://www.cancer.gov/about-cancer/treatment/cam/patient/mistletoe-pdq

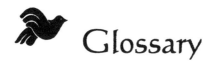

Glossary

Akashic records: Repository of all human events, thoughts, words, emotions, and intentions, eternally.

amulet: Any object believed to confer protection on the bearer.

aura: An energy field that encloses a living being; the subtle body.

Chakra: Focal points of the subtle body; literally "wheels."

cronewort: A new common name for mugwort (*Artemisia vulgaris*).

Entrainment: A state that occurs when rhythmic physiological or behavioral events match their period to that of an environmental oscillation. An interaction between the circadian rhythms and the environment.

Grandmother/father Spider (Sussistanako, Tse-che-nako, Ananssi): An archetype of wholeness found amoung many First Nations peoples, from the Cherokee of the eastern forests to the Hopi of the desert southwest to the Akan of Africa.

Mandala: A geometric pattern that represents wholeness/holiness/health metaphysically and symbolically.

meta-study: Also **meta-analysis**. A combination of multiple scientific studies. There are often rigorous standards that a study must adhere to in order to be included in a meta-study.

Talisman: Any object believed to bring good luck. To increase the power, the talisman may be magically "charged."

telomeres: Like the tip of a shoe-lace, this region of repetitive nucleotide sequences at the end of each chromosome prevents deterioration of the genetic material. Senescence and age-related problems are the result of shortened or missing telomeres.

thangka: A Tibetan Buddhist painting, usually on silk or cotton cloth, of a deity, scene, or a mandala; often used in meditation.

Tree of Life: A symbol used world-wide, found in the Christian bible, and also a scientific premise and metaphor denoting the interlinked relationships among all living things.

Using the Seven Medicines

The Seven Medicines, used step-by-step or globally, guide us in using complementary, integrated medicine. They are not just for when we have time to stop and consider; they work when we suffer a traumatic injury, too. Some of the stories collected here show thoughtful planning, others are reactions in the heat of the moment.

These are stories of the Seven Medicines in action. Each one is a unique story of an individual who seeks to be abundantly well. Your story may be different; your choices will be different. May these stories help you become your own expert and see your problems as allies, as expressions of wholeness and perfection.

It is with awe and wonder at the amazing abilities we have to grow and expand, to experience love and gratitude in the face of daunting challenges, that I share these stories with you.

If you wish to share your Seven Medicines story, please visit me at https://www.facebook.com/AbundantlyWellSusunWeed/

 Alternative Medicine as First Aid
Dismembered Finger
Buzz, 28, orchardist

Alternative medicine offers ways to care for our health while waiting for the doctors to figure out what to do.

Buzz says: "I cut off the tip of my finger last year. It's fine now. It has sensation and there's a small fingernail. If I hadn't used herbal first aid, I don't think that would be the case.

"I didn't intend to cut off the top of my finger. Actually, the apple sorting machine did it, not me. Okay. I guess I put my fingertip where it could get cut off. At any rate, it did, and there it was. I picked it up from among the apples, stuck it back on my finger, and wrapped my bandana around it.

"I was in shock, which slowed the bleeding, prevented me from feeling much pain, and gave me the energy to run home and awaken my partner. She sat me down, unwound the bandana, and poured yarrow tincture over my finger. Ouch!

"That shook me out of the shock. She soaked a fresh bandana in yarrow tincture and rewrapped my re-membered finger. Then off we went to the nearest emergency room, an hour away. There we waited for over an hour before they could see me.

"And when they did, they said: 'This is too severe for us. You need a big hospital; they can reattach the tip of your finger.'

"It took two hours to get to the big hospital. All the while, my maimed finger was still wrapped in a yarrow-tincture-soaked bandana. There we waited another hour. And when they looked at my finger, they said: 'If you had come earlier, we might have been able to do something. It is too late now.' Too late for surgery, too late for modern medicine.

"Not too late for pain-killing, infection-fighting, wound-healing yarrow. Seriously. The fingertip just grew back on without surgery. Herbal medicine saved my finger, I am sure."

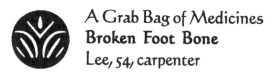

A Grab Bag of Medicines
Broken Foot Bone
Lee, 54, carpenter

Lee smiles and begins: "I stepped off the ladder onto a rock. My ankle bent and made an odd sound. I sat down, took off my shoe and sock, and applied arnica gel lavishly. An hour later, the places I missed were swollen and purple.

"Fearing a broken bones, I learned how to use sonic 'x-rays.' A vibrating tuning fork placed first at one end, and then the other, of a bone makes the edges of a broken bone rub against each other in a sharply painful way. No breaks. Time for RICE and comfrey.

"The Seven Medicines helped me take care of myself in a simple and satisfying way. My foot is just fine."

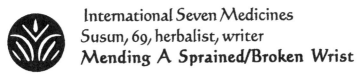

International Seven Medicines
Susun, 69, herbalist, writer
Mending A Sprained/Broken Wrist

This story takes place in Costa Rica in 2015. All the names are actual people who have consented to be part of this tale.

It hurt so much I thought I would faint. Or throw up. Or shit myself. Actually, thought was impossible. My world narrowed down to my rapidly swelling, grossly distorted, painful, but not bleeding, wrist. It HURT!!! It hurt too much to cry.

I willed myself to breathe out, a long breath, like blowing out the candles on a birthday cake. Again. And again. Long . . . slow . . . breaths . . . out, until the pain diminished, ever so slightly . . . but enough for me to remember: I am spacious.

I am made of atoms. Atoms are mostly space. Atoms are spacious. I am made of atoms. I am spacious. The volcanic rocks of this river are made of atoms, which are mostly space. They are spacious. I am spacious. My spaciousness passes through their spaciousness. The space of my wrist passing through the space of the rocks. Spaciousness passing though spaciousness.

Alex and EagleSong sit on either side of me as I lie in the water. They hold me and support me for an eternity as I remind myself again and again of my spaciousness. Their calmness is a balm, and a counter to the panic trying to grab me. Yet I need to be alone.

"My glasses are gone." At my words, my friends leap into action and begin to search the river. Alone, I find the strength to twist over onto my belly, rest, then push up onto my elbows and knees, and finally, swaying, put my feet down and rise to a squat.

"My glasses are gone. No point in searching," I hear myself say out loud. Alex and EagleSong stop searching, come back, and help me to my feet. Clinging to them, I make the quarter-mile walk back to the car. There the women of our Healing Adventure wait for us, unsure of how our adventure will continue.

At top speed! No, not to an emergency room, but back home, for first aid: out of my wet clothes, and into dry ones. Arnica gel to moderate the rapid swelling and bruising; my wrist now several times its normal size. A glass of nourishing herbal infusion with seven drops of skullcap helped cut the pain.

R.I.C.E. for traumatic injuries. I can't stand – still dizzy – so **Rest** was easy: lying flat on my back with my injured arm held out to the side. **Ice** was too hard and edgy, but a kitchen towel soaked in ice water felt good on my wrist. An Ace bandage offered **Compression**. Pulling on my fingers felt great, as did hanging from door frames, but **Elevation** increased my pain.

Time for my class on the healing power of natural minerals. "My wrist is injured," I told the women, "but my mind and mouth work just fine. If you are willing to accept teaching from a teacher lying on her back, I am happy to teach!"

They were. I did.

While that takes place, let's look at what we did so far from the model of the Seven Medicines.

We began with **Serenity Medicine**. Alex and EagleSong attended to me quietly. They did not ask me questions. They did not voice fears that may have been in their minds. I focused on breathing out. Breathing in deeply can increase pain and anxiety. Breathing out calms the vagus nerve, helping it diminish pain and limit swelling from trauma.

It can be difficult to stay with Serenity Medicine. The urge to get answers brings us to **Story Medicine**. We assessed the situation, saw that it was not life-threatening, understood that we had as much time as we wanted. I was conscious. I could ambulate. I was moaning, but not crying or screaming. There was serious swelling, but no blood.

My frightened/curious child-self wanted (demanded) to know "What has happened? Are any bones broken? Is it sprained?" To answer that question would require x-rays. And once I agree to Step 6 for diagnosis, it requires super-human willpower to resist the pressure to use Step 6 treatments as well. So I said "No."

Not only is Step 6 damaging in and of itself, it usually curtails or demolishes our interest in the foundation medicines (Steps 0-3).

The nearest x-ray facility was far away: several hours of travel on rough roads, a ferry ride of an hour, then more miles on paved roads. A round trip of at least 10 hours. So I said "No." (Step 0)

Without access to their story, I had to create my own, or find a way to be comfortable without one (Step 1).

My left hand held and cradled my hurt wrist, suffusing it with **healing chi.** I took some pellets of **Arnica 200x.** I used homeopathic **arnica gel** on my unbroken, though swollen and bruised, skin. And I am eternally grateful for the beautiful wishes for my well-being that the group shared with me (Step 2).

As is often the case, there was no time for Step 3. I relied on the strong bones I had built by my daily consumption of nourishing herbal infusions and my commitment to walking, yoga, tai chi.

Thank goodness for Step 4 allies that counter pain and swelling: anodynes, analgesics, and anti-inflammatories. They work just as well as drugs, with far fewer side effects. I used them both internally and externally to heal the injury to my wrist. And they worked so well I had no need to use over-the-counter pain killers.

I alternated between two herbal tinctures – skullcap and high CBD cannabis – that reduce traumatic and chronic pain through non-addiction-forming pathways. Small, 5-8 drop doses – of fresh, flowering plant in 100-proof vodka – eases pain without sedation. (Larger doses can bring sleep.)

Class was over, dinner done, I went to my cabina. That first night, pain woke me every two hours. I took a sip of water and a dose of skullcap or CBD tincture from the supplies on my bedside table, and went back to sleep. The second night, I woke up every four hours, took some tincture and resumed my sleep. As the swelling receded and the pain lessened, I slept longer at a time and took my pain-relieving tinctures less frequently.

Countering swelling was a main goal. I began with liberal applications of homeopathic Arnica, then added Step 4 remedies: vinegar compresses, comfrey soaks, and cold poultices.

Alex offered to poultice my arm with the Costa Rican plant that his mother used when he hurt himself. "It grows by the river," he said. Thumbing through his iPhone, he pulled up a picture and the botanical name: *Anthurium salvinii.* "I will get a leaf and poultice your arm tonight."

 I heal quickly and well.

My body has a map of its own perfection; it recreates and heals itself perfectly.

Injury is an opening to greater wholeness.

Our crone from Slovakia soaked cotton kitchen towels in apple cider **vinegar** and bound them to my arm with an old Ace bandage, covered with a plastic bag to contain the vinegar fumes and protect against drips. My torn tissues felt cooled and revived as the vinegar soaked into them.

EagleSong was the queen of the **comfrey leaf infusion**. We had enough dried herb to make a quart of nourishing herbal infusion for each woman every day, so we had plenty of comfrey. In addition to drinking a quart of nourishing herbal infusion daily, I also drank at least two cups of comfrey infusion every day.

Cold reduces swelling. I applied frozen things to my wrist off and on all day long for about six weeks of the healing cycle because it felt really good. Some of that first batch of comfrey infusion went into the freezer just long enough to get deeply chilled, then I soaked my wrist in a shallow bowl of it. Wet comfrey leaves in ice water provided another healing soak. Kitchen towels saturated with infusion and partially frozen were a favorite cold compress, held in place with that Ace bandage covered by a plastic bag.

After straining off the infusion, we added cold water (2 cups for each ounce of dried herb initially used) to the unsqueezed, wet comfrey leaves, heated that up to boiling, and let it steep for 4-6 hours. That was strained, the liquid drunk and used for compresses and the squeezed comfrey leaves retained for poultices.

Even so, since I had my arm in a sling up against my chest, the comfrey applications did stain my shirts. Perhaps that wouldn't have happened if I had stayed at home, sitting still. But, really! My legs and my brain were working fine. The next afternoon, about 24 hours after the initial trauma, I led our first weed walk in Costa Rica, with a smile. A near-sighted, no glasses, smile.

After dinner that night, Alex appeared, holding out for my inspection a large, and I mean LARGE – well over a meter/yard long – shiny, dark green leaf.

"A bandana, a knife, some oil, a frying pan, and this leaf is all we need. Come, let's poultice your arm," he invited.

He got the oil so hot, water popped when flicked into it. He cut sections of leaf the width of my swollen wrist and dropped them, one at a time, into the hot oil, and applied them (pretty hot) directly to my skin. One section on the front, one on the back, and one wrapping around. All held in place and covered by that useful Ace bandage. "My mother used a bandana," Alex muttered.

"Keep it on all night, very important," were his parting words. And I did, though it itched a little. I made sure my pain-relief remedy was at hand with some water to drink, lay down, propped up my stretched-out arm, turned off the light, and slept, awakening every few hours to take a few drops of skullcap.

In the morning, when I removed the poultice, we were amazed. The area not covered by the leaf – my fingers and mid-hand – were twice as swollen as those covered by the poultice!

"More. Tonight," said Alex with a smile.

All through the day, we applied cold comfrey compresses. When night came, Alex and the *Anthurium salvinii* came out to play.

The second night was like the first, but Alex cut bigger pieces of leaf, and used more of them. Did I only imagine they were hotter? "Keep it on all night, very important," Alex said and left. And I did, though it itched. I slept with my arm stretched out and propped up, awakening only to pee and take a little skullcap.

The third night, repeat. More leaf, hotter oil, itchier skin.

"All night, important!" Alex repeated. "All night, important!"

No way. Not all night, not even five minutes. No sooner had Alex departed than a fierce burning and itching erupted on my skin where the hot leaf touched it. Maybe, I thought, it will calm down if I take some of the plant material away. My left hand was great at unwrapping the poultice but not very adept at rewrapping it. I admitted failure, hung from the doorframe for a minute to stretch my wrist, and went to sleep *sans* poultice.

Next morning, when I admitted that I had failed to keep the poultice on all night, Alex grinned.

"Ah, now I understand why Mama only did it three times!"

This is **herbal medicine as people's medicine**, the medicine that grows outside your door. This is people's medicine, which is also story medicine, for it weaves us back into wholeness. The plants are aware of our interest, our use. They talk to one another.

They come to our dreams. The Old Ones bend an ear. They respect self-sufficiency.

Everything works. I don't ask "Does it work?" because the answer is always "Yes!" To counter swelling and pain in a traumatic injury, vinegar works, comfrey works, ice works, arnica ointment works, and a plant I never heard of before works. They all work.

Instead, I ask: "Does it make the family as well as the person healthier? Does it make the community as well as the family healthier? Does it keep the ecology healthy too?" Only in the case of the healing leaf of Costa Rica, *Anthurium salvinii*, are all answers: "Yes, indeed." (Back at home, in the Catskills, the best answer would be comfrey, which I grow, and vinegar, which I make.)

The Alternative Medicine remedies we were using – especially homeopathy – were not "home grown." We had to go out of our home, out of our family, to the marketplace, to procure them. They work. They heal. But they are loose threads. They have come undone from the healing cloak of the Ancients and cannot weave us back into wholeness.

Using *Anthurium salvinii* in this place, for this injury, is the true beating heart of herbal medicine, the shuttle of the reweaving of abundant health. Plant and planet, community, family and individual are woven together by the use of this local plant, this local story, becoming more whole, more holy, more healthy.

Eight weeks later, with most of the swelling receded, I quit using cold applications. I celebrated the end of that phase by going through the freezer, taking out frozen comfrey leaves and turning them into the compost heap. Then I washed out the cloths I'd

used for poultices and compresses and hung them on the line to dry in the sun. Big smile.

Once or twice a week, I apply a comfrey poultice. I use herbal oils daily. I am healing. I can hold two pounds unassisted in my injured hand. I can type with two hands, but I can't milk the goats with both hands yet.

Story Medicine is central to the Wise Woman Tradition of healing by nourishing. Stories nourish us; we become our stories. And, as with anything we use for nourishment, there are "junk foods" in story medicine, too: blame, shame, and guilt.

Unfortunately, many of us are raised on this junk. It is fed to us by parents, teachers, religious figures, even our friends. We internalize their voices, and now heap shame and blame and guilt on ourselves, especially when we are sick or in an accident.

We may unconsciously believe that we are never supposed to get sick or injured, and that, if we do, something is wrong with us. The shame and guilt we feel for being unwell prevents us from seeking help; we don't deserve it. Or, we may believe that we are the victim of our misbehaving body, which we blame and punish. These ideas have deep historical roots and lots of modern offshoots.

The Heroic Tradition is exceptionally fond of blame, shame, and guilt. You are the victim of environmental toxins. It is your fault if you are sick. You have to get worse to get better. And if you are injured, there is a lesson to be learned.

I asked my mentor Elisabeth Kübler-Ross why people blame themselves for accidents, for cancer, for a terminal diagnosis.

"Because guilt is preferable to chaos," she replied. "The world is fundamentally chaotic. Bad things just happen. Blame and guilt imply that we can control our lives and that seems safer."

When EagleSong pulled me up out of the river, I did not blame myself, the rock, the water, or anyone or anything. Blame looks backward, to a time that we cannot change. Because I had already changed my story, I was ready to jump into Mind Medicine and affirm my ability to heal easily and well.

Affirmations take us into the future, into a time that we can change. Affirmations replace blame, shame, and guilt. They help us avoid looking for the reason we are hurt. Affirmations short circuit our desire to blame. Affirmations can create a new story.

Every day my hands and wrists are healthier and more flexible.

Around ten weeks after the injury, my fear rises up and insists that I cannot take care of this injury myself. It seems to be taking so long to get better. So I seek stories to calm and reassure myself.

I ask Sandra, a massage therapist who focuses on sports injuries, how long it will take for my wrist to heal. "Third-degree ligamentous sprains can take three or more months to heal fully."

I ask my doctor friend Aviva. "Worst thing that can happen is the circulation to that hand could be impaired." My right hand was paler at first, but, I reassure her, full blood flow has returned and it is now a healthy pink. Big smile.

"Your body has a miraculous ability to heal itself," she affirms.

Talking with others allows me to tell my story. Telling my story is important. It changes my perception. It has an impact on others. It gives us all support to be proactive about health.

Telling my story is part of my return to health. Trauma threw me over the Great Divide and into Alternative, Pharmaceutical, and Deep Medicines. Telling my story builds a bridge to guide me back to the safety of the first four medicines.

Three months since the injury. Time for another trip to Costa Rica, to a conference at Termales del Bosque, where thermal pools from a nearby volcano provide a perfect opportunity to use **heat for healing**. Heat therapies can increase inflammation, so I have waited until all the swelling is gone.

I submerge my wrist and body in steaming water, I dangle my wrist in the hot water, I float my arm in the bubbling heat of Mama Earth. The heat and the water expand my mind and spirit, relax my muscles and nerves. I remember that I am spacious.

When I return home, I continue healing with heat by using **moxibustion**: the therapeutic burning (bustion) of the white fuzz (moxa) from the leaves of *Artemisia chinensis* or the weedy American *Artemisia vulgaris.* I buy ready-made moxa sticks in Chinatown.

To apply moxibustion, I remove the paper from one end of the moxa stick and light it, then I blow on it until the moxa is glowing. I bring the glowing end of the moxa stick very near to, but not touching, my skin and move it in spirals and circles around the area being treated. It is time to quit when the sensation goes from warm to TOO HOT. Sand is handy for quenching the burning end of the moxa stick to be sure it is completely out.

Moxibustion is a tonifying technique that is used to "fill empty chi." It is at home both in Lifestyle Medicine and in Alternative Medicine.

I seek out the help of a physical therapist. She puts some physiotape on my arm, from elbow to wrist, and does some massage. She asks me to get an x-ray, to buy and wear a wrist brace, and to do some (slightly painful) exercises to regain more flexibility.

I am coming home to Lifestyle Medicine, but first, a visit to high-tech diagnosis and a curious result.

At the walk-in urgent care center, I get an x-ray after filling out the forms and showing my insurance and repeating my birth date.

Looking at the x-ray of my wrist, the doctor says two things. One, the bone *was* broken and two, based on how well it is healed, I didn't break it three months ago, but three *years* ago. (Not true.) Hooray for comfrey! Hooray for *Anthurium*.

The suggested treatment? Deep Medicine. Make an appointment to have my wrist broken and set with pins, "as it should have been in the first place, so you won't develop arthritis."

When I ask the physical therapist what she thinks of this suggestion, she laughs. Me too. We concur that surgery would increase, not decrease, the likelihood of arthritis in my wrist.

The bone healing is complete. Now it is time to focus on muscles and connective tissues, strength and flexiblity. Ligaments, tendons, and joints heal slowly, the physical therapist says. I need to build flexibility before increasing strength. My green allies are happy to help.

Comfrey ointment, applied, and worked in well, to the area of my wrist that hurts the most, strengthens ligaments and tendons.

Arnica oil, used liberally and often, is a specific for healing after trauma, and so kind to overused and strained muscles.

St. Joan's wort oil, a favorite of mine, not only eases muscle aches, it soothes nerve pain, like those shooting pains I get in my wrist when I try to pull the covers up in bed.

Plantain oil, perhaps the best of them all, is renowned for healing sprains that are years old. It helps the skin and fascia heal smoothly after trauma.

One hundred weeks since the injury. Two years have passed. I have full strength and flexibililty in my wrist and hand, for both delicate work and hard work. I can turn a doorknob, twist the lid off the smallest jar, support my weight on my wrist in yoga poses, lift bales of hay without the slightest twinge of pain, and milk the goats with *both* hands.

My body does indeed heal rapidly and well, with the aid of **Green Blessings** and the Seven Medicines.

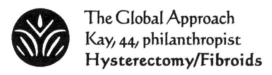

The Global Approach
Kay, 44, philanthropist
Hysterectomy/Fibroids

It was a bright spring morning with the scent of lilacs in the air when Kay called. *It begins in beauty.*

"I have a fibroid, a big one. I started spotting Saturday, eleven days before my period was due. I made time to sit and meditate (Step 0). I asked my uterus what it wanted [Step 1]. It felt heavy, weighty, ponderous, trapped.

"I envisioned the bleeding slowing [Step 2]. I brewed and drank some raspberry leaf tea [Step 3]. The bleeding continued; it got heavier. I felt tired. *Beauty beside me.*

"Tuesday I took shepherd's purse tincture every few hours. I continued to flood. I felt weak. Wednesday I tried a witch hazel sitz bath, to no avail [Step 4]. Thursday I tried some herbal capsules someone suggested, but that didn't help [Step 5].

"Friday, still bleeding heavily, feeling utterly exhausted, I went to the emergency room. A sonogram showed a large mass on top of my uterus. I saw my doctor yesterday; he recommends a hysterectomy as soon as possible, in a few days [Step 6]."

I waited in lilac-scented silence.

"I'm scared, but I know this surgery is right for me right now. I am a woman of extremes, a warrior woman. I am willing to let go of this weight, this mass weighing my womb down. Will you help me do this? Will you support me?"

"Yes," I replied, focusing my attention keenly on her.

"I'm interviewing surgeons and anesthesiologists [Step 6], creating the best team for my abundant health. I want you to guard my chakras so I don't leave my body under anesthesia [Step 2]."

"I won't let you get away," I reassure her.

"Do you think they'll let me set up an altar with some crystals in the operating room [Step 1]?" *Beauty before me.*

"It's worth asking," I replied, with a smile.

"I've been drinking nettle infusion to build my blood [Step 3]. What else can I do?"

"Eat blackstrap molasses on orange sections to get iron into your blood fast. Suck on kelp when you can't eat."

"I can hardly eat, I'm so nervous."

"Nervous? Take some . . ."

"Motherwort. I am. It's in my pocket so I can take some whenever I start to feel anxious. And I'm taking four dropperfuls of echinacea tincture several times a day so I will be ready to fend off those nasty hospital bacteria [Step 4]." *Beauty within me.*

Three days later, all her preparations in order, every one of the Seven Medicines working for her, Kay was sedated in preparation for full anesthesia and surgery. Before the tube went into her throat, her voice rang out, jarringly clear: "The fibroid is not attached to any major blood vessels. Make an incision just big enough to get a couple of fingers in, and slide them behind the fibroid. Then you will know it is safe to proceed with the hysterectomy via my vagina as we discussed. Remember: Leave my ovaries."

Amazed, the surgeon complied. Kay was out of surgery in record time, out of the recovery room in a few hours, and out of the hospital the next morning. *Beauty all around me.*

"With the Seven Medicines at hand, I was able to heal and strengthen myself during a frightening time. Not just physically, but emotionally, symbolically, and psychically. The ordering of the Seven Medicines guided me through the tangles of my fear to my deep roots. My hysterectomy was transformative.

"And now, I share this story with you, completing my healing, making it whole." *It ends in beauty.*

Deep Medicine/Story Medicine
Jess, 47, bank executive
Breast Reconstruction

Jess tells me: "Six surgeons said I was the perfect candidate for trans-flap breast reconstruction done with skin-sparing surgery.

"I asked a lot of questions. I thought I understood. But I didn't. They didn't tell me the whole truth.

"They said fat from my belly would be made into a breast. But they took the belly muscle too. Now I can't sit up in bed, and when that muscle in my breast goes into spasm, which is frequently, the pain in my chest is excruciating.

"It feels like a fist where my breast used to be. The cancer surgery took one hour. The reconstruction surgery took seven.

"That was eight years ago, and I regret my choice of reconstruction every day. I wish I had known about the Seven Medicines then. I thought the doctors knew more than I did about my breasts.

"It is too late fror me to change my mind, but sharing my story might save another woman."

Story Medicine/Deep Medicine
Catherine Guthrie [*Flat*. Skyhorse, 2018]
Breast Reconstruction Refused

In her book *Flat*, Catherine shares with us her post-operative fear that her muscles wouldn't support her as she lifts her legs and feet to the ceiling in an inverted yoga pose.

"What if my decision to sacrifice my breast [reconstruction] in order to keep my muscle intact, to maintain the integrity and power of my back muscle, had been for nothing?

"[My back] muscle worked in ways I imagined would have been impossible had it been severed for reconstruction purposes. My muscles harmonized in familiar ways, engaging, supporting, and stabilizing my pose. . . . My body was strong and whole."

"When discussing reconstruction post-breast cancer, plastic surgeons often say, 'Most women want to feel whole.' And by whole, they mean breasted.

"To me 'whole' means freedom to inhabit my body without pain or discomfort, to feel strong enough to support myself physically and mentally.

"But medicine is myopic in its desire to return a woman's body to the shape it was before cancer – just maybe with bigger breasts and a tummy tuck.

"Pretty quickly, the definition of 'whole' starts to drift into 'better than before'. . . ."

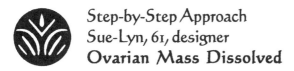

Step-by-Step Approach
Sue-Lyn, 61, designer
Ovarian Mass Dissolved

Sue-Lyn recalls: "Seeing a large mass on my ovary during a well-woman ultrasound, my doctor urged me to schedule surgery immediately to counter the threat of ovarian cancer [Step 6].

"I was frightened, but I asked for a month to think it over.

"I began a daily period of silent meditation [Step 0]. My inner guide affirmed my gut feeling that I didn't have cancer, as did a medical psychic I consulted, who said the mass was scar tissue from appendicitis surgery [Step 1].

"I took a homeopathic remedy recommended after a long consultation, and I prayed [Step 2]. I started drinking nourishing herbal infusions every day, especially violet leaf and red clover, and I rubbed calendula oil on the area several times a day to help break up the adhesion [Step 3].

"Within three weeks, the mass began to shrink. That was enough for me, but my doctor was impatient and pushing me, so I sped things along with several dropperfuls of chickweed tincture internally morning and evening and castor oil packs several times a week [Step 4]. The mass is still shrinking. My surgery is postponed indefinitely."

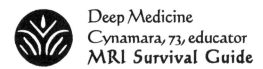
Deep Medicine
Cynamara, 73, educator
MRI Survival Guide

Cynamara educates me: "Magnetic resonance imaging allows us to see inside without radiation or surgery. MRI is really quite safe. Metals in and on the body will react; and there are rare reactions to contrast dyes like gadolinium; nothing else.

"An MRI is however loud and tedious, and being absolutely still *is* difficult. Loud music, an eye mask, and meditation help some. Others prefer to visulalize encircling bands of love-light.

"Gadolinium, a heavy metal, may be injected to make soft tissues visible. Protect your liver and your brain by taking dropperful doses of milk thistle and St. Joan's wort tinctures every four hours for 1-3 days beforehand.

"Everyone says: 'Drink lots of water after the scan.' This is not based on facts or studies, just the general belief that peeing more must help you get rid of unwanted things. Nonetheless, drink afterward: Nourishing herbal infusion. Water with fresh lemon. Hot green tea. Warm sake. Steaming miso soup. Even a cup of coffee.

"Seaweed and burdock, especially when eaten after the scan, also help clear the gadolinium from your body.

"I think you will find this site helpful:
https://www.radiologyinfo.org/en/info.cfm?pg=safety-contrast
"Be well."

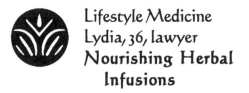
Lifestyle Medicine
Lydia, 36, lawyer
Nourishing Herbal Infusions

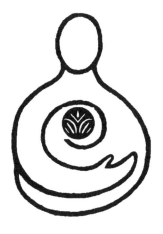

Lydia says she works too much. " I don't eat well [Step 3], so I take nutritional supplements [Step 5]. I wanted to substitute a quart of nourishing herbal infusion daily, but was afraid. I would return to my supplements after six weeks if I didn't see results.

"My energy took off almost immediately. Within a week I was feeling a lot better than usual. After two weeks, my habitual craving for sweets was gone. In fact, I found myself craving a bowl of brown rice or almonds instead of cookies or ice cream. Amazing! Incredible! This is what it is to be abundantly nourished and abundantly well. Good-bye supplements. I love you infusions."

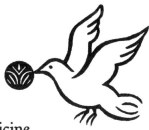

 Story Medicine
Sandra, 55, mother of three
children in college
ArtLife Personal Drama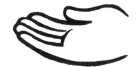

This is a ritual of reclamation.
"I speak the words, the pieces of my life. I tell my story. The words are written on a sheet. They make sentences. The sentences are written strips of sheeting tied into one long strip. It is wound around me as I speak the words that bind me. I tell the limiting stories I was told. Strips of knotted sheet bind my hips, my hands, my waist. I am wrapped up in the story of being a victim.

"I will speak the words. I will tell my story. My story is everywoman's story. My neck, my mouth, my eyes, my entire head are wound up and knotted. I am too wrapped up to speak. I cannot speak, see, hear. Cannot tell my truth, speak my story.

"There are scissors in my hand. They have always been there. I can cut the knots. I can cut the stories out. I can cut myself free.

"I do it. I cut the knots. I am unbound. I tell my own story."

"Difficult, despised areas of life, like addiction and depression, are not just problems to be resolved. They actually point to treasure. They are signposts, indicators that something valuable and positive is hidden away, waiting to return to one's wholeness."
Ann Weiser Cornell, *The Radical Acceptance of Everything*

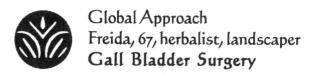

Global Approach
Freida, 67, herbalist, landscaper
Gall Bladder Surgery

Freida's to-do list as she prepared for her elective surgery:

Step 0:
- o   Sleep more in the weeks leading up to my surgery.

Step 1:
- o   Gather more information on the surgery I will be having. Get specifics.

Step 2:
- o   Buy homeopathic remedies for before and after: *Arnica* (both tablets and gel), *Hypericum* tablets, *Nux vomica* tablets.
- o   Find/use self-guided imagery/trances before, during, and after the surgery to calm myself and to encourage rapid healing.
- o   Ask for good wishes from family and beloved friends during the procedure.
- o   Put together a kit for my hospital room with my favorite images, icons of health, and a live plant.
- o   Have Reiki sessions before, during, and after the surgery.
- o   Endeavor to have music I like played during the surgery and in the recovery room.

Step 3:
- o   Drink a quart of nourishing herbal infusion daily for a week before and after surgery to increase protective antioxidants, healing proteins, and electrolyte minerals.
- o   Eat miso soup with lots of seaweed and burdock root four times a week for two weeks before and after surgery.
- o   Eat more well-cooked vegetables, fruit, and whole grains to strengthen my ability to heal.
- o   Ask if I can wear socks during the procedure.
- o   Make sure my advocate has my glasses and wedding ring.
- o   Ask for hugs. Whenever I need them. From whoever is near.

During my recovery, I ask my husband/advocate to:
- ♥ Hold my hand unless I don't want you to.
- ♥ Pet me. Hug me. Kiss my forehead. Kiss me softly on the lips.
- ♥ Tell me you love me. Often.
- ♥ Read the pain meditation on page 134 in *Who Dies* (by Stephen Levine) to me.
- ♥ If you leave the room, please be sure music is playing for me.
- ♥ Thank the doctors and the nurses; be sweet to them, but be sure they wash their hands.
- ♥ Have ginger tea with honey, miso broth, and nourishing herbal infusion available for me when I want to drink.

Step 4:
- o Pre-surgery: Take hawthorn berry and gotu kola tinctures, a dropperful of each daily for several weeks to strengthen connective tissue and assist in repair after surgery.
- o Book a massage once a week for the two weeks before and two weeks after my surgery.
- o Schedule an acupuncture session for no later than two weeks after surgery.
- o Ginger tea with lots of honey will be the last food I consume before surgery; and the first afterward.

Collect and get ready the herbal remedies I want to have at the hospital:
- o Candied ginger. Chocolate covered ginger.
- o Homeopathic remedies.
- o Immune helping herbs: reishi, echinacea, ginseng, osha, astragalus, and eleuthero tinctures.
- o Liver-loving herbs: milk thistle, dandelion, yellow dock tinctures.
- o Skin healing ointments: calendula, yarrow, plantain, comfrey.
- o Calming motherwort tincture.
- o Pain-killing CBD and skullcap tinctures.
- o Honey to soothe my throat.
- o Shepherd's purse tincture to stop bleeding.
- o Yarrow tincture as a disinfectant.
- o Elderberry tincture because it is magic.
- o Elecampane or mullein tincture to help my lungs recover from the anesthesia.

Step 5:
o Zinc supplements okay. Stop taking all others; esp. C and E.
o Discuss pain-killing options with my surgeon, anesthesiologist.
o Discuss antibiotic options with my surgeon.

Step 6:
o Access the symbolic power of Deep Medicine.
o See this as an expansive experience. Affirm that I will be healthier as a result of this surgery.
o Write a note to the recovery room nurse outlining my wishes.

Return to Health, Go Back Across the Gap

Step 6:
o Remove stitches. Use yarrow tincture to disinfect area daily.

Step 5:
o Stop using prescription pain-killers and NSAIDs as soon as possible. Integrate CBD and skullcap tinctures (2-5 drops every two hours) to keep dosage of drugs low.
o Stop using antibiotics (or don't use at all) as soon as possible. Take echinacea and eleuthero (3-6 dropperfuls every two hours) alone, or to increase effectiveness of drugs (if used).

Step 4:
o Use herbal remedies as needed. Listen to my body.

Steps 3 and 2:
o Continue to eat well and drink nourishing herbal infusions.
o Continue to use affirmations and visualizations.

Step 1:
o Create a healing story about my surgery that increases my sense of health. I am giving up my gall bladder. What else wants to be given up now? What wants to come into the opening that is being created? How does my gall bladder relate to my anger? Is it hardened bile that is causing my pain? Do I need to be angrier now? How does my gall bladder relate to my ability to digest what I experience?

Step 0: OOOOOMMMMMmmmmmmm

Appendix 1
Cholesterol-Reducing Foods

Cholesterol-reducing foods are eaten every day, at every meal.
(daily recommended amount in parentheses)

o **Almonds** (2 handfuls): Lowers total cholesterol 12 percent; LDL cholesterol 9.4 percent.
o **Almond oil** (up to half of daily fat intake): Reduces total cholesterol 4 percent; LDL, 6 percent.
o **Apple** (½ cup dried): Lowers LDL 23 percent; total cholesterol, 14 percent. (1 raw): Lowers LDL 40 percent.
o **Apple juice** (1.5 cups): Lowers LDL; counters lipid oxidation.
o **Avocado** (1): Lowers total cholesterol 16 percent; LDL and triglycerides, 22 percent. Raises HDL 11 percent.
o **Beans, peas, lentils** (¾ cup): Lowered LDL at least 5 percent in 26 large randomized trials. Two servings a day reduce cholesterol levels by 19 percent.
o **Carrots** (2 medium): Reduces total cholesterol 20 percent in three weeks.
o **Cayenne** (½ teaspoon) and **chili peppers** contain substances that reduce total and LDL cholesterol, dissolve plaque already in the blood vessels, and have a relaxing effect on the heart and circulatory system. *Do not exceed recommended dose.*
o **Chocolate, dark** (½-3 ounces): Increases HDL; counters LDL oxidation; lowers total cholesterol.
o **Cocoa powder** (¾ ounce): Reduces LDL; counters oxidation.
o **Cinnamon** (½ tablespoon, in food or as a tea): Reduces total cholesterol up to 26 percent; LDL reduced by 33 percent.
o **Cooked leafy greens** (½-1 cup): Binds cholesterol.
o **Fatty fish** (2-4 ounces of salmon, mackerel, sardines at least twice a week): Reduces triglyceride levels by 25-30 percent; lowers incidence of coronary artery calcification by a factor of three.
o **Flaxseed** (1-2 tablespoons, best ground and cooked): Lowers LDL and total cholesterol; excellent for postmenopausal women.
o **Garlic** (1-4 cloves): Lowers total cholesterol.
o **Hibiscus** (1 cup infusion): Lowers LDL.

o **Nourishing herbal infusions** (1-4 cups): Polyphenols and phytosterols reduce total cholesterol; counter LDL oxidation.

o **Nuts** (handful): Lower LDL an average of 5 percent.

o **Oats** (½-1 cup): Soluble fiber lowers total cholesterol.

o **Olive oil** (2-4 tablespoons): Reduces total cholesterol when used as the primary dietary fat.

o **Oranges/orange juice** (3 glasses): Increases HDL 21 percent after 1 month; reduces LDL/HDL ratio 16 percent. Benefits persisted for 5 weeks after the trial ended.

o **Pears** (1, dried or fresh): Soluble fiber (more than apples) soaks up and eliminates cholesterol, especially LDL.

o **Roots** (½ cup cooked): Beets, parsnips, burdock, turnips, rutabaga, and other roots contain phytosterols and polyphenols which reduce total cholesterol and improve cholesterol ratios.

o **Shiitake** (dried or fresh, 1 ounce or more a day):
  • Women on a low-fat diet who ate 3½ ounces of shiitake a day lowered their cholesterol by 12 percent in 7 days.
  • Women who ate 2 ounces of butter daily had a 14 percent increase in total cholesterol, unless they were eating shiitake, in which case, their total cholesterol *decreased* by 4 percent.
  • Mice on high-cholesterol diets who ate shiitake (5 percent of diet) had total cholesterol 45 percent lower than those who did not get shiitake.

o **Soy** (2 cups beverage): Reduces LDL 5 percent; increases HDL.

o **Strawberries** (1 pound/500 grams): Reduces total cholesterol 9 percent, LDL cholesterol 14 percent, and triglycerides 21 percent. Improves platelet function, too. But who can eat a pound of strawberries in a day, let alone every day!

o **Tea, green** or **black** (2-5 cups): Reduces LDL cholesterol 11 percent; total cholesterol as much as 6.5 percent after 3 weeks.

o **Whole grains** (1-4 servings of ½ cup): Unrefined amaranth, barley, corn, kasha, millet, oats, quinoa, rice, spelt, teff, and wheat are great sources of cholesterol-lowering fiber.

o **Vegetables** that lower total cholesterol: okra, eggplant, gobo/burdock.

o **Avoid:** coffee creamer, white sugar, white flour, corn syrup, soda pop, vegetable oils, processed meats, eating out.

Appendix II

Foods that Lower Blood Pressure

o **Fruits:** apple, banana, blueberry, cranberry, fig, grape, orange

✓ **Pomegranate juice** mimics the effects of ACE inhibitors. Two ounces a day lowers systolic pressure 12 percent.

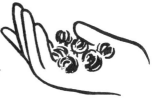

o **Vegetables:** broccoli, celery, dandelion greens, garlic, all mushrooms, parsley, potato, seaweed, spinach

✓ Drinking 4-8 ounces of **beet root juice** or **cooking liquid** daily decreases blood pressure about as quickly and about as much as most drugs. Beet juice and cooking water are loaded with nitrate, which turns into nitric oxide in the body, widening blood vessels and increasing blood flow.

✓ Eating two half-cup servings of **purple potatoes** daily provides plant compounds that act like ACE inhibitors. Increase the heart health effects by soaking potatoes in water for an hour before cooking. This increases the amount of available vitamin C, an antioxidant that heals and relaxes the blood vessels.

o **Fats:** avocado and avocado oil, olive oil, fatty fish like salmon, herring, sardines, anchovy, and mackerel.

✓ Changing your cooking fat to **sesame oil** can cause a drop in blood pressure comparable to the decrease caused by drugs. Sesamin, sesamol, and sesamolin are special fatty acids and antioxidants found in sesame.

o **Whole grains/seeds/beans:** oats, buckwheat (kasha), flaxseed, sesame seeds, lentils.

✓ Eating two tablespoons of **flaxseed** cooked into

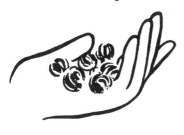

muffins or bread can cause significant lowering of blood pressure within six months. The effect is strong enough to lower risk of heart attack by 30 percent and risk of stroke by 50 percent. (Also reduces breast cancer risk.)

Appendix III
Sources for Herbs

- Avena Botanicals: 866-at-avena; www.avenabotanicals.com
- Blessed Herbs: 800-489-herbs; www.blessedherbs.com
- Catskill Mt. Herbals: 845-657-2943;
                                www.catskillmountainherbals.com
- Frontier: 800-669-3275; www.frontiercoop.com
- HerbPharm: 800-348-4372; www.herb-pharm.com
- Herbalist & Alchemist: 908-689-9020;
                                www.herbalist-alchemist.com
- Mountain Rose Herbs: 800-879-3337;
                                www.mountainroseherbs.com
- Pacific Botanicals: 541-479-7777; www.pacificbotanicals.com
- Red Moon Herbs: 888-929-0777; www.redmoonherbs.com

A Word About Simples

I am a simpler. A simpler uses one herb at a time rather than mixtures. Using simples builds relationships with individual plants, and I am all for that. Choosing simples helps highlight herbs that may not agree with us individually. Relying on simples reminds us that herbal medicine is people's medicine: as near as your back door and easy enough for a three-year-old to do. Having simples at hand puts the power of health care back into our own hands.

Herbs don't need to be combined to be effective. Mushrooms are more effective in combinations, it is true, and some herbs do work very well together. For safety's sake, use single herb remedies rather than combinations.

It is fine to drink an infusion of one herb, use an herbal vinegar of another, and take tinctures of others all at the same time.

Herbal combinations are an important part of our herbal history, a window into how previous generations used plants, but I suggest you keep it simple.

Using Herbs Safely

Use one herb at a time.
Learn about each plant from several sources.
Avoid herbs in capsules.
Respect the power of the plants; those strong enough to act as medicines can affect the body and spirit in powerful ways.
Remember, every plant, person, and situation is unique.

Nourishing herbs are the safest; side effects are rare. Brew in water or vinegar. Safe to take in quantity, for extended periods of time. They offer high levels of protein, minerals, vitamins, and antioxidants. Nourishing herbs are safe to take with drugs.

Nourishing herbs in this book include: amaranth, astragalus, bladderwrack, burdock root, chickweed, comfrey leaf, cornsilk, dandelion leaf, elderberry, hibiscus, mallow, mullein, mushrooms, nettle, oatstraw, plantain, purslane, red clover, seaweed, self-heal, slippery elm, violet leaves/flowers.

Tonic herbs act slowly and have cumulative effects. They are best used consistently for long periods. Tonics are safe to take with drugs. Prepare in water, vinegar, or alcohol (tincture).

• **Food tonics** may be used as often as desired. Food tonics in this book: berries (black, blue, cran, elder, goji, hawthorn, rasp, straw), flaxseed, garlic, ginger, leafy greens, mushrooms, nettle, seaweed, turmeric.

• **Adaptogenic tonics**, sometimes called alteratives, are used daily to protect against stress, normalize all functions, and aid longevity, stamina, and essential energy. Adaptogenic herbs in this book: amla, ashwagandha, American ginseng, astragalus, Chinese ginseng, codonopsis, cordyceps, eleuthero, fo ti, hawthorn, jiao gulan, reishi, schisandra, shiitake, shiso, tulsi, turkey tail.

• **Soothing tonics** are used in large quantity for a limited time, or in small doses for longer periods. Soothing tonics in this book: amla, bitterroot, burdock, calendula, cleavers, cornsilk, echinacea, fennel seed, fenugreek seeds, goldenrod, hibiscus, jewelweed, linden, marshmallow, passionflower, red clover, St. Joan's wort.

- **Bitter tonics** aid digestion and influence hormones. Bitter tonics in this book: angelica, boneset, buchu, chicory, chocolate, coffee, cronewort/mugwort, Culver's root, dandelion, dill seed, elecampane, garlic mustard, gentian, gotu kola, ground ivy, milk thistle, motherwort, saw palmetto, tea, vitex, wild yam, yellow dock.
- **Astringent tonics** are used externally, or in small amounts internally. Astringent tonics in this book: arnica, barberry, birch, coptis, cranesbill, horsetail, myrrh, oak bark, Oregon grape root, quaking aspen, raspberry leaf, witch hazel, yarrow.

Stimulating/sedating herbs act quickly and have powerful effects and may have side effects. They are used in the smallest effective dose, and only for as long as needed. They are problematic when combined with drugs. Daily use of stimulating/sedating herbs can undermine health. Stimulating/sedating herbs are used most often as tinctures. *Avoid capsules.*

Stimulating/sedating herbs in this book: aloes, black cohosh, black pepper, blue cohosh, buchu, California poppy, cannabis, cardamom, catnip, cayenne, chamomile, Chinese skullcap, cinchona, cinnamon, cloves, coca leaves, crampbark, ephedra, eucalyptus, galangal, ginkgo, guarana, hops, horseradish, hyssop, kava kava, kola nut, lavender, lemon balm, licorice, lobelia, maté, meadowsweet, mint, moxa, oregano, osha, parsley, peppermint, rosemary, sage, skullcap, thyme, usnea, valerian, wild carrot seed, wild cherry, wild lettuce, willow, wintergreen.

Potentially poisonous herbs can cause severe side effects; they are unsafe to use with drugs. They are used in the smallest effective dose and only for as long as needed. Potentially poisonous herbs are usually prepared as tinctures.

Potentially poisonous herbs in this book: essential oils, any herb in a capsule, dried St. John's/Joan's wort (but not the tincture or oil of fresh flowers); ayahuasca, belladonna, black walnut hulls, bitter orange, brugmansia, cascara, datura, feverfew, foxglove, golden seal, henbane, horse chestnut, liferoot, mandrake, mistletoe, myrrh, *Nux vomica,* peyote, puke weed, poke root, poppy, psilocybin, ragweed, rose geranium, saffron, tea tree oil, tobacco, Turkey rhubarb root.

Note: Some herbs appear in more than one list.

Your Herbal Pharmacy

 ## Make A Nourishing Herbal Infusion

I create abundant health by drinking a quart of nouishing herbal infusion every day. I switch around what I drink, enjoying the benefits of many herbs, one at a time.

Nettle leaf builds energy, mineralizes, restores adrenals.
Oatstraw herb nourishes nerves and hormones.
Comfrey leaf builds strength and flexibility in all tissues.
Linden flowers soothe inflammation, bring cheer.
Red clover blossoms restore health to hormones and nerves.
Mullein rebuilds and strengthens respiratory function.
Hawthorn herb and berries nourish a healthy heart.

Place 1 ounce/30 grams dried herb in a quart/liter jar. Fill jar with boiling water. Cap tightly. Steep for four hours or overnight. Strain, squeezing well. Refrigerate liquid; compost herb. To make linden flower infusion, use ½ ounce of herb.

 ## Make A Tincture/Fresh Herb

Tinctures last for a long time. The best tinctures are made from fresh plants. Tonic tinctures may be taken daily. Others, only as needed.

These tinctures require fresh plants, no exceptions.
St. Joan's wort flowers mean trouble for viruses and frowns.
Poke root stirs up the lymphatic and immune systems.
Bloodroot in tiny amounts counters periodontal disease.
Chickweed herb dissolves cysts, esp. on the ovaries.
Motherwort calms anxiety, eases the heart.
Skullcap eases pain and brings deep sleep.

Fill any size jar to the top with chopped-up fresh, just harvested, herb of your choice. Fill jar to the top with 100-proof vodka. Put on a tight lid. Label the jar: herb, vodka, date. Your tincture is ready to use in six weeks.

Alcohol pulls out more active, medicinal, potentially poisonous constituents than water, so 5-25 drops is a full dose.

Make A Tincture/Dried Herb

If fresh herbs are not available, use dried herbs, but use less.

Roots: Echinacea, eleuthero, ginseng, codonopsis
Berries: Amla, vitex, elder, hawthorn, schisandra

Put 4 ounces/115 grams of dried berries or cut root in a quart/liter jar. Fill the jar to the top with 100-proof vodka. Cap tightly, label. Wait at least six weeks before use; best after a year.

 ## Make An Infused Oil/Fresh Herb

Oil and animal fat coax a variety of healing compounds out of fresh plants. Dried plants, with a few exceptions, never make great oils.

Calendula flower oil calms inflammation and irritation.
Chickweed herb oil softens and dissolves cysts and scars.
Comfrey oil from fresh roots/leaves heals tears and breaks.
Plantain leaf oil stops itching, hastens deep wound recovery.
St. Joan's wort oil eases burns, muscle soreness, nerve pain.

Fill a dry jar almost full with finely-chopped fresh herb, then fill with any edible oil/fat. Cap tightly. Label (on lid). Put in a small bowl to catch ooze. Steep, out of direct sunlight, for six weeks. Sieve plant material from oil, squeeze well. Store cool and dark.

 ## Make An Infused Oil/Dried Herb

The easiest and most fool-proof way of extracting dried herbs into oil is to use a crockpot with a temperature gauge.

Fill a crockpot or dry jar half full of chopped dried herb. Add oil or animal fat nearly to the top; leave a breathing space. Heat gently – 110° F/43° C is perfect – for a week or two. Strain.

 ## Make An Ointment

Gently warm infused oil. Melt about a tablespoon of beeswax into each ounce of oil. To check consistency, drip some on a china plate. If too stiff, add more oil; if too loose, more beeswax. Lip balm needs lots of beeswax. Pour into container and let harden.

Make an Herbal Vinegar

Use herbal vinegars on salads, in marinades, on beans, on greens.

Dandelion leaf/root/flower vinegar prevents heartburn.
Mint vinegar aids digestion.
Garlic vinegar builds immunity.
Burdock root vinegar clears the skin, improves memory.
Blueberry vinegar prevents cancer, dementia.

Fill any size jar to the top with cut-up pieces of fresh, just harvested herb, then add pasteurized vinegar, right to the top of the jar. Use any lid but a metal one. Label. Ready to use in six weeks.
Vinegar concentrates minerals, which build strong bones.

Make Your Own Placebo

There are many ways to make placebos.

Most start with **water**, often with a bit of brandy added. Placebo effect is heightened by **ritual**, so use special sacred water.

Then, try one or more of these: Imbue your special water with your **intention** by meditating on it. Charge the water with **color** frequencies by adding a brightly-hued flower to it. Infuse it with the qualities of the **moon** or the **sun** or a special place by leaving the water where it can absorb those energies. Put a **crystal** or gemstone in the water. Label the water with a special **word**.

You can also make a simple homeopathic remedy to counter allergens and addictions. You need alcohol, fresh or dried plants, and a strong arm to shake the remedy daily.

First, make a tincture of the offending substance by soaking the fresh or dried plant, chopped, in vodka for six weeks. If you sneeze when ragweed (*Ambrosia artemisifolia*) blooms, make a tincture of that. If you are addicted to tobacco, make a tincture of your brand.

When the tincture is ready, put ten drops of it in one cup of pure water in a pint jar. Shake the jar for 5-10 minutes. Then put ten drops of the liquid from that jar into a new jar with one cup of water; shake for 5-10 minutes. Repeat at least once more.

The greater the dilution, the stronger the remedy.

Dandelion Italiano

Keeps refrigerated for two weeks. Eat with meals for great digestion.

Fill a quart kettle with water and bring it to a boil.

Wash a big bunch of fresh **dandelion greens**. If necessary, cut
away root crowns.

Chop washed greens into one inch pieces and put in a saucepan.

Add boiling water to just cover greens; bring to a boil.

Refill kettle and put back on the burner.

Cook greens 3-5 minutes. Drain. Return to pan. Add boiling
water to just cover the greens; return to a boil.

Cook greens 3-5 minutes again. Drain. Return to pan. Add boiling water to barely cover greens; return to a boil again.

Reduce heat; simmer 25-45 minutes, until tender.

While greens cook, peel and mince 5-15 cloves of **garlic**.

Drain greens and add minced garlic to hot greens.

Add ¼ cup extra virgin **olive oil** and mix well.

Add 2 tablespoons shoyu (**tamari**) and mix well. Chill.

Dried Tomato Paté

Spread on crackers, spoon into soup, add to omelets

Pack dried **tomatoes** into a one-cup measure.

Add boiling water to just barely cover.

When tomatoes are soft, strain out the soaking liquid; save.

Put half the tomatoes in a blender or Cuisinart mini-prep.

Add ¼ cup extra virgin **olive oil**.

Add 1-2 cloves **garlic**, chopped.

Add a little **sea salt**.

Blend well.

Add the rest of the soaked tomatoes.

Add 1-2 more cloves of chopped garlic.

Add a little more salt.

And enough olive oil or soaking liquid to enable blending.

Blend very well.

You can eat this immediately or keep it in a tightly covered jar
in the refrigerator for up to a month.

Simple Green Pesto

This simple pesto has only four ingredients. It keeps up to three years in the refrigerator. Pesto preserves the herbs' antioxidant power.

Dandelion leaf pesto is bitter and tangy.
Chickweed pesto is mellow and grassy; use new growth.
Shiso or **tulsi** pesto is aromatic and romantic.
Garlic mustard pesto is bitter and spicy and delicious.
Garlic scape pesto is heaven on earth.

There are no specific amounts; use what is abundant.
Chop **herb** coarsely with a knife. Peel **garlic** and mince.
Half fill a mini-prep or blender with herb.
Add extra virgin olive oil to cover well.
Add minced garlic and some salt.
It is important to use salt. It acts as a preservative and it helps turn the green leaves into a paste (pesto).
Puree/blend well. Add more oil as needed.
Add more herb, more salt, and more garlic, too.

Pack almost to the top of a tall jar. Tap lightly to remove air bubbles. Pour more olive oil over the top. Label on lid, refrigerate.

 ## Cheesy Seaweed Quiche

Serves 15-25. Travels well. Leftovers disappear quickly.

In a large bowl beat 6 **eggs**.
Add 2 cans **organic corn** (save the liquid).
Add 2 tablespoons **cornstarch** mixed into the **corn liquid**.
Add 2 sticks (½ pound) of melted **butter**.
Add 2/3 cup **cornmeal**.
Add cup **sour cream**.
Add ¾ teaspoon **salt**.
Mix well.
Stir in ½ pound firm **goat cheese**, cut into ¾-inch cubes.
Stir in ½ pound **cheddar cheese**, cut into ¾-inch cubes.
Stir in ½ cup minced *Nereocystis* **kelp** (or toasted dulse).
Pour into 3 **whole wheat pie shells**.
Bake for one hour at 350° F or until firm in the center. Serve.

Hot/Cold Herb Pillow

A craft project that provides innumerable benefits

Heat 1 pound or more **flaxseed**, buckwheat, *or* short-grain rice in a slow oven (250°F) for one hour to kill the insect eggs present in all organic grains and to ensure that the moisture content is as low as possible.

Allow seeds to cool completely.

Mix with 1 ounce or more of dried **herb**: lavender, hops, lemon balm, cronewort, sage, or any favorite mint.

Create a case for your pillow. Keep it small: no more than 18 inches/45cm long and 6 inches/15cm wide. Or use an old sock or the pocket from worn-out pants or the bottom six inches of an old pillowcase. Heavy-weight cotton or silk are ideal fabrics.

Fill your case – not too full – with the herb/seed mix.

Sew or safety-pin it shut.

To reduce inflammation: Place in the freezer, then apply.

To reduce pain: Wrap in foil; heat in oven; remove foil; apply.

Purslane Gazpacho

A late summer favorite. Serves 6-8. Purslane brings joy.

In a large bowl place:

6 cups **tomatoes** cut into into ½-inch squares; include juice
4 cups **cucumbers**, peeled, seeded, cut into ½-inch squares.
1 tablespoon **sea salt**
2-3 teaspoons **granulated garlic**
2 tablespoons **lemon juice**
½ cup **extra virgin olive oil**
Mix, cover, and refrigerate for several hours. Then add
4 cups **purslane** tender tips, chopped
20 fresh **basil leaves**, chopped
10 fresh **shiso leaves**, chopped
Adjust seasoning and serve, garnished with edible flowers.

Gratitude

Penelope Goat gave me the idea for this book as I sat vigil by her graveside. My goats continue to inspire and teach me.

Michael Dattorre, beloved consort and strong support, fielded phone calls, milked the goats, made dinner – *and* did the dishes – and brought me countless cups of nourishing herbal infusion. My gratitude and love are eternal.

Justine Smythe, daughter extraordinaire, has pushed, prodded, supported, succored, nourished and noodled me with finesse and infinite care. It is so fine to be loved by you. Love you, too.

Betsy Grace Sandlin, my oldest, bestest friend, always makes certain every word is as it should be and every nit-picking detail is nailed. You B the one for me.

Marie Summerwood wove decades of discussions with me about the Seven Medicines into infinite chants that spiral through me as I write. You are with me every day, Daughter of the Void.

My friends, apprentices, correspondence course students, and readers have also had twenty years to comment on and criticize my words and ideas. Your suggestions, annoyances, desires, smiley faces and hearts in red made me reach deeper and deeper inside to find simpler and simpler ways to express complicated thoughts.

A huge thank you to: Karen Battese, Brenda Bordogna, Elizabeth Carver, Candace Cave, Jonathan Delson, Marie Frohlich, Julia Gleize, Gretchen Gould, Astrid Grove, Vic Hernández, Kutira (Maui), Lauren Lesser, Belinda Lindroos, Molly Hall, Melissa Hammond, Larch Hansen, Evelyn Heyd, Holly Hughes, Casandra Kaiser, Dawn Marie Kay, Lata Kennedy, Janice Knapik, Yvette Lewis, Lindsay McRae, Kristin Moore, Ann/Inanna Moss, Lisa Natoli, Dunk One, Joel and Tish Packman, Dr. JoAnn Quattrone, Chan Siefert, Molly Scott, and Barbara Volk.

The trees give their lives to the making of these books. May you thrive, standing ones. May you prosper, green nations.

May it be in beauty. May it be in peace. So mote it be.

Index

Index   329

Index   **329**

osteoarthritis 79, 106, 114, 165, 189
osteopathy 162
osteoporosis 23, 165, 186, 211
ovaries 124, 128, 238
  cyst/mass/tumor 32, 237, 296
oxytocin 122, 199

Pain 3, 8, 74, 122, 154
  arm, shoulder, neck 74, 160, 164
  back 79, 162, 164, 165, 234,
  chronic 79, 85, 156, 160, 162, 165,
    199, 251, 248, 251, 260
  to counter 5, 6, 14, 55, 156, 198
  drugs that cause 215, 220
  emotional 165
  hip, knee, wrist 79
  joint 162, 165, 212, 216
  and LSD 267
  menstrual 162
  musculo-skeletal 78, 198, 251
  neck, ease 14, 73, 74
  nerve 251
  to prevent 103, 110
  psychic 76
  relief 3, 11, 73, 79, 104, 111, 112,
    114, 116, 117, 148, 149, 154, 162,
    163, 165, 193, **198-199**, 216, 236,
    250-251, 284, 307
  stomach 213
pain-spasm cycle 119
painful treatments, relief 119
Paleo diet 96, 100
Panax ginseng 126, 158, 193, 194,
    235, 236, 299, 305, 308
pancreas 124, 128
panic 149, 208
Pap smear 230
papaya (*Carica papaya*) 108, 212
parabens 191
paralysis 117
paranoia 201, 264
parasites 93, 161
parasympathetic nerves 13

parietal lobe 7
Parkinson's 21, 55, 76, 103, 104,
    114, 117, 154, 221
parsley (*Petroselinum*) 99, 303
passionflower (*Passiflora incarnata*)
    128, 158, 200, 204, 208, 305
pellagra 32
pelvic health 160
pelvic organs 115
  pain, chronic, ease 39
penethylamine 105
pennyroyal 149, 153, 306
peppermint (*Mentha piperita*) 49,
    158, 162, 306
peptic ulcer disease 197
peristalsis 258
PET scan 33, 234, 273
pet therapy **122**, 249
peyote (*Lophophora willamsii*) 263,
    265, 266
phage therapy 202, **276**
phagocytes 102
phobias 166, 169
phosphate 241
photobiology 64
phthalates 191
Phyllanthus emblica is amla
physical disabilities 117
phytates 130
phytoestrogen 106
phytosterols 302
piercings 259
Pierrakos, Eva 54
pineal 128
Piper methysticum is kava kava
Piper nigrum is black pepper
pituitary 128
placebo effect **55-59**
Placebo, How to Make a 309
plant spirits 266
plantain (*Plantago majus*) 299, 305,
    292, 308
  seeds 162, 258

serotonin 7, 105, 122, 207, 263, 266, 278
Serratia marcescens 202
sex/ual 11
  dysfunction 199, 207, 209
  responsiveness 125, 213
  -transmitted infections, less 102
shamanic trance/healing 63, 228
shea butter 191
shellfish 98
shepherd's purse (*Bursa capsella pastoris*) 292, 299, 306
shiatsu 149, 153, 154, 160
shiitake (*Lentinus edodes*) 107, 126, 194
  and cholestrerol 302
shingles 214, 215
Shinrin Yoku 9, 71
shiso (*Perilla fructescens*) 305, 311, 312
shoyu 235
Siberian ginseng *is eleuthero*
Siegel, Bernie MD xix, 65
sigmoidoscopy 230
Simple Green Pesto 311
sinus infections 74, 215, 234
skin 128, 210
  cancer, less 104
  clearer, healthier 101, 106, 309
  problems 78, 165
skullcap (*Scutellaria lateriflora*) 128, 158, 198, 200, 208, 214, 251, 284, 285, 287, 299, 300, 306, 307
sleep 3, 11, 64, 79, 110, 114, 124, 133, 158, 198, 204, 298
  disorders 124
  deepen 101, 113, 114, 117, 127, 163
  deprivation, and depression 206
  on the ground 70
  herbs for **200**
  improve/increase 14, 64, 71, 74
  induce 39, 56, 307
  and light 11, 18
  and noise 11
  pills 158, 201

slippery elm (*Ulmus fulva*) 128, 196, 197, 210, 305
  balls 250
SMILES 132
smoking 63, 90
social anxiety disorder 208
social network, benefits 53
soft drinks 149
soft tissue strains 160
Solanum nigrum is black nightshade
solar plexus 123
solitude 19
sonic x-rays 282
sonogram 237, 292
soy 235
  beverage 94, 130
  cheese 130
  milk 184
spices 105
spinal adjustment 153, 164
spinal/soft-tissue manipulation 161
spiral xx
spirulina 131
sprains 210, 290
sprouts 93
SSRIs 207, 216
St. John's/St. Joan's wort (*Hypericum perforatum*) 112, 128, 191, 206, 214, 251, 296, 298 305, 306, 307, 308
  oil 215, 235, 291
stamina 127, 305
standardized tincture 142, 159
Staphylococcus/staph 165, 202, 214
statin/s 192, 194, 195, 216, 221
Statue of Liberty 66
steam room 166
steroids 183, 211, 218
stimulant/s 105, **158**
stinging nettle *is nettle*
stomach 128
story/telling 27, 39, 40, 41, 44, 45, 54, 67, 204, 208
strength 53, 113, 114, 160

Notes

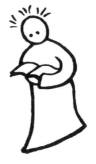